T0362329

Bone Disorders

Editor

ALBERT SHIEH

ENDOCRINOLOGY AND METABOLISM CLINICS OF NORTH AMERICA

www.endo.theclinics.com

Consulting Editors
ANAT BEN-SHLOMO
MARIA FLESERIU

March 2017 • Volume 46 • Number 1

ELSEVIER

1600 John F. Kennedy Boulevard • Suite 1800 • Philadelphia, Pennsylvania, 19103-2899

http://www.theclinics.com

ENDOCRINOLOGY AND METABOLISM CLINICS OF NORTH AMERICA Volume 46, Number 1
March 2017 ISSN 0889-8529, ISBN 13: 978-0-323-50976-3

Editor: Stacy Eastman
Developmental Editor: Meredith Clinton

Endocrinology and Metabolism Clinics of North America (ISSN 0889-8529) is published quarterly by Elsevier Inc., 360 Park Avenue South, New York, NY 10010-1710. Months of issue are March, June, September, and December. Periodicals postage paid at New York, NY and additional mailing offices. Subscription prices are USD 337.00 per year for US individuals, USD 674.00 per year for US institutions, USD 100.00 per year for US students and residents, USD 423.00 per year for Canadian individuals, USD 834.00 per year for Canadian institutions, USD 490.00 per year for international individuals, USD 834.00 per year for international institutions, and USD 245.00 per year for international and Canadian and foreign students/residents. To receive student/resident rate, orders must be accompanied by name of affiliated institution, date of term, and the signature of program/residency coordinator on institution letterhead. Orders will be billed at individual rate until proof of status is received. Foreign air speed delivery is included in all *Clinics* subscription prices. All prices are subject to change without notice. **POSTMASTER:** Send address changes to *Endocrinology and Metabolism Clinics of North America*, Elsevier Health Sciences Division, Subscription Customer Service, 3251 Riverport Lane, Maryland Heights, MO 63043. **Customer Service: Telephone: 1-800-654-2452** (U.S. and Canada); **1-314-447-8871** (outside U.S. and Canada). **Fax: 1-314-447-8029. E-mail: journalscustomerservice-usa@elsevier.com (for print support)**; **journalsonlinesupport-usa@elsevier.com (for online support)**.

Reprints. For copies of 100 or more, of articles in this publication, please contact the Commercial Rights Department, Elsevier Inc., 360 Park Avenue South, New York, NY 10010-1710; phone: +1-212-633-3874; fax: +1-212-633-3820; E-mail: reprints@elsevier.com.

Endocrinology and Metabolism Clinics of North America is covered in *MEDLINE/PubMed (Index Medicus), EMBASE/Excerpta Medica, Current Contents/Clinical Medicine, Current Contents/Life Sciences, Science Citation Index, ISI/BIOMED, BIOSIS,* and *Chemical Abstracts*.

Contributors

CONSULTING EDITORS

ANAT BEN-SHLOMO, MD
Pituitary Center, Division of Endocrinology Diabetes, and Metabolism, Cedars Sinai Medical Center, Los Angeles, California

MARIA FLESERIU, MD, FACE
Division of Endocrinology, Diabetes, and Clinical Nutrition, Departments of Medicine and Neurological Surgery, Northwest Pituitary Center, Oregon Health and Science University, Portland, Oregon

EDITOR

ALBERT SHIEH, MD, MSCR
Clinical Instructor, Divisions of Geriatrics, and Endocrinology, Diabetes, and Hypertension, Department of Medicine, David Geffen School of Medicine, University of California, Los Angeles, Los Angeles, California

AUTHORS

RAFIA AFZAL, MBBS
Department of Anesthesiology, Aga Khan University Hospital, Karachi, Pakistan

JOHN F. ALOIA, MD
Professor, Department of Medicine, Bone Mineral Research and Treatment Center, Chief Academic Officer, Dean Winthrop University Hospital Clinical Campus, Stony Brook University School of Medicine, Mineola, New York

LEONARDO BANDEIRA, MD
Department of Medicine, College of Physicians and Surgeons, Columbia University, New York, New York

JOHN P. BILEZIKIAN, MD
Department of Medicine, College of Physicians and Surgeons, Columbia University, New York, New York

ROBERT D. BLANK, MD, PhD
Professor of Medicine and Chief, Division of Endocrinology, Metabolism, and Clinical Nutrition, Department of Medicine, Medical College of Wisconsin, Staff Endocrinologist, Medical Service, Clement J. Zablocki VAMC, Milwaukee, Wisconsin

LYNDA F. BONEWALD, PhD
Professor, Departments of Anatomy and Cell Biology and Orthopaedic Surgery, Director, Indiana Center for Musculoskeletal Health, Indianapolis, Indiana

ANGELA M. CHEUNG, MD, PhD, FRCPC
Professor of Medicine, University of Toronto, Toronto, Ontario, Canada

ADI COHEN, MD, MHS
Associate Professor of Medicine, Division of Endocrinology, Department of Medicine, Columbia University Medical Center, Columbia University, College of Physicians & Surgeons, New York, New York

ANDA R. GONCIULEA, MD
Division of Endocrinology, Diabetes and Metabolism, Johns Hopkins University School of Medicine, Baltimore, Maryland

DONA L. GRAY, MD
Endocrinology Clinic, Indiana University Health Arnett, Lafayette, Indiana

NAINA SINHA GREGORY, MD
Assistant Professor of Medicine, Division of Endocrinology, Department of Medicine, New York Presbyterian Hospital, Weill Cornell Medical College, New York, New York

SUZANNE M. JAN DE BEUR, MD
Associate Professor of Medicine; Division of Endocrinology, Diabetes and Metabolism, Johns Hopkins University School of Medicine, Baltimore, Maryland

MICHAEL G. JOHNSON, PhD
Research Scientist, Department of Medicine, University of Wisconsin, Madison, Wisconsin

ALIYA A. KHAN, MD, FRCPC, FACP, FACE
Professor of Clinical Medicine, McMaster University, Hamilton, Ontario, Canada

MOIN KHAN, MD, MSc, FRCSC
McMaster University, Hamilton, Ontario, Canada

JASMIN KRISTIANTO, PhD
Postdoctoral Fellow, Division of Endocrinology, Metabolism, and Clinical Nutrition, Department of Medicine, Medical College of Wisconsin, Milwaukee, Wisconsin

WILLIAM D. LESLIE, MD, MSc, FRCPC
Professor, Department of Medicine, University of Manitoba, Winnipeg, Manitoba, Canada

DOROTHY S. MARTINEZ, MD
Clinical Professor, David Geffen School of Medicine, University of California, Los Angeles, Los Angeles, California

ELIZABETH RENDINA-RUEDY, PhD
Research Fellow, Maine Medical Center Research Institute, Scarborough, Maine

CLIFFORD J. ROSEN, MD
Senior Scientist, Maine Medical Center Research Institute, Scarborough, Maine

G. ISANNE SCHACTER, MD, FRCPC
Assistant Professor, Department of Medicine, University of Manitoba, Winnipeg, Manitoba, Canada

YANG SHEN, MD
Endocrinology Clinic, Huntington Health Physicians, Pasadena, California

ALBERT SHIEH, MD, MSCR
Clinical Instructor, Divisions of Geriatrics, and Endocrinology, Diabetes, and Hypertension, Department of Medicine, David Geffen School of Medicine, University of California, Los Angeles, Los Angeles, California

BARBARA C. SILVA, MD, PhD
Department of Medicine, UNI-BH, Santa Casa Hospital, Belo Horizonte, Minas Gerais, Brazil

MICHAEL W. YEH, MD
Associate Professor of Surgery and Medicine, Chief, Section of Endocrine Surgery, David Geffen School of Medicine, University of California, Los Angeles, Los Angeles, California

KYLE A. ZANOCCO, MD, MS
Assistant Professor of Surgery, Section of Endocrine Surgery, David Geffen School of Medicine, University of California, Los Angeles, Los Angeles, California

Contents

Foreword xiii

Anat Ben-Shlomo and Maria Fleseriu

Preface: An Introduction to the Bone Disorders Issue xvii

Albert Shieh

Erratum xix

The Role of the Osteocyte in Bone and Nonbone Disease 1

Lynda F. Bonewald

When normal physiologic functions go awry, disorders and disease occur. This is universal; even for the osteocyte, a cell embedded within the mineralized matrix of bone. It was once thought that this cell was simply a placeholder in bone. Within the last decade, the number of studies of osteocytes has increased dramatically, leading to the discovery of novel functions of these cells. With the discovery of novel physiologic functions came the discoveries of how these cells can also be responsible for not only bone diseases and disorders, but also those of the kidney, heart, and potentially muscle.

Fibroblast Growth Factor 23–Mediated Bone Disease 19

Anda R. Gonciulea and Suzanne M. Jan De Beur

Fibroblast growth factor 23 (*FGF23*) is an important regulator of phosphate and vitamin D metabolism and its excessive or insufficient production leads to a wide variety of skeletal disorders. This article reviews the *FGF23*-α-Klotho signaling pathway, highlighting the latest developments in *FGF23* regulation and action, and describes the disorders associated with *FGF23* excess or deficiency.

Bone–Fat Interaction 41

Elizabeth Rendina-Ruedy and Clifford J. Rosen

Marrow adipose tissue (MAT) is a recently identified endocrine organ capable of modulating a host of responses. Given its intimate proximity to the bone microenvironment, the impact marrow adipocytes exert on bone has attracted much interest and scientific inquiry. Although many questions and controversies remain about marrow adipocytes, multiple conditions/disease states in which alterations occur have provided clues about their function. The consensus is that MAT is associated inversely with bone density and quality. While further investigation is warranted, MAT has clearly been demonstrated as an active dynamic depot that contributes to bone turnover and overall metabolic homeostasis.

Endothelin Signaling in Bone 51

Jasmin Kristianto, Michael G. Johnson, Rafia Afzal, and Robert D. Blank

The endothelin (ET) system includes 3 small peptide hormones and a pair of G-protein–coupled receptors. This review first outlines the ET signaling pathway and ET metabolism. Next, it summarizes the role of ET1 signaling in craniofacial development. Then, it discusses observations relating ET signaling to osteoblastic and other osteosclerotic processes in cancer. Finally, it describes recent work in our laboratory that points to endothelin signaling as an upstream mediator of WNT signaling, promoting bone matrix synthesis and mineralization. It concludes with a statement of some remaining gaps in knowledge and proposals for future research.

Diabetes and Bone Disease 63

G. Isanne Schacter and William D. Leslie

The World Health Organization estimates that diabetes mellitus occurs in more than 415 million people; this number could double by the year 2040. Epidemiologic data have shown that the skeletal system may be a target of diabetes-mediated damage, leading to the development of diabetes-induced osteoporosis. T1D and T2D have been associated with an increased risk of fracture. Bone mineral density and fracture risk prediction tools developed for the general population capture some of the risk associated with diabetes. Recent adaptations to these tools have improved their efficacy in patients with diabetes.

Primary Hyperparathyroidism: Effects on Bone Health 87

Kyle A. Zanocco and Michael W. Yeh

Primary hyperparathyroidism (PHPT) is the most common cause of chronic hypercalcemia. With the advent of routine calcium screening, the classic presentation of renal and osseous symptoms has been largely replaced with mild, asymptomatic disease. In hypercalcemia caused by PHPT, serum parathyroid hormone levels are either high, or inappropriately normal. A single-gland adenoma is responsible for 80% of PHPT cases. Less frequent causes include 4-gland hyperplasia and parathyroid carcinoma. Diminished bone mineral density and nephrolithiasis are the major current clinical sequelae. Parathyroidectomy is the only definitive treatment for PHPT, and in experienced hands, cure rates approach 98%.

The Effects of Bariatric Surgery on Bone Metabolism 105

Naina Sinha Gregory

Most metabolic effects following bariatric surgery are favorable. One area in which the consequences seem to be detrimental is on skeletal health. Mechanisms that have been cited include malabsorption of calcium and vitamin D, decrease in mechanical loading, and changes in gastrointestinal and fat-derived hormone levels. It is important that the impact of these procedures on bone metabolism is closely examined. The significance of the bone loss that occurs, and its possible effect on future fracture risk, should also be evaluated.

Premenopausal Osteoporosis 117

Adi Cohen

Most premenopausal women with low trauma fracture(s) or low bone mineral density have a secondary cause of osteoporosis or bone loss. Where possible, treatment of the underlying cause should be the focus of management. Premenopausal women with an ongoing cause of bone loss and those who have had, or continue to have, low trauma fractures may require pharmacologic intervention. Clinical trials provide evidence of benefits of bisphosphonates and teriparatide for bone mineral density in several types of premenopausal osteoporosis, but studies are small and do not provide evidence regarding fracture risk reduction.

Assessing Vitamin D Status in African Americans and the Influence of Vitamin D on Skeletal Health Parameters 135

Albert Shieh and John F. Aloia

In the United States, there is a significant disparity in vitamin D status among individuals of African versus European descent. Despite having lower total 25-hydroxyvitamin D levels compared with white Americans, African Americans have higher bone mineral density and lower fracture risk. This article reviews classical and nonclassical vitamin D physiology, describes whether total versus free 25-hydroxyvitamin D is a better marker of vitamin D status in African Americans, and summarizes the influence of vitamin D status and vitamin D supplementation on markers of vitamin D bioactivity (intestinal calcium absorption, parathyroid hormone secretion, bone mineral density, fracture) in African Americans.

Trabecular Bone Score: A New DXA–Derived Measurement for Fracture Risk Assessment 153

Barbara C. Silva and William D. Leslie

Trabecular bone score (TBS) is a novel method that assesses skeletal texture from spine dual-energy X-ray absorptiometry (DXA) images. TBS improves fracture-risk prediction beyond that provided by DXA bone mineral density (BMD) and clinical risk factors, and can be incorporated to the Word Health Organization Fracture Risk Assessment tool (FRAX®) to enhance fracture prediction. There is insufficient evidence that TBS can be used to monitor treatment with bisphosphonates. TBS may be particularly helpful to assess fracture risk in diabetes. This article reviews technical and clinical aspects of TBS and its potential utility as a clinical tool to predict fracture risk.

Drug-Related Adverse Events of Osteoporosis Therapy 181

Moin Khan, Angela M. Cheung, and Aliya A. Khan

Postmenopausal osteoporosis is associated with microarchitectural deterioration and increased risk of fracture. Osteoporosis therapy effectively reduces the risk of vertebral, nonvertebral, and hip fracture and has been associated with increased survival. Currently approved treatments for osteoporosis include bisphosphonates, denosumab, selective estrogen receptor modulators, and teriparatide. This article reviews the adverse events of therapy associated with these medical interventions. Hormone replacement therapy is not included, because it is no longer indicated for the treatment of osteoporosis in all countries. Calcitonin and strontium ranelate are also not included, because their indication for osteoporosis has recently been limited or withdrawn.

Combined Pharmacologic Therapy in Postmenopausal Osteoporosis **193**

Yang Shen, Dona L. Gray, and Dorothy S. Martinez

Antiresorptive agents for treating postmenopausal osteoporosis include selective estrogen receptor modulator (SERM), bisphosphonates and denoumab. Teriparatide is the only Food and Drug Administration-approved anabolic agent. Synergistic effects of combining teriparatide with an antiresorptive agent have been proposed and studied. This article reviews the trial designs and the outcomes of combination therapies. Results of the combination therapy for teriparatide and bisphosphonates were mixed; while small increases of bone density were observed in the combination therapy of teriparatide and estrogen/SERM and that of teriparatide and denosumab. Those clinical studies were limited by small sample sizes and lack of fracture outcomes.

Novel Therapies for Postmenopausal Osteoporosis **207**

Leonardo Bandeira and John P. Bilezikian

Recently discovered mechanisms have assisted in developing new therapies for osteoporosis. New classes of drugs have been developed for the treatment of postmenopausal osteoporosis. Although there have been numerous advances over the past 2 decades, the search for newer therapies continues.

Index **221**

ENDOCRINOLOGY AND METABOLISM CLINICS OF NORTH AMERICA

FORTHCOMING ISSUES

June 2017
Genetics in Endocrine Disorders
Constantine A. Stratakis, *Editor*

September 2017
Biochemical and Imaging Diagnostics in Endocrinology
Richard J. Auchus, Barry D. Pressman, Adina F. Turcu, and Alan D. Waxman, *Editors*

December 2017
Vitamin D
J. Chris Gallagher and Daniel Bikle, *Editors*

RECENT ISSUES

December 2016
Diabetes
S. Sethu K. Reddy, *Editor*

September 2016
Obesity
Caroline M. Apovian & Nawfal W. Istfan, *Editors*

June 2016
Pediatric Endocrinology
Robert Rapaport, *Editor*

ISSUE OF RELATED INTEREST

Foot and Ankle Clinics of North America, December 2016 (Vol. 21, Issue 4)
Bone Grafts, Bone Graft Substitutes, and Biologics in Foot and Ankle Surgery
Sheldon Lin, *Editor*
http://www.foot.theclinics.com/

Foreword

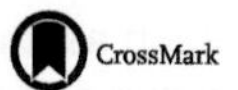

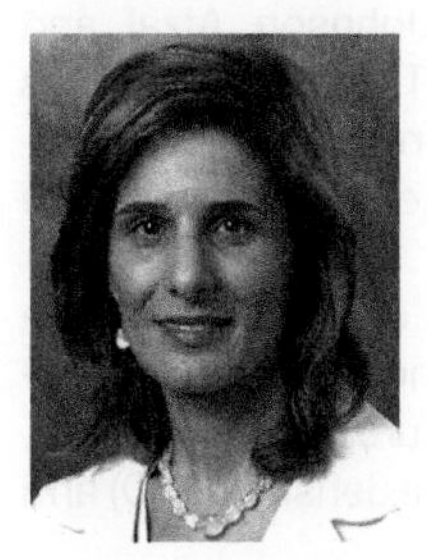

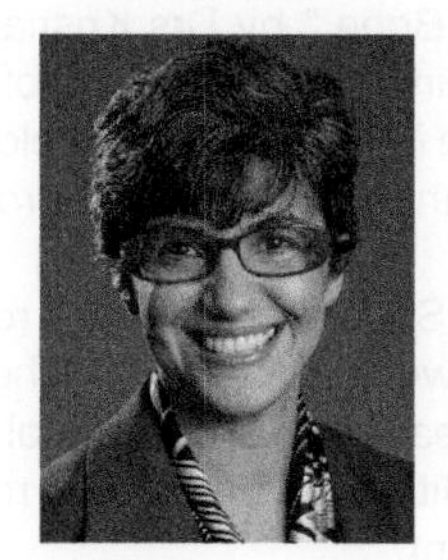

Anat Ben-Shlomo, MD   Maria Fleseriu, MD, FACE
Consulting Editors

Low bone mass and osteoporosis affect more than 50 million people in the United States, and fractures continue to be a frequent cause of morbidity and increased mortality. Furthermore, medical and hospitalization costs in the United States associated with osteoporotic fractures are high, especially in the elderly and with hip fractures. Over the last decade, bone research has significantly progressed and new pharmacotherapies have evolved, making this issue particularly timely. "Bone Diseases" in *Endocrinology and Metabolism Clinics of North America* summarizes key issues in the field of skeletal pathophysiology, including skeletal fragility and metabolic bone disease.

Our distinguished guest editor, Dr Albert Shieh, from University of California, Los Angeles, a recognized expert in the field, has gathered an outstanding group of clinicians with expertise in various aspects of bone disease, comorbidities, treatment guidelines, and management approaches.

Osteocytes comprise more than 90% of bone cells in the adult human skeleton and have been the subject of multiple studies, as summarized in "The Role of the Osteocyte in Bone and Non-bone Disease" by Dr Bonewald. The multiple normal functions of osteocytes are presented, including mechanosensation, calcium hemostasis, bone repair, and their newly recognized function as endocrine cells. The role of osteocytes in bone diseases, including osteoporosis, aging, and hypophosphatemic rickets, is also reviewed, as well as genetic disorders of high and low bone mass. The role of osteocytes in nonbone diseases, including kidney, heart, and muscle abnormalities, as well as pharmacotherapy targeting osteocyte factors is discussed as well.

In "Fibroblast Growth Factor 23-Mediated Bone Disease," Drs Gonciulea and Jan De Beur review the effect of osteocyte-derived FGF23 on the kidneys and parathyroid glands, where it regulates phosphate homeostasis and vitamin D synthesis and metabolism. Causes of Fibroblast Growth Factor 23 excess or deficiency associated with hypophosphatemia and bone demineralization and fractures or hyperphosphatemia and ectopic calcifications, respectively, are also described.

In "Bone-Fat Interaction," Drs Rendina-Ruedy and Rosen discuss the inverse relationship between bone marrow adipose tissue and bone density and quality. They review how bone marrow behaves as an endocrine organ producing hormones such as leptin and adiponectin and consider how this inverse relationship manifests in diseases

Endocrinol Metab Clin N Am 46 (2017) xiii–xv
http://dx.doi.org/10.1016/j.ecl.2016.12.002
0889-8529/17/© 2016 Published by Elsevier Inc.

such as anorexia nervosa, type 1 diabetes mellitus, and hypogonadism, as well as in aging and immobility.

The article, “Endothelin Signaling in Bone,” by Drs Kristianto, Johnson, Afzal, and Blank highlights the role of the endothelin system in bone biology. The authors discuss the critical role of the endothelin system in craniofacial development, bone matrix synthesis, and mineralization and review the osteosclerotic processes seen in prostate and breast cancer.

In “Diabetes and Bone Disease,” Drs Schacter and Leslie review epidemiologic data connecting type 1 and type 2 diabetes with osteoporosis. The pathophysiology of diabetes-mediated osteoporosis and increased risk for skeletal fractures are discussed, as is the utility of commonly used modalities to assess bone mineral density (BMD) and fracture risk and the benefit of treatment.

Drs Zanocco and Yeh discuss congenital and acquired causes and diagnosis of primary hyperthyroidism in “Primary Hyperparathyroidism: Effects on Bone Health.” Skeletal pathogenesis in primary hyperparathyroidism is highlighted along with therapeutic options, including surgery and pharmacotherapy.

In “The Effects of Bariatric Surgery on Bone Metabolism,” Dr Gregory reviews skeletal health in patients after bariatric surgery. The effects of malabsorption of vitamin D and calcium and the altered secretion of adipokines and gut hormones on bone density and fracture risk are emphasized.

In “Premenopausal Osteoporosis,” Dr Cohen notes that low BMD and low trauma fractures in premenopausal women are often driven by secondary causes. Premenopausal women with low BMD or fracture should undergo a thorough clinical, laboratory, and imaging evaluation to search for and treat secondary causes. Although treatment to increased bone density is necessary in the presence of deteriorating bone density and recurrent bone fractures, the ideal treatment in premenopausal women is unclear.

African Americans have higher BMD and lower fracture risk compared with Caucasians, despite having lower total 25-hydroxyvitamin D levels. The physiologic mechanisms behind these observations are reviewed in “Assessing Vitamin D Status in African Americans and the Influence of Vitamin D on Skeletal Health Parameters” by Drs Shieh and Aloia. The authors discuss classical endocrine and nonclassical intracrine vitamin D physiology, vitamin D bioactivity markers, and the effects of vitamin D supplements on these markers.

Drs Silva and Leslie review a new lumbar spine DXA-derived measurement to assess skeletal structure and predict fracture risk in “Trabecular Bone Score (TBS): A New DXA-Derived Measurement for Fracture Risk Assessment.” TBS predicts the risk of major osteoporotic fracture and hip fractures in women and men older than 40 to 50 years of age and can be used to adjust FRAX probability of fracture in postmenopausal women and older men, assisting in treatment decisions in clinical practice.

Drs M Khan, Cheung, and A Khan discuss the clinically available pharmacotherapies for osteoporosis in “Drug-Related Adverse Events of Osteoporosis Therapy.” Indications for as well as risk and benefits of treatment with bisphosphonates, denosumab, teriparatide, raloxifene, and bazedoxifene are detailed. The authors conclude that when no contraindications for therapy exist, the benefits of treatment outweigh the risks.

Drs Bandeira and Bilezikian summarize current and future osteoporosis pharmacotherapies in “Novel Therapies for Osteoporosis.” They discuss the clinically available RANK ligand denosumab and parathyroid hormone (PTH) analogue teriparatide, as well as pharmacotherapies in development including odanacatib, a highly selective cathepsin K inhibitor, PTH analogues, and romosozumab, an antisclerostin antibody.

The search for a better drug for osteoporosis that restores microarchitectural deterioration of the osteoporotic bone and eliminates fracture risk continues.

In "Combined Pharmacologic Therapy in Postmenopausal Osteoporosis," Drs Shen, Gray, and Martinez discuss combination therapy for postmenopausal therapy. The results and limitations of studies exploring effects on bone density using antiresorptive agents, such as estrogen and raloxifene, bisphosphonates, and denosumab, together with anabolic agents such as teriparatide, are presented.

We hope you will find this issue on Bone Diseases in *Endocrinology and Metabolism Clinics of North America* useful in your practice. We thank Dr Albert Shieh for guest editing this exciting and timely issue and the Elsevier editorial staff for their invaluable help.

Anat Ben-Shlomo, MD
Pituitary Center
Division of Endocrinology Diabetes, & Metabolism
Cedars Sinai Medical Center
8700 Beverly Boulevard
Los Angeles, CA 90048, USA

Maria Fleseriu, MD, FACE
Northwest Pituitary Center
Division of Endocrinology, Diabetes
& Clinical Nutrition
Departments of Medicine and
Neurological Surgery
Oregon Health & Science University
3138 SW Sam Jackson Park Road
Portland, OR 97239, USA

E-mail addresses:
benshlomoa@cshs.org (A. Ben-Shlomo)
fleseriu@ohsu.edu (M. Fleseriu)

Preface
An Introduction to the Bone Disorders Issue

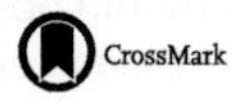

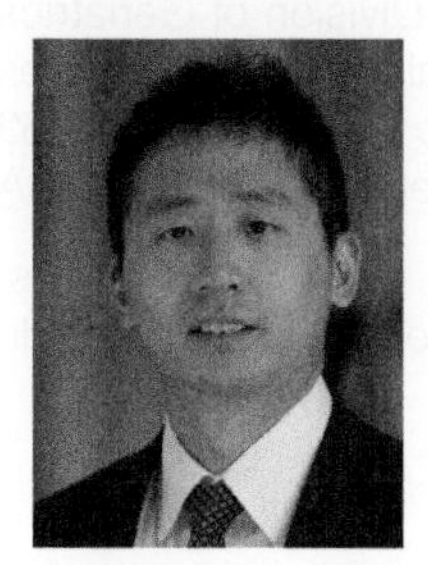

Albert Shieh, MD, MSCR
Editor

It is my distinct pleasure to serve as guest editor for the Bone Disorders Issue of *Endocrinology and Metabolism Clinics of North America*. This issue is especially timely for several reasons. Low bone mass and osteoporosis affect over 50 million US adults. As our population continues to age, the incidence and prevalence of osteoporosis are expected to increase further. Since the clinical consequence of skeletal fragility, fracture, is associated with increased debilitation and even mortality, effective recognition and treatment of individuals with osteoporosis are critical for helping aging US adults maintain their independence and health. Importantly, recent lay media coverage of certain safety concerns related to some osteoporosis pharmacotherapy has understandably led to widespread patient concern. It is therefore especially important for clinicians to be comfortable discussing the risks and benefits of available treatments to provide optimal counsel.

This issue covers advances in, and controversies surrounding, (1) skeletal physiology, (2) conditions associated with skeletal fragility, (3) diagnosis of metabolic bone disease, and (4) treatment of metabolic bone disease. These articles were written with a clinical focus to provide clinicians with up-to-date and balanced overviews on key topics. I would like to conclude by offering my thanks to those who made this issue possible. First, I would like to express my tremendous gratitude to all contributing authors, each a recognized expert in his or her respective field. Without their commitment and hard work, this issue would not have been possible. Second, I would like to thank Dr Richard Bockman, who introduced me to the field of metabolic bone disease, and who was instrumental in helping me create the table of contents and identifying

Endocrinol Metab Clin N Am 46 (2017) xvii–xviii
http://dx.doi.org/10.1016/j.ecl.2016.12.003
0889-8529/17/© 2016 Published by Elsevier Inc.

potential authors. Finally, I would like to recognize the diligence of the *Endocrinology and Metabolism Clinics of North America* staff, whose efforts made this endeavor a smooth operation.

Please enjoy.

Albert Shieh, MD, MSCR
Department of Medicine
Division of Geriatrics
University of California, Los Angeles
10945 Le Conte Avenue, Suite 2339
Los Angeles, CA 90095, USA

E-mail address:
ashieh@mednet.ucla.edu

Erratum

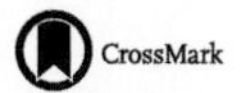

An error was made in the December 2016 issue of *Endocrinology and Metabolism Clinics of North America* on page 959 in "Evidence-based Mobile Medical Applications in Diabetes" by Andjela Drincic, Priya Prahalad, Deborah Greenwood and David C. Klonoff. The sentence "An instant feedback message tells the patient whether the BG level is in range, and provides tailored educational messages from the American Association of Diabetes Educators (AADE) curriculum," has been updated to the following: "An instant feedback message tells the patient whether the BG level is in range, and provides tailored educational messages based upon the AADE-7 self-care behaviors."

Endocrinol Metab Clin N Am 46 (2017) xix
http://dx.doi.org/10.1016/j.ecl.2016.12.001

The Role of the Osteocyte in Bone and Nonbone Disease

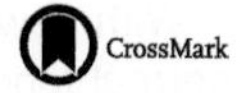

Lynda F. Bonewald, PhD[a,b,c,*]

KEYWORDS

• Osteocyte • Bone disease • Sclerostin • FGF23 • Therapeutics

KEY POINTS

- Within the last decade, the number of studies of osteocytes has increased dramatically leading to the discovery of novel functions of these cells.
- These cells can also be responsible for not only bone diseases and disorders, but also those of the kidney, heart, and potentially muscle.
- Osteocytes have entered the realm of therapeutic targets for bone disease and now potentially kidney disease.
- It will be important not to overlook these cells with regard to the health of other systems and organs.

INTRODUCTION

Before osteocytes were recognized as active essential bone cells necessary for bone health, it was assumed that all the action took place on the bone surface and not within the bone. Osteoblasts and osteoclasts were the major players, osteoblasts making bone and osteoclasts resorbing bone to maintain bone homeostasis. It was assumed that osteoblasts and osteoclasts were regulated by external factors such as parathyroid hormone (PTH) or 1,25 dihydroxyvitamin D_3, and other external regulatory factors. It has also been proposed that osteoblasts make factors that regulate osteoclast activity and, conversely, that osteoclasts make factors that could regulate osteoblast activity. Therapeutics were generated that would target either osteoclasts or osteoblasts. Osteocytes were left out of the picture.

The author is funded by NIH NIA grants PO1AG039355.

[a] Indiana Center for Musculoskeletal Health, VanNuys Medical Science Building, MS 5055, 635 Barnhill Drive, Indianapolis, IN 46202, USA; [b] Department of Anatomy and Cell Biology, VanNuys Medical Science Building, MS 5035, Indianapolis, IN 46202, USA; [c] Department of Orthopaedic Surgery, 1120 West Michigan Street, Suite 600, Indianapolis, IN 46202, USA
* Indiana Center for Musculoskeletal Health, VanNuys Medical Science Building, MS 5055S, 635 Barnhill Drive, Indianapolis, IN 46202.
E-mail address: lbonewal@iu.edu

Endocrinol Metab Clin N Am 46 (2017) 1–18
http://dx.doi.org/10.1016/j.ecl.2016.09.003
0889-8529/17/

With new technology and new tools, it became possible to study osteocytes. The normal functions of osteocytes expanded rapidly to include regulation of osteoblast and osteoclast activity to control bone remodeling, as regulators of both phosphate and calcium homeostasis, as mechanosensory cells that coordinate the skeleton's response to loading or unloading, and as endocrine cells targeting other tissues such as kidney. These cells are also one of the longest lived cell types in the body, with some living for decades; therefore, survival and normal function is paramount (**Box 1**). A number of pathologic or disease conditions can now be ascribed to abnormal or missing osteocyte functions, including sclerosteosis, hypophosphatemic rickets, osteoporosis, necrotic bone, and aging (**Fig. 1**). Now therapeutics are being generated that target osteocyte factors (for reviews see[1,2]).

NORMAL OSTEOCYTE FUNCTIONS

Mechanosensation

When early histomorphomists peered through their microscopes and began to visualize osteocytes in bone, the morphology and connectedness suggested a network perhaps similar to the neural system. One of the earliest functions ascribed to osteocytes was mechanosensation based on Julius Wolff's descriptions of the capacity of bone to adapt to mechanical loading or lack of loading by adding or removing bone.[3]

Box 1
Normal functions of osteocytes

- Control mineralization through *Phex*,[123] *Dmp1*,[56] and *MEPE*.[124,125]
- Regulate phosphate homeostasis through *FGF23*.[56,84]
- Play a role in calcium homeostasis in response to parathyroid hormone/parathyroid hormone-related protein.[40,126]
- Can recruit osteoclasts through expression of *RANKL* with or without cell death.[24,113,114]
- Can regulate osteoblast activity through *Sclerostin*.[127,128]
- Are mechanosensory cells through β-catenin signaling.[14,129]
- Have autocrine/paracrine effects through *prostaglandin* production.[6,130,131]
- Under calcium restriction, osteocytes remove calcium from bone through the vitamin D receptor.[132]
- Osteocytes regulate myelopoiesis/hematopoiesis through *G-CSF*.[63]
- *G-CSF* targets osteocytes that mediate mobilization of hematopoietic stem/progenitor cells and is prevented by surgical sympathectomy.[64]
- Osteocytes regulate primary lymphoid organs and fat metabolism[65]
- Osteocytes can dedifferentiate to become a source of matrix-producing osteoblasts.[133]
- Can increase muscle myogenesis and muscle function[60,62,134] and can inhibit muscle mass with aging.[107]
- Can have effects on heart[120,135] and liver[136] through fibroblast growth factor 23.
- Play a role in fracture healing through insulinlike growth factor-1.[137,138]
- Regulate bone formation through Bmpr1a signaling,[139] Notch activation,[140] and ERα signaling.[141,142]
- Suppress breast cancer growth and bone metastasis.[143]

Data from Ref.[1,2,122]

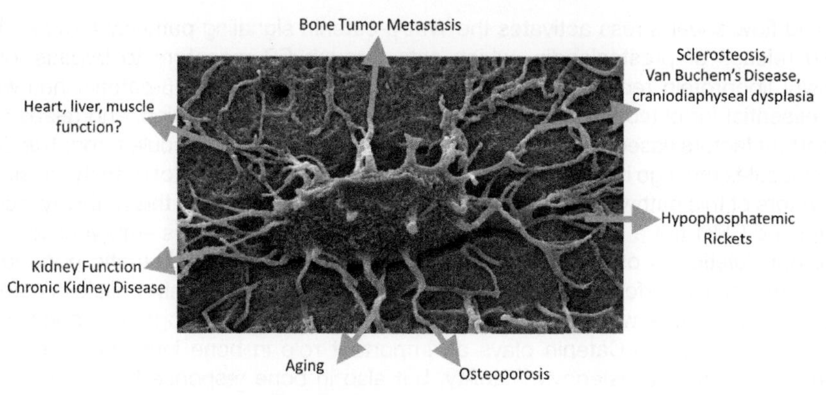

Fig. 1. Defective osteocyte function and disease.

More than a century later, experiments have been performed supporting the hypothesis that osteocytes are responsible for bone adaption in response to loading. By performing targeted deletion of osteocytes in mice expressing the diphtheria toxin receptor specifically in osteocytes, it was shown that these mice were resistant to unloading-induced bone loss.[4]

The osteocyte and its dendritic processes are exposed constantly to canalicular fluid that flows through the lacunocanalicular system. A baseline flow of canalicular fluid flow is driven by the extravascular pressure and intermittent mechanical loading superimposes rapid alterations in canalicular fluid flow.[5] This process results in the cells being exposed to different types and magnitudes of fluid flow shear stress. Almost every cell responds to mechanical loading; however, osteocytes seem to be most sensitive when compared with osteoblasts and fibroblasts.[6,7]

In both primary osteocytes and MLO-Y4 osteocyte-like cells, fluid flow shear stress has been shown to have numerous sequential effects.[2] The first event is the release of intracellular calcium followed by the release of nitric oxide, adenosine triphosphate, and prostaglandins, and the opening of connexin 43 hemichannels enhancing gap junction functions. Soon after the rapid change in calcium signaling (within seconds) nitric oxide, adenosine triphosphate, and prostaglandin (within seconds to minutes) are released. Deleting any 1 of these 3 early small molecules will inhibit bone's anabolic response to loading. Shear stress has also been shown to induce the bending of osteocyte cilia, and to initiate signaling pathways such as the wnt/β-catenin and protein kinase A pathways. Shear stress also activates gene transcription and translation, and promotes dendrite elongation. One very important effect of fluid flow shear stress is the protection of osteocytes against apoptosis and cell death. Ideally, it would be important to identify early regulators of anabolic signaling in osteocytes in addition to calcium, nitric oxide, adenosine triphosphate, and prostaglandin E_2 (PGE_2) to develop new therapeutics (For review see[8]).

A major source of prostaglandin in the body seems to be from bone. Osteocytes are prodigious producers of prostaglandin in response to loading,[9] and PGE_2 has paracrine effects on osteocytes to enhance gap junction function,[10] protects and maintains osteocyte viability,[11] and seems to be one of the key initiators of anabolic bone formation. Administration of prostaglandin increases bone mass and inhibitors of prostaglandin production, such as indomethacin, block the effects of anabolic loading.[12,13] One of the most important effects of prostaglandin released in response to loading may be to activate a very important signaling pathway in the osteocyte, the Wnt/β-catenin signaling pathway.

Fluid flow shear stress activates the Wnt/β-catenin signaling pathway through the rapid release of prostaglandin, which acts through EP receptors to bypass low-density lipoprotein receptor activation.[14,15] Components of the β-catenin pathway are essential for osteocyte viability, mechanosensation, transduction, and release of important factors essential for bone homeostasis. The central molecule through which all molecules must go is β-catenin. β-Catenin regulates expression of both the positive activators of this pathway, the wnts, and the negative regulators of this pathway, sclerostin and Dkk1 (for a review see[16]). Global deletion of β-catenin is embryonically lethal, but deletion in osteocytes using the Dmp1-Cre results in dramatic bone loss characterized by perforated cortises.[17] Interestingly, deletion of only 1 allele in osteocytes results in mice with a normal skeleton but a completely abrogated response to anabolic loading.[18] β-Catenin plays an important role in bone integrity, osteocyte communication, and osteocyte viability, but also in bone response to loading. This role extends to other components of this signaling pathway.

Two of the most famous and well-studied components of this pathway are the Lrp5 receptor and the negative regulator of the β-catenin pathway, sclerostin encoded by the gene *Sost*. Lrp5, a major coreceptor for Wnt signaling is expressed by many cells in the body, but sclerostin is relatively osteocyte specific. Deletion of Lrp5 results in mice with impaired response to anabolic loading.[19] Because sclerostin is expressed in mature osteocytes and mechanical loading reduces sclerostin levels, the downregulation of sclerostin most likely creates a permissive environment in which the Wnt proteins already present can activate the Wnt/β-catenin pathway. The role of the β-catenin pathway in disease is discussed elsewhere in this article.

It has been shown that osteocyte-specific or -selective genes are regulated by loading or unloading. These genes include the markers for early osteocytes, E11/gp38, phosphate regulating neutral endopeptidase on chromosome X (PHEX), dentin matrix protein 1 (DMP1), and the markers for late osteocytes, sclerostin, matrix extracellular phosphoglycoprotein (MEPE), and fibroblast growth factor (FGF23). (The function of these and their relationship to disease are discussed elsewhere in this article.) Regulators of mineralization and phosphate homeostasis such as PHEX, MEPE, and DMP1 are upregulated in response to mechanical loading,[20–22] as is E11/gp38, a marker for the early osteocyte.[23] It would be expected that genes involved in bone formation would be upregulated in response to anabolic load and genes responsible for resorption would be downregulated. It has been shown that unloading increases receptor activator of nuclear factor κB ligand (RANKL), an essential promoter of osteoclast formation, in osteocytes,[24] that may be responsible for the bone loss associated with unloading. *Sost*/sclerostin, a marker for the late osteocyte and an inhibitor of osteoblast function, is downregulated by anabolic mechanical loading and is increased in response to hindlimb unloading.[25,26]

The osteocyte's response to mechanical loading may be one of the major cellular mechanisms responsible for the positive effects of exercise, not only on bone but on the function of other tissues and organs in the body.

Calcium homeostasis

Probably the earliest proposed function of osteocytes was a capacity to remove their perilacunar matrix, a process referred to by Belanger as "osteocytic osteolysis."[27] In 1910, Von Recklinghausen described enlarged lacunae in patients with rickets or osteomalacia suggesting "pericellular digestion."[28] Belanger and associates[27,29,30] created the term "osteocytic osteolysis" for the enlarged lacunae induced by PTH or a by low-calcium diet. "Osteocytic osteolysis" was viewed as being a feature of pathologic conditions, especially owing to high or continuous PTH.[27,29,30] The stimulating effects of PTH on lysosomal vesicles in osteocytes was described in the 1970s[31,32] and in 1977, "perilacunar osteolysis" was described in rats sent into space[33] and alveolar bone of hibernating ground squirrels.[34] However, the number of publications began to decrease for various reasons[35] until technology had advanced sufficiently to address critics of this concept. Wergedal and Baylink[36] had described tartrate resistant acid phosphatase activity in osteocytes in 1969, which was criticized as being a diffusion artifact from osteoclasts but later validated by in situ hybridization, a technology not yet available in the 1960s and 1970s.[37]

Baylink and Wergedal[38] also showed tetracycline binding to the perilacunar matrix, which led to the hypothesis that osteocytes can replace their perilacunar matrix, which was later reproduced in egg-laying hens.[39] This suggested that under nonpathologic conditions osteocytes could remove and replace their perilacunar matrix. Qing and colleagues[40] proposed that the term "perilacunar modeling" be used in place of "osteocytic osteolysis" for nonpathologic conditions such as lactation. These investigators showed an increase in lacunar area with lactation, that the PTH type 1 receptor was responsible and described a return to normal lacunar area with weaning. They showed that genes thought to be osteoclast specific such as tartrate resistant acid phosphatase and cathepsin K were increased in osteocytes during lactation and returned to normal with weaning. This study shows that healthy osteocytes can both remove and replace their perilacunar matrix, thereby playing a role in mineral homeostasis during calcium demanding conditions. Recently, it has been shown that the calcitonin receptor may also play a role by inhibiting perilacunar remodeling with lactation.[41]

Because the PTH type 1 receptor is most highly expressed in osteocytes, the osteocyte may be the target of PTH in hyperparathyroidism and, conversely, the positive effects of intermittent PTH on bone formation may also be owing to effects on the osteocyte. The target of the therapeutic teriparatide recombinant human (Forteo) may be osteocytes in the mature skeleton.

Bone repair

Repair of microdamage and bone fatigue in bone is a normal, physiologic process. Bone is constantly sustaining damage in the form of microcracks that are repaired by osteoclasts targeting the damaged bone. Osteoclasts are responsible for initiating a cutting cone, but how does the osteoclast know the location of the microdamage? It seems that the osteocyte sends signals to the osteoclast providing information on where to resorb and where not to resorb bone (for a review see[42]). Microdamage and bone fatigue are associated with osteocyte apoptosis where an antiapoptotic factor, BAX, is found in osteocytes around the cutting cone, whereas the proapoptotic factor, Bcl2, is found in osteocytes in the path of the cutting cone.[43] The suggests that the osteocytes in the path are undergoing programmed cell death, whereas those in the periphery are preserving viability.[44] A number of in vitro studies using MLO-Y4 osteocyte-like cells have investigated potential mechanisms. Apoptotic bodies are released by MLO-Y4 cells and primary osteocytes, but not osteoblasts,[45] serum-starved MLO-Y4 cells will secrete soluble RANKL, which is necessary for osteoclast formation,[46] and damaged MLO-Y4 cell networks in 3-dimensional gels express increased RANKL and lesser osteoprotegerin, an inhibitor of the RANK receptor.[47]

Pathologic osteocyte cell death is associated with thiazolidinediones,[48] high-dose alcohol,[49] and methotrexate used for cancer treatment.[50] Osteocytes express markers of apoptosis in response to withdrawal of estrogen,[51] to oxygen deprivation as occurs during immobilization,[52] and in response to glucocorticoid treatment.[53] Tumor necrosis factor-α and interleukin-1 are potent inducers of osteocyte apoptosis.[54] Osteonecrosis, or dead bone, is owing to osteocyte cell death but the mechanisms responsible are still debated. Aging is associated with increased numbers of empty osteocyte lacunae. Therefore, a major research focus has been on osteocyte viability and approaches to prevent osteocyte cell death.

Osteocytes are endocrine cells

Potentially, osteoblasts have the capacity to release factors into the circulation, but they compose approximately 3% to 5% of bone cells compared with 1% osteoclasts, whereas 90% to 95% of bone cells in the adult human skeleton are osteocytes. It has not been appreciated that the total mass of osteocytes and their dendritic processes in bone that are equivalent to or greater than the mass of the brain[55]; therefore, these cells are most likely a major source of circulating bone factors. Bone is highly vascularized and secretes factors such as FGF23 into the bloodstream to affect distant targets,[56] it must be defined as an endocrine organ.[2] Interestingly, FGF23 is also able to act on the parathyroid gland to decrease PTH secretion, identifying the parathyroid gland as another endocrine target of osteocyte signaling.[57,58] The vascular system has a close, connecting association with the osteocyte lacuna–canalicular system with its bone fluid. Osteocytes also produce other circulating factors such as sclerostin. Osteocytes may also target muscle. It has recently been shown that 2 factors, PGE_2 and Wnt3a, both produced by osteocytes in response to shear stress support myogenesis and muscle function.[59–62] Therefore, mechanical loading of the skeleton, especially in the form of exercise, is important to ensure that osteocyte factors are released into the circulation.

In addition to cross-talk with muscle, osteocytes may also send signals to hematopoietic cells. Studies showed that osteocytes and G-protein-coupled receptor signaling were important in controlling myeloid cells proliferation[63] and mice lacking osteocytes were shown to have defective hematopoietic stem cell mobilization and lymphopenia.[64,65] Osteocyte may also have a role in regulating fat. Using a mouse model in which osteocytes can be ablated by use of diphtheria toxin, it was shown that osteocytes may also regulate adipose tissue.[65] Studies have shown that sclerostin may play a role in inducing adipocyte differentiation.[66] Osteocytes may be an important reservoir of factors that target other unknown organs and tissues.

ROLE OF OSTEOCYTES IN BONE DISEASE

Osteoporosis

Estrogen deficiency, glucocorticoid treatment, oxidative stress caused by disuse, and oxidative stress associated with aging may be responsible for osteocyte cell death and, therefore, bone fragility and osteoporosis.[67] As described, osteocyte cell death is important for repair of damaged bone[43,44,68] so any condition that compromises osteocyte health and function most likely compromises the skeleton. A number of factors and cytokines have been shown to induce osteocyte cell death including glucocorticoids, interleukin-1, and tumor necrosis factor-α, and conversely, a number of molecules have been shown to protect osteocytes from cell death such as estrogen, PTH, bisphosphonates (for review see[69–71]), and secreted muscle factors.[59] Osteocyte viability is crucial not only for the normal functioning of the skeleton, but for other organs such as kidney as discussed and muscle as discussed elsewhere in this article. Because osteocytes seem to have multiple, very important functions, it is important to maintain the normal viability and function of these cells.[2]

Aging

The osteocyte is a long-lived, nondividing, aging cell headed for senescence. Although some osteocytes are removed from bone with remodeling, many osteocytes can reside in human bone for decades, in contrast with osteoblasts and osteoclasts that live for only days or weeks. Recently, it has been shown that primary osteocytes from old mice (22 months of age) have 6-fold more telomere dysfunction-induced foci than osteocytes from young mice (6 months of age).[72] Senescent osteocytes predominately develop the senescence-associated secretory phenotype compared with other bone cells types, which may contribute to age-related bone loss. Once the cell dies, micropetrosis can result where mineral fills the lacuna, resulting in a cell that becomes a "living fossil."[73] Fewer numbers of osteocyte lacunae were found in patients suffering from fractures compared with controls[74] and an age-dependent decrease occurs in osteocyte lacunar density with an increased amount of hypermineralized calcium phosphate occlusions caused by micropetrosis.[75] The aging and dying osteocyte in a compromised lacunocanalicular system is less likely to produce secretory factors, less likely to repair bone, and less likely to respond to anabolic load. Therefore, it is important to maintain osteocyte viability with age.

Hypophosphatemic Rickets

Several phosphate-regulating hormones and enzymes—namely, PHEX, DMP1, MEPE, and FGF23—are produced mainly by late osteoblasts and by early and late osteocytes. PHEX is the earliest regulator of phosphate homeostasis to be expressed in the late osteoblast/early osteocyte. PHEX is the mutated gene in the Hyp mouse, which is also widely used as a model of X-linked hypophosphatemic rickets,[76] which leads to increased levels of FGF23 and hypophosphatemia.[77] Hypophosphatemic rickets in humans is caused by inactivating mutations of *Pex (HYP Consortium Nat Gen 1995)*. PHEX also interacts with DMP1 to regulate phosphate homeostasis by mechanisms that still have not been elucidated clearly. DMP1 is produced by early osteocytes and mice lacking DMP1 are hypophosphatemic and have increased FGF23 levels.[56] Two teams of investigators independently showed that autosomal-recessive hypophoshatemic rickets was caused by a mutation in DMP1 that affected FGF23 circulating levels.[56,78] Both PHEX and DMP1 are negative regulators of FGF23, but again the mechanisms have not been determined clearly. MEPE is expressed predominantly by osteocytes[79] and is not believed to act on FGF23 directly but through PHEX.[80] The ASARM peptide of MEPE can bind to PHEX, inhibiting its activity, which results in an increase in FGF23.[80,81]

The molecule at the center of phosphate regulation is FGF23. FGF23 was identified in 2000[82] as the phosphate-regulating hormone responsible for autosomal-dominant hypophosphatemic rickets, and for phosphate-wasting in tumor-induced osteomalacia and X-linked hypophosphatemia. Osteocytes are also a main source of FGF23 and recent work has shown that targeted ablation of FGF23 in bone cells recapitulates the hypophosphatemia observed in FGF23 null mice.[83] Clinkenbeard and colleagues[84,85] targeted FGF23 deletion using Col2.3-cre in osteoblasts and using DMP1-cre in early osteocytes and showed that most likely both osteoblasts and osteocytes are the physiologic source of FGF23. FGF23 is not normally expressed at high levels in osteocytes in the healthy state, but is upregulated dramatically in both DMP1- and PHEX-associated hypophosphatemic rickets,[77] and osteocytes seem to be the main source of the increased circulating levels of FGF23.

Genetic High and Low Bone Mass Diseases

Many of the mutations resulting in high or low bone mass are owing to mutations in components of the wnt/β-catenin signaling pathway. Among the most well-known are mutations in SOST, which is highly expressed in mature osteocytes, but also expressed in articular chondrocytes (Hinton and colleagues[86], 2009, Chan et al,[87]

2011). As stated, the protein sclerostin is an inhibitor of bone formation and the gene *Sost* is increased in response to unloading, decreased in response to loading, but also decreased in response to PTH.[88] Patients with sclerosteosis carry a point mutation in the *SOST* gene, whereas patients with van Buchem disease are characterized by a 52-kb deletion downstream of the gene.[89] Recently, craniodiaphyseal dysplasia, a rare and severe bone dysplasia characterized by sclerosis of the skull and facial bones has also been linked to a "de novo" mutation in the SOST gene.[83] The pathologic role of mutations in sclerostin has been reproduced in knockout and transgenic animal models that also show the high bone mass phenotype of sclerosteosis and van Buchem patients.[26,90] Sclerostin binds to low-density lipoprotein-related proteins 5, 6, and 4 to inhibit Wnt/β-catenin signaling.[91]

Genetic mutations in the receptors for sclerostin have also been shown to result in bone disease. Loss of function of LRP5 results in the condition osteoporosis pseudoglioma.[92] The condition is homozygous recessive and affected individuals had a *Z*-score of −4.7. Conversely, gain of function of LRP5 results in greatly increased bone mass.[93] The condition is autosomal dominant and individuals had bone mineral densities of 5 to 8, yet had normally shaped bones. These individuals never broke bones and could not float in water. Mutations in Lrp4 have also resulted in bone overgrowth.[94] Genetically modified mice have replicated these human phenotypes.

ROLE OF OSTEOCYTES IN NONBONE DISEASE

Chronic Kidney Disease

FGF23 secreted from osteocytes plays a pathologic role in chronic kidney disease (CKD). FGF23 is increased in osteocytes in CKD[95] and serum levels of FGF23 are increased, particularly in the later stages of the disease.[96,97] FGF23 levels predict cardiovascular events before but not after dialysis and FGF23 is a risk factor for adverse outcomes in patients with CKD and end-stage renal disease (for a review see[98]). Therefore, considerable effort is being put toward blocking or reducing FGF23 levels in these patients.

Cardiac Function

High circulating levels of FGF23 have negative effects on cardiac muscle (for a review see[99]). Increased levels of circulating FGF23 have been linked to increased risk of heart disease and independently associated with left ventricular hypertrophy in human population studies.[100,101] Increased serum FGF23 has also been linked with impaired vascular function,[100] vascular calcification,[102] and increased fat mass.[103]

Sarcopenia?

It is not clear if osteoporosis and sarcopenia are concurrent or if one precedes the other. Dogma has been that the main interaction between muscle and bone is the mechanical loading of bone through muscle contraction. Osteocytes secrete factors that regulate muscle mass and function. MLO-Y4 osteocyte-like cells and primary osteocyte factors induce muscle myogenesis and activate the Wnt/β-catenin pathway.[60,61] Two factors produced by osteocytes in response to shear stress, PGE_2 and Wnt3a, were found to enhance myogenesis and ex vivo primary muscle function.[62] The hypothesis that osteocytes can support myogenesis and muscle function is now supported by several lines of evidence.

Very recently, in vivo data have been published to support the concept that bone regulates muscle mass and function. In 2015, it was shown that osteocalcin partially restored muscle mass in a model of deletion of Cx43 in osteocytes.[104] In 2016, it was shown that osteocalcin can have positive effects on muscle mass.[105] Also in 2015, it was shown that cancer induced release of transforming growth factor-β from bone was responsible for muscle cachexia.[106] That same year it was shown that deletion of a protease, MBTPS1, in osteocytes had little effect on bone but significantly increased muscle mass and function with aging.[107] A reduction in members of the transforming growth factor-β superfamily was observed. This suggests that bone produces osteocalcin, which has positive effects on muscle, but also that bone and in particular osteocytes can produce negative regulators of muscle. It is not known if osteocyte dysfunction will play a role in sarcopenia.

Conversely, muscle also seems to secrete factors that affect osteocyte viability and function. In 2007, Pedersen coined the term "myokines" for muscle-secreted factors, opening the door to new concepts regarding muscle interaction with bone. Conversely, secreted factors from electrically stimulated skeletal muscle and from myotubes but not from myoblasts was shown to protect MLO-Y4 osteocyte-like cells from dexamethasone induced cell death.[108] Other muscle factors are being identified that have positive effects on bone.

THERAPEUTICS TARGETING OSTEOCYTE FACTORS

Antisclerostin Antibody

In animal studies, antisclerostin antibody has been shown consistently to increase bone mass. Inhibition of sclerostin by monoclonal antibody increases bone formation, bone mass, and bone strength in aged male rats.[109] Neutralizing antibody to sclerostin is being developed as a therapeutic to treat osteoporosis (for a review see[110]). The antibody blocks or reduces bone loss and supports bone formation, promotes fracture healing,[111] and is a potential therapeutic for a number of conditions of low bone mass such as osteogenesis imperfecta.[112] AMG 785 (Romosozumab) has been tested in phase I and II and blosozumab has been tested in phase I clinical trial with good results. These antibodies increase bone mass to a greater extent than any previously developed therapeutic for osteoporosis including bisphosphonates, teriparatide recombinant human, and denosumab. Phase III clinical trials are in progress.

Anti–receptor Activator of Nuclear Factor κB Ligand Antibody

MLO-Y4 osteocyte-like cells support osteoclast formation[113] and apoptotic bodies released from MLO-Y4 cells express RANKL.[45] Primary osteocytes express RANKL.[17] Osteocytes express greater amounts of RANKL than osteoblasts and are better supporters of osteoclast formation.[24,114] Deletion of RANKL using the 10-kb Dmp1-Cre results in mice with increased bone mass. This suggests that anti-RANKL antibody is mainly targeting osteocytes. Human anti-RANKL monoclonal antibody, denosumab, is now available for the treatment of osteoporosis. The antibody decreases osteoclast differentiation, function, and survival. It reduces risk of spine, hip, and nonvertebral fractures and does not require dose adjustment for decreased kidney function. For treatment of osteoporosis, subcutaneous dosing every 6 months is applied and the effect is reversible within 6 to 12 months of stopping.[115]

Anti–fibroblast Growth Factor 23 Antibody

There are several conditions that could potentially benefit from treatment with anti-FGF23 antibody. In bone, autosomal-dominant hypophosphatemic rickets, caused by gain-of-function mutations in FGF23 that prevent proteolytic cleavage[82] and homozygous mutation in FAM20, a regulatory molecule of FGF23, resulting in hypophosphatemic osteomalacia[116] may benefit from anti-FGF23 antibody. In the kidney, because

FGF23 is increased in osteocytes[95] and in serum in CKD,[96,97] these would also benefit from reducing FGF23 circulating levels. In heart disease, studies have linked increased levels of circulating FGF23 to an increased risk of heart disease, left ventricular hypertrophy in human population studies,[101,117] impaired vascular function, vascular calcification, and increased fat mass.[102] All of these conditions could potentially benefit from FGF receptor inhibitors and anti-FGF23 antibody. Treatment with FGF23 antibody restored serum phosphate levels and corrects bone defects in the Hyp mouse and Dmp1 null model[118] and treatment with anti-FGF23 antibody KR23 increases serum phosphate in X-linked hypophosphatemic rickets.[119] (for a review see[120]).

Other Therapeutics to Treat Bone Disease

Could other therapeutics targeted to either osteoclasts or osteoblasts be also having effects on osteocytes? The is a distinct possibility. Calcitonin, bisphosphonates (alendronate [Fosamax], ibandronate [Boniva], etc), anti-RANKL (denosumab), and cathepsin K inhibitors (odanacatinb) have been developed to target osteoclasts. However, bisphosphonates have also been shown to reduce osteocyte apoptosis,[69] osteocytes can also express cathepsin K under certain conditions[40] and, as shown, the anti-RANKL antibody may be targeting osteocytes. Hormone replacement therapy, selective estrogen receptor modulators (Raloxifene [Evista]), and parathyroid hormone peptides (teriparatide recombinant human) have been thought to mainly target osteoblasts, but these could also be having significant effects on osteocytes.

Are There Other Osteocyte Factors?

Much attention has focused on osteocalcin produced by osteoblasts. This bone-specific factor has been shown to have effects on glucose metabolism, fertility, calcification, and others.[121] The osteoblast has been ascribed the production of osteocalcin and the osteoclast as the releaser of uncarboxylated, the "active" form of osteocalcin from the bone matrix to target other tissues. However, in the adult skeleton, osteoclasts make up less than 1% of bone cells, and osteoblasts less than 5%. Osteocytes have been shown to also produce osteocalcin, so it will be interesting to see if osteocalcin production by osteocytes has a role in normal physiology and pathophysiology. Gene arrays have been performed on primary osteocytes and osteocyte cell lines. As with any gene arrays analysis, it is difficult to identify specific genes. It is likely that there are osteocyte factors responsible for normal function that may also play a role in disease that have not yet been identified.

SUMMARY

When normal physiologic functions go awry, disorders and disease occurs. This is universal and, as discussed herein, even for the osteocyte, a cell thought to not be in contact with the rest of the body. It was once thought that this cell was simply a placeholder in bone. The early functions proposed for this type of bone cell were mechanosensation and the capacity to remove their perilacunar matrix called "osteocytic osteolysis." Considerable skepticism existed even for these ascribed functions for decades. Within the last decade, the number of studies of osteocytes has dramatically increased leading to the discovery of novel functions of these cells. Along with these discoveries came the discoveries of how these cells can also be responsible for not only bone diseases and disorders, but also those of the kidney, heart, and potentially muscle. Osteocytes have entered the realm of therapeutic targets for bone disease and now potentially kidney disease. It will be important not to overlook these cells with regard to the health of other systems and organs.

REFERENCES

1. Bonewald LF. The amazing osteocyte. J Bone Miner Res 2011;26(2):229–38.
2. Dallas SL, Prideaux M, Bonewald LF. The osteocyte: an endocrine cell... and more. Endocr Rev 2013;34(5):658–90.
3. Wolff J. Das Gesetz der Transformation der Knochen. Berlin: A Hirschwald; 1982.
4. Tatsumi S, Ishii K, Amizuka N, et al. Targeted ablation of osteocytes induces osteoporosis with defective mechanotransduction. Cell Metab 2007;5(6):464–75.
5. Weinbaum S, Cowin SC, Zeng Y. A model for the excitation of osteocytes by mechanical loading-induced bone fluid shear stresses. J Biomech 1994;27(3):339–60.
6. Klein-Nulend J, van der Plas A, Semeins CM, et al. Sensitivity of osteocytes to biomechanical stress in vitro. FASEB J 1995;9(5):441–5.
7. Klein-Nulend J, Semeins CM, Ajubi NE, et al. Pulsating fluid flow increases nitric oxide (NO) synthesis by osteocytes but not periosteal fibroblasts–correlation with prostaglandin upregulation. Biochem Biophys Res Commun 1995;217(2):640–8.
8. Klein-Nulend J, Bakker AD, Bacabac RG, et al. Mechanosensation and transduction in osteocytes. Bone 2013;54(2):182–90.
9. Kamel MA, Picconi JL, Lara-Castillo N, et al. Activation of beta-catenin signaling in MLO-Y4 osteocytic cells versus 2T3 osteoblastic cells by fluid flow shear stress and PGE(2): Implications for the study of mechanosensation in bone. Bone 2010;47(5):872–81.
10. Cherian PP, Siller-Jackson AJ, Gu S, et al. Mechanical strain opens connexin 43 hemichannels in osteocytes: a novel mechanism for the release of prostaglandin. Mol Biol Cell 2005;16:3100–6.
11. Kitase Y, Jiang JX, Johnson ML, et al. The anti-apoptotic effects of mechanical strain on osteocytes are mediated by PGE_2 and monocyte chemotactic protein-3 (MCP-3); SElective protection by MCP-3 against glucocorticoid (GC), but not TNF-a Induced apoptosis. J Bone Miner Res 2006;21(Suppl 1):S48.
12. Forwood MR. Inducible cyclo-oxygenase (COX-2) mediates the induction of bone formation by mechanical loading in vivo. J Bone Miner Res 1996;11(11):1688–93.
13. Pead MJ, Lanyon LE. Indomethacin modulation of load-related stimulation of new bone formation in vivo. Calcif Tissue Int 1989;45(1):34–40.
14. Bonewald LF, Johnson ML. Osteocytes, mechanosensing and Wnt signaling. Bone 2008;42(4):606–15.
15. Johnson ML, Picconi JL, Recker RR. The gene for high bone mass. Endocrinologist 2002;12:445–53.
16. Baron R, Kneissel M. WNT signaling in bone homeostasis and disease: from human mutations to treatments. Nat Med 2013;19(2):179–92.
17. Kramer I, Halleux C, Keller H, et al. Osteocyte Wnt/beta-catenin signaling is required for normal bone homeostasis. Mol Cell Biol 2010;30(12):3071–85.
18. Javaheri B, Dallas M, Zhao H, et al. b-catenin haploinsufficiency in osteocytes abolishes the osteogenic effect of mechanical loading in vivo. J Bone Miner Res 2014;29:705–15.
19. Sawakami K, Robling AG, Pitner ND, et al. Site-specific osteopenia and decreased mechanoreactivity in Lrp5 mutant mice. J Bone Miner Res 2004;19(Suppl 1):S38.

20. Yang W, Lu Y, Kalajzic I, et al. Dentin matrix protein 1 gene cis-regulation: use in osteocytes to characterize local responses to mechanical loading in vitro and in vivo. J Biol Chem 2005;280(21):20680–90.
21. Gluhak-Heinrich J, Ye L, Bonewald LF, et al. Mechanical loading stimulates dentin matrix protein 1 (DMP1) expression in osteocytes in vivo. J Bone Miner Res 2003;18(5):807–17.
22. Gluhak-Heinrich J, Pavlin D, Yang W, et al. MEPE expression in osteocytes during orthodontic tooth movement. Arch Oral Biol 2007;52(7):684–90.
23. Zhang K, Barragan-Adjemian C, Ye L, et al. E11/gp38 selective expression in osteocytes: regulation by mechanical strain and role in dendrite elongation. Mol Cell Biol 2006;26(12):4539–52.
24. Xiong J, Onal M, Jilka RL, et al. Matrix-embedded cells control osteoclast formation. Nat Med 2011;17(10):1235–41.
25. Robling AG, Niziolek PJ, Baldridge LA, et al. Mechanical stimulation of bone in vivo reduces osteocyte expression of Sost/sclerostin. J Biol Chem 2008; 283(9):5866–75.
26. Lin C, Jiang X, Dai Z, et al. Sclerostin mediates bone response to mechanical unloading through antagonizing Wnt/beta-catenin signaling. J Bone Miner Res 2009;24(10):1651–61.
27. Belanger LF, Belanger C, Semba T. Technical approaches leading to the concept of osteocytic osteolysis. Clin Orthop Relat Res 1967;54:187–96.
28. Von Recklinghausen F. Untersuchungen uber Rachitis und Osteomalacia. Jena Gustav Fischer; 1910.
29. Belanger LF. Osteocytic osteolysis. Calcif Tissue Res 1969;4(1):1–12.
30. Belanger LF, Robichon J. Parathormone-induced osteolysis in dogs. A microradiographic and alpharadiographic survey. J Bone Joint Surg Am 1964;46: 1008–12.
31. Bonucci E, Gherardi G. Osteocyte ultrastructure in renal osteodystrophy. Virchows Arch A Pathol Anat Histol 1977;373(3):213–31.
32. Bonucci E, Gherardi G, Mioni G, et al. Clinico-morphological correlations in uremic osteodystrophy of patients with conservative and hemodialytic treatment with special regard to the ultrastructure. Minerva Nefrol 1975;22(2–3):99–108 [in Italian].
33. Iagodovskii VS, Triftanidi LA, Gorokhova GP. Effect of space flight on rat skeletal bones (an optical light and electron microscopic study). Kosm Biol Aviakosm Med 1977;11(1):14–20 [in Russian].
34. Haller AC, Zimny ML. Effects of hibernation on interradicular alveolar bone. J Dent Res 1977;56(12):1552–7.
35. Qing H, Bonewald L. Osteocyte remodeling of the perilacunar and pericanalicular matrix. Int J Oral Sci 2009;1(2):59–65.
36. Wergedal JE, Baylink DJ. Distribution of acid and alkaline phosphatase activity in undermineralized sections of the rat tibial diaphysis. J Histochem Cytochem 1969;17(12):799–806.
37. Nakano Y, Toyosawa S, Takano Y. Eccentric localization of osteocytes expressing enzymatic activities, protein, and mRNA signals for type 5 tartrate-resistant acid phosphatase (TRAP). J Histochem Cytochem 2004;52(11):1475–82.
38. Baylink DJ, Wergedal JE. Bone formation by osteocytes. Am J Physiol 1971; 221(3):669–78.
39. Zambonin Zallone A, Teti A, Primavera MV, et al. Mature osteocytes behaviour in a repletion period: the occurrence of osteoplastic activity. Basic Appl Histochem 1983;27(3):191–204.

40. Qing H, Ardeshirpour L, Pajevic PD, et al. Demonstration of osteocytic perilacunar/canalicular remodeling in mice during lactation. J Bone Miner Res 2012; 27(5):1018–29.
41. Clarke MV, Russell PK, Findlay DM, et al. A role for the calcitonin receptor to limit bone loss during lactation in female mice by inhibiting osteocytic osteolysis. Endocrinology 2015;156(9):3203–14.
42. Schaffler MB, Cheung WY, Majeska R, et al. Osteocytes: master orchestrators of bone. Calcif Tissue Int 2013;94(1):5–24.
43. Verborgt O, Gibson GJ, Schaffler MB. Loss of osteocyte integrity in association with microdamage and bone remodeling after fatigue in vivo. J Bone Miner Res 2000;15(1):60–7.
44. Verborgt O, Tatton NA, Majeska RJ, et al. Spatial distribution of Bax and Bcl-2 in osteocytes after bone fatigue: complementary roles in bone remodeling regulation? J Bone Miner Res 2002;17(5):907–14.
45. Kogianni G, Mann V, Noble BS. Apoptotic bodies convey activity capable of initiating osteoclastogenesis and localized bone destruction. J Bone Miner Res 2008;23(6):915–27.
46. Al-Dujaili SA, Lau E, Al-Dujaili H, et al. Apoptotic osteocytes regulate osteoclast precursor recruitment and differentiation in vitro. J Cell Biochem 2011;112(9): 2412–23.
47. Mulcahy LE, Taylor D, Lee TC, et al. RANKL and OPG activity is regulated by injury size in networks of osteocyte-like cells. Bone 2011;48(2):182–8.
48. Mabilleau G, Mieczkowska A, Edmonds ME. Thiazolidinediones induce osteocyte apoptosis and increase sclerostin expression. Diabet Med 2010;27(8): 925–32.
49. Maurel DB, Jaffre C, Rochefort GY, et al. Low bone accrual is associated with osteocyte apoptosis in alcohol-induced osteopenia. Bone 2011;49(3):543–52.
50. Shandala T, Ng YS, Hopwood B, et al. The role of osteocyte apoptosis in cancer chemotherapy-induced bone loss. J Cell Physiol 2011;227(7):2889–97.
51. Tomkinson A, Reeve J, Shaw RW, et al. The death of osteocytes via apoptosis accompanies estrogen withdrawal in human bone. J Clin Endocrinol Metab 1997;82(9):3128–35.
52. Dodd JS, Raleigh JA, Gross TS. Osteocyte hypoxia: a novel mechanotransduction pathway. Am J Physiol 1999;277(3 Pt 1):C598–602.
53. Weinstein RS, Nicholas RW, Manolagas SC. Apoptosis of osteocytes in glucocorticoid-induced osteonecrosis of the hip. J Clin Endocrinol Metab 2000;85(8):2907–12.
54. Pacifici R, Brown C, Puscheck E, et al. Effect of surgical menopause and estrogen replacement on cytokine release from human blood mononuclear cells. Proc Natl Acad Sci U S A 1991;88(12):5134–8.
55. Buenzli PR, Sims NA. Quantifying the osteocyte network in the human skeleton. Bone 2015;75:144–50.
56. Feng JQ, Ward LM, Liu S, et al. Loss of DMP1 causes rickets and osteomalacia and identifies a role for osteocytes in mineral metabolism. Nat Genet 2006; 38(11):1310–5.
57. Krajisnik T, Bjorklund P, Marsell R, et al. Fibroblast growth factor-23 regulates parathyroid hormone and 1alpha-hydroxylase expression in cultured bovine parathyroid cells. J Endocrinol 2007;195(1):125–31.
58. Ben-Dov IZ, Galitzer H, Lavi-Moshayoff V, et al. The parathyroid is a target organ for FGF23 in rats. J Clin Invest 2007;117(12):4003–8.

59. Jahn K, Lara-Castillo N, Brotto L, et al. Skeletal muscle secreted factors prevent glucocorticoid-induced osteocyte apoptosis through activation of beta-catenin. Eur Cell Mater 2012;24:197–210.
60. Mo C, Romero-Suarez S, Bonewald L, et al. Prostaglandin E2: from clinical applications to its potential role in bone- muscle crosstalk and myogenic differentiation. Recent Pat Biotechnol 2012;6(3):223–9.
61. Mo CL, Romero-Suarez S, Bonewald LF, et al. Evidence for biochemical and functional communication from the MLO-Y4 osteocyte-like cell to the C2C12 muscle cells. Cell Cycle 2015;14:1507–16.
62. Huang J, Mo C, Bonewald L, et al. Wnt3a potentiates myogenesis in C2C12 myoblasts through changes of signaling pathways including Wnt and NFkB. ASBMR 2014 Annual Meeting. 2014. SU0190:s266. Houston (TX), September 14, 2014.
63. Fulzele K, Krause DS, Panaroni C, et al. Myelopoiesis is regulated by osteocytes through Gsalpha-dependent signaling. Blood 2013;121(6):930–9.
64. Asada N, Katayama Y, Sato M, et al. Matrix-embedded osteocytes regulate mobilization of hematopoietic stem/progenitor cells. Cell Stem Cell 2013;12(6): 737–47.
65. Sato M, Asada N, Kawano Y, et al. Osteocytes regulate primary lymphoid organs and fat metabolism. Cell Metab 2013;18(5):749–58.
66. Ukita M, Yamaguchi T, Ohata N, et al. Sclerostin enhances adipocyte differentiation in 3T3-L1 cells. J Cell Biochem 2016;117(6):1419–28.
67. Almeida M. Aging mechanisms in bone. Bonekey Rep 2012;1.
68. Kennedy OD, Herman BC, Laudier DM, et al. Activation of resorption in fatigue-loaded bone involves both apoptosis and active pro-osteoclastogenic signaling by distinct osteocyte populations. Bone 2012;50(5):1115–22.
69. Bellido T, Plotkin LI. Novel actions of bisphosphonates in bone: preservation of osteoblast and osteocyte viability. Bone 2011;49:50–5.
70. Jilka RL, Noble B, Weinstein RS. Osteocyte apoptosis. Bone 2013;54(2):264–71.
71. Jilka RL, O'Brien CA. The role of osteocytes in age-related bone loss. Curr Osteoporos Rep 2016;14(1):16–25.
72. Farr JN, Fraser DG, Wang H, et al. Identification of senescent cells in the bone microenvironment. J Bone Miner Res 2016. [Epub ahead of print].
73. Bell LS, Kayser M, Jones C. The mineralized osteocyte: a living fossil. Am J Phys Anthropol 2008;137(4):449–56.
74. Qiu S, Rao DS, Palnitkar S, et al. Reduced iliac cancellous osteocyte density in patients with osteoporotic vertebral fracture. J Bone Miner Res 2003;18(9):1657–63.
75. Qiu S, Rao DS, Palnitkar S, et al. Age and distance from the surface but not menopause reduce osteocyte density in human cancellous bone. Bone 2002; 31(2):313–8.
76. Strom TM, Francis F, Lorenz B, et al. Pex gene deletions in Gy and Hyp mice provide mouse models for X-linked hypophosphatemia. Hum Mol Genet 1997; 6(2):165–71.
77. Liu S, Tang W, Zhou J, et al. Distinct roles for intrinsic osteocyte abnormalities and systemic factors in regulation of FGF23 and bone mineralization in hyp mice. Am J Physiol Endocrinol Metab 2007;293(6):E1636–44.
78. Lorenz-Depiereux B, Bastepe M, Benet-Pages A, et al. DMP1 mutations in autosomal recessive hypophosphatemia implicate a bone matrix protein in the regulation of phosphate homeostasis. Nat Genet 2006;38(11):1248–50.

79. Igarashi M, Kamiya N, Ito K, et al. In situ localization and in vitro expression of osteoblast/osteocyte factor 45 mRNA during bone cell differentiation. Histochem J 2002;34(5):255–63.
80. Liu S, Rowe PS, Vierthaler L, et al. Phosphorylated acidic serine-aspartate-rich MEPE-associated motif peptide from matrix extracellular phosphoglycoprotein inhibits phosphate regulating gene with homologies to endopeptidases on the X-chromosome enzyme activity. J Endocrinol 2007;192(1):261–7.
81. Rowe PS, Garrett IR, Schwarz PM, et al. Surface plasmon resonance (SPR) confirms that MEPE binds to PHEX via the MEPE-ASARM motif: a model for impaired mineralization in X-linked rickets (HYP). Bone 2005;36(1):33–46.
82. ADHR Consortium. Autosomal dominant hypophosphataemic rickets is associated with mutations in FGF23. Nat Genet 2000;26(3):345–8.
83. Kim SJ, Bieganski T, Sohn YB, et al. Identification of signal peptide domain SOST mutations in autosomal dominant craniodiaphyseal dysplasia. Hum Genet 2011;129(5):497–502.
84. Clinkenbeard EL, Cass TA, Ni P, et al. Conditional deletion of murine Fgf23: interruption of the normal skeletal responses to phosphate challenge and rescue of genetic hypophosphatemia. J Bone Miner Res 2016;31(6):1247–57.
85. Clinkenbeard EL, White KE. Systemic control of bone homeostasis by FGF23 signaling. Curr Mol Biol Rep 2016;2(1):62–71.
86. Hinton RJ, Serrano M, So S. Differential gene expression in the perichondrium and cartliage of the neonatal mouse temporomandibular joint. Orthod Craniofac Res 2009;12(3):168–77.
87. Chan BY, Fuller ES, Russell AK, et al. Increased chondrocyte sclerostin may protect against cartilage degradation in osteoarthritis. Osteoarthritis Cartliage 2011;19(7):874–85.
88. Bellido T, Ali AA, Gubrij I, et al. Chronic elevation of PTH in mice reduces expression of sclerostin by osteocytes: a novel mechanism for hormonal control of osteoblastogenesis. Endocrinology 2005;146(11):4577–83.
89. Balemans W, Patel N, Ebeling M, et al. Identification of a 52 kb deletion downstream of the SOST gene in patients with van Buchem disease. J Med Genet 2002;39(2):91–7.
90. Li X, Ominsky MS, Niu QT, et al. Targeted deletion of the sclerostin gene in mice results in increased bone formation and bone strength. J Bone Miner Res 2008; 23(6):860–9.
91. Li X, Ominsky MS, Warmington KS, et al. Sclerostin antibody treatment increases bone formation, bone mass, and bone strength in a rat model of postmenopausal osteoporosis. J Bone Miner Res 2009;24(4):578–88.
92. Gong Y, Slee RB, Fukai N, et al. LDL receptor-related protein 5 (LRP5) affects bone accrual and eye development. Cell 2001;107(4):513–23.
93. Little RD, Carulli JP, Del Mastro RG, et al. A mutation in the LDL receptor-related protein 5 gene results in the autosomal dominant high-bone-mass trait. Am J Hum Genet 2002;70(1):11–9.
94. Leupin O, Piters E, Halleux C, et al. Bone overgrowth-associated mutations in the LRP4 gene impair sclerostin facilitator function. J Biol Chem 2011;286(22): 19489–500.
95. Pereira RC, Juppner H, Azucena-Serrano CE, et al. Patterns of FGF-23, DMP1, and MEPE expression in patients with chronic kidney disease. Bone 2009;45(6): 1161–8.
96. Larsson T, Nisbeth U, Ljunggren O, et al. Circulating concentration of FGF-23 increases as renal function declines in patients with chronic kidney disease,

but does not change in response to variation in phosphate intake in healthy volunteers. Kidney Int 2003;64(6):2272–9.
97. Imanishi Y, Inaba M, Nakatsuka K, et al. FGF-23 in patients with end-stage renal disease on hemodialysis. Kidney Int 2004;65(5):1943–6.
98. Kovesdy CP, Alrifai A, Gosmanova EO, et al. Age and outcomes associated with BP in patients with incident CKD. Clin J Am Soc Nephrol 2016;11(5):821–31.
99. Bonewald LF, Kiel DP, Clemens TL, et al. Forum on bone and skeletal muscle interactions: summary of the proceedings of an ASBMR workshop. J Bone Miner Res 2013;28(9):1857–65.
100. Mirza MA, Larsson A, Lind L, et al. Circulating fibroblast growth factor-23 is associated with vascular dysfunction in the community. Atherosclerosis 2009; 205(2):385–90.
101. Faul C, Amaral AP, Oskouei B, et al. FGF23 induces left ventricular hypertrophy. J Clin Invest 2011;121(11):4393–408.
102. Desjardins L, Liabeuf S, Renard C, et al. FGF23 is independently associated with vascular calcification but not bone mineral density in patients at various CKD stages. Osteoporos Int 2011;23(7):2017–25.
103. Mirza MA, Alsio J, Hammarstedt A, et al. Circulating fibroblast growth factor-23 is associated with fat mass and dyslipidemia in two independent cohorts of elderly individuals. Arterioscler Thromb Vasc Biol 2011;31(1):219–27.
104. Shen H, Grimston S, Civitelli R, et al. Deletion of connexin43 in osteoblasts/osteocytes leads to impaired muscle formation in mice. J Bone Miner Res 2015; 30(4):596–605.
105. Mera P, Laue K, Ferron M, et al. Osteocalcin signaling in myofibers is necessary and sufficient for optimum adaptation to exercise. Cell Metab 2016;23(6): 1078–92.
106. Waning DL, Mohammad KS, Reiken S, et al. Excess TGF-beta mediates muscle weakness associated with bone metastases in mice. Nat Med 2015;21(11): 1262–71.
107. Gorski JP, Huffman NT, Vallejo J, et al. Deletion of Mbtps1 (Pcsk8, S1p, Ski-1) gene in osteocytes stimulates soleus muscle regeneration and increased size and contractile force with age. J Biol Chem 2016;291(9):4308–22.
108. Brakenhoff JPJ, Hart M, De Groot ER, et al. Structure-function analysis of human IL-6: epitope mapping of neutralizing monoclonal antibodies with amino- and carboxyl- terminal deletion mutants. J Immunol 1990;145:561–8.
109. Li X, Warmington KS, Niu QT, et al. Inhibition of sclerostin by monoclonal antibody increases bone formation, bone mass, and bone strength in aged male rats. J Bone Miner Res 2010;25(12):2647–56.
110. Clarke BL. Anti-sclerostin antibodies: utility in treatment of osteoporosis. Maturitas 2014;78(3):199–204.
111. Morse A, Yu NY, Peacock L, et al. Endochondral fracture healing with external fixation in the Sost knockout mouse results in earlier fibrocartilage callus removal and increased bone volume fraction and strength. Bone 2015;71:155–63.
112. Roschger A, Roschger P, Keplingter P, et al. Effect of sclerostin antibody treatment in a mouse model of severe osteogenesis imperfecta. Bone 2014;66: 182–8.
113. Zhao S, Zhang YK, Harris S, et al. MLO-Y4 osteocyte-like cells support osteoclast formation and activation. J Bone Miner Res 2002;17(11):2068–79.
114. Nakashima T, Hayashi M, Fukunaga T, et al. Evidence for osteocyte regulation of bone homeostasis through RANKL expression. Nat Med 2011;17(10):1231–4.

115. Miller PD. A review of the efficacy and safety of denosumab in postmenopausal women with osteoporosis. Ther Adv Musculoskelet Dis 2011;3(6):271–82.
116. Takeyari S, Yamamoto T, Kinoshita Y, et al. Hypophosphatemic osteomalacia and bone sclerosis caused by a novel homozygous mutation of the FAM20C gene in an elderly man with a mild variant of Raine syndrome. Bone 2014;67:56–62.
117. Mirza MA, Hansen T, Johansson L, et al. Relationship between circulating FGF23 and total body atherosclerosis in the community. Nephrol Dial Transplant 2009;24(10):3125–31.
118. Aono Y, Yamazaki Y, Yasutake J, et al. Therapeutic effects of anti-FGF23 antibodies in hypophosphatemic rickets/osteomalacia. J Bone Miner Res 2009;24(11):1879–88.
119. Carpenter TO, Imel EA, Ruppe MD, et al. Randomized trial of the anti-FGF23 antibody KRN23 in X-linked hypophosphatemia. J Clin Invest 2014;124(4):1587–97.
120. Bonewald LF, Wacker MJ. FGF23 production by osteocytes. Pediatr Nephrol 2013;28(4):563–8.
121. Wei J, Karsenty G. An overview of the metabolic functions of osteocalcin. Rev Endocr Metab Disord 2015;16(2):93–8.
122. Plotkin LI, Bellido T. Osteocytic signalling pathways as therapeutic targets for bone fragility. Nat Rev Endocrinol 2016. http://dx.doi.org/10.1038/nrendo.2016.71.
123. Yuan B, Takaiwa M, Clemens TL, et al. Aberrant Phex function in osteoblasts and osteocytes alone underlies murine X-linked hypophosphatemia. J Clin Invest 2008;118(2):722–34.
124. Gowen LC, Petersen DN, Mansolf AL, et al. Targeted disruption of the osteoblast/osteocyte factor 45 gene (OF45) results in increased bone formation and bone mass. J Biol Chem 2003;278(3):1998–2007.
125. Addison WN, Nakano Y, Loisel T, et al. MEPE-ASARM peptides control extracellular matrix mineralization by binding to hydroxyapatite: an inhibition regulated by PHEX cleavage of ASARM. J Bone Miner Res 2008;23(10):1638–49.
126. Divieti PP. PTH and osteocytes. J Musculoskelet Neuronal Interact 2005;5(4):328–30.
127. Winkler DG, Sutherland MK, Geoghegan JC, et al. Osteocyte control of bone formation via sclerostin, a novel BMP antagonist. EMBO J 2003;22(23):6267–76.
128. Van Bezooijen RL, Roelen BA, Visser A, et al. Sclerostin is an osteocyte-expressed negative regulator of bone formation, but not a classical BMP antagonist. J Exp Med 2004;199(6):805–14.
129. Duan P, Bonewald LF. The role of the wnt/beta-catenin signaling pathway in formation and maintenance of bone and teeth. Int J Biochem Cell Biol 2016;77(Pt A):23–9.
130. Lara-Castillo N, Kim-Weroha NA, Kamel MA, et al. In vivo mechanical loading rapidly activates beta-catenin signaling in osteocytes through a prostaglandin mediated mechanism. Bone 2015;76:58–66.
131. Cheng B, Kato Y, Zhao S, et al. PGE(2) is essential for gap junction-mediated intercellular communication between osteocyte-like MLO-Y4 cells in response to mechanical strain. Endocrinology 2001;142(8):3464–73.
132. Lieben L, Masuyama R, Torrekens S, et al. Normocalcemia is maintained in mice under conditions of calcium malabsorption by vitamin D-induced inhibition of bone mineralization. J Clin Invest 2012;122(5):1803–15.

133. Torreggiani E, Matthews BG, Pejda S, et al. Preosteocytes/osteocytes have the potential to dedifferentiate becoming a source of osteoblasts. PLoS One 2013; 8(9):e75204.
134. Brotto M, Bonewald LF. Bone and muscle: interactions beyond mechanical. Bone 2015;80:109–14.
135. Touchberry CD, Green TM, Tchikrizov V, et al. FGF23 is a novel regulator of intracellular calcium and cardiac contractility in addition to cardiac hypertrophy. Am J Physiol Endocrinol Metab 2013;304(8):E863–73.
136. Singh S, Grabner A, Yanucil C, et al. Fibroblast growth factor 23 directly targets hepatocytes to promote inflammation in chronic kidney disease. Kidney Int 2016;90(5):985–96.
137. Lau KW, Rundle CH, Zhou XD, et al. Conditional deletion of IGF-I in osteocytes unexpectedly accelerates bony union of the fracture gap in mice. Bone 2016;92: 18–28.
138. Sheng MH, Zhou XD, Bonewald LF, et al. Disruption of the insulin-like growth factor-1 gene in osteocytes impairs developmental bone growth in mice. Bone 2013;52(1):133–44.
139. Lim J, Shi Y, Karner CM, et al. Dual function of Bmpr1a signaling in restricting preosteoblast proliferation and stimulating osteoblast activity in mouse. Development 2016;143(2):339–47.
140. Canalis E, Bridgewater D, Schilling L, et al. Canonical notch activation in osteocytes causes osteopetrosis. Am J Physiol Endocrinol Metab 2016;310(2): E171–82.
141. Kondoh S, Inoue K, Igarashi K, et al. Estrogen receptor alpha in osteocytes regulates trabecular bone formation in female mice. Bone 2014;60:68–77.
142. Windahl SH, Borjesson AE, Farman HH, et al. Estrogen receptor-alpha in osteocytes is important for trabecular bone formation in male mice. Proc Natl Acad Sci U S A 2013;110(6):2294–9.
143. Zhou JZ, Riquelme MA, Gu S, et al. Osteocytic connexin hemichannels suppress breast cancer growth and bone metastasis. Oncogene 2016. [Epub ahead of print].

Fibroblast Growth Factor 23–Mediated Bone Disease

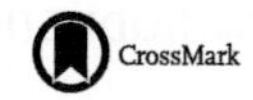

Anda R. Gonciulea, MD, Suzanne M. Jan De Beur, MD*

KEYWORDS

- *FGF23* • α-Klotho • Hypophosphatemia • Hyperphosphatemia • Rickets
- Osteomalacia

KEY POINTS

- Fibroblast growth factor (FGF) 23, one of the circulating FGFs, is produced by osteocytes and exerts its action on the kidney and parathyroid glands to maintain phosphate homeostasis and regulate vitamin D synthesis and metabolism.
- *FGF23* is regulated by systemic factors such as 1,25-dihydroxyvitamin D3 ($1,25(OH)_2D_3$), phosphate, calcium, parathyroid hormone, iron, and local factors expressed in bone, such as *PHEX* (phosphate-regulating gene with homologies to endopeptidases on the X chromosome), matrix extracellular phosphoglycoprotein (MEPE), dentin matrix protein 1 (*DMP1*), and ectonucleotide pyrophosphatase/phosphodiesterase 1 (*ENPP1*); *FGF23* requires the presence of α-Klotho for interaction with and activation of the FGF receptor (FGFR) 1c.
- *FGF23* excess results in hypophosphatemia secondary to reduced renal phosphate reabsorption and dysregulated vitamin D synthesis, which lead to bone demineralization and fractures.
- Causes of *FGF23* excess include ectopic production of *FGF23* (tumor-induced osteomalacia), *FGF23* missense mutations that prevent *FGF23* protein degradation (autosomal dominant hypophosphatemic rickets), and overproduction of *FGF23* in bone through either overgrowth of dysplastic bone (fibrous dysplasia, osteoglophonic dysplasia) or deficiency in local regulatory factors, such as *PHEX* (X-linked hypophosphatemic rickets), *DMP1* (autosomal recessive hypophosphatemic rickets [ARHR] 1), *ENPP1* (ARHR2).
- *FGF23* deficiency results in hyperphosphatemia secondary to renal phosphate retention and increased $1,25(OH)_2D_3$ level, which lead to ectopic calcification in various tissues known as tumoral calcinosis. Mechanisms of *FGF23* deficiency include inactivating mutations in the *FGF23* gene, defective *FGF23* glycosylation due to N-Acetylgalactosaminyl transferase-3 (*GALNT3*) mutations that render *FGF23* more susceptible to proteolytic cleavage and inactivation, and *FGF23* resistance due to mutations in α-Klotho, the *FGF23* co-receptor.

Disclosures: Dr A.R. Gonciulea has no conflict of interests. Dr S.M. Jan de Beur is site PI for clinical trials for KRN23 in tumor-induced osteomalacia and X-linked hypophosphatemic rickets and is a consultant to Ultragenyx.
Division of Endocrinology, Diabetes and Metabolism, Johns Hopkins University School of Medicine, Baltimore, MD, USA
* Corresponding author. 5200 Eastern Avenue, Mason F. Lord Center Tower, Suite 4300, Baltimore, MD 21224.
E-mail address: sjandebe@jhmi.edu

Endocrinol Metab Clin N Am 46 (2017) 19–39
http://dx.doi.org/10.1016/j.ecl.2016.09.013
endo.theclinics.com

INTRODUCTION

The fibroblast growth factors (FGFs) are a family of proteins with numerous important functions in both embryonic and adult tissues. Based on their mechanism of action, they have been classified into 2 main groups: the canonical FGFs, which exert their function by binding to and activating FGF receptors (FGFRs); and the noncanonical FGFs, which exert their actions intracellularly, independent of FGFRs. Although most FGFs are membrane-bound proteins exerting their effects in an autocrine or paracrine fashion, a subgroup of FGFs, including FGF19, FGF21, *FGF23*, circulate in the bloodstream to affect distant target organs in a true endocrine fashion.

The discovery and characterization of *FGF23* has significantly improved the understanding of phosphate and vitamin D homeostasis and many clinical disorders of phosphate homeostasis.

PATHOPHYSIOLOGY

Fibroblast Growth Factor 23 and Klotho

The *FGF23* gene is located on human chromosome 12p13 and consists of 3 coding exons. The full-length *FGF23* is a 32-kDa glycoprotein (251 amino acids) with an N-terminal hydrophobic region and a C-terminal domain. The N-terminus contains the FGFR binding domain and the C-terminus is important for interaction with its coreceptor, α-Klotho. Cleavage of *FGF23* occurs at the 176RXXR179/S180 motif, a subtilisin-like proprotein convertase proteolytic site, resulting in 2 inactive cleavage products (**Fig. 1**). Glycosylation at the S129 residue by UDP-N-acetyl-alpha-D-galactosamine: polypeptide N-acetylgalactosaminyl transferase-3 (*GALNT3*) results in resistance to proteolytic cleavage and inactivation.[1] For activation of the FGFR, *FGF23* requires the presence and direct interaction with its obligate coreceptor, α-Klotho. The equal importance of both molecules is suggested by the finding of a similar phenotype with increased serum phosphate levels in both Klotho[2] and *FGF23* knockout mice.[3]

Although FGFRs are ubiquitously distributed in the body, α-Klotho expression is limited to certain tissues, such as the proximal and distal renal tubules, parathyroid, pituitary, heart, and testis. Here, the membrane-bound α-Klotho interacts with several FGFRs, such as FGFR1c, FGFR3c, and FGFR4, therefore it determines tissue specificity for *FGF23*.[4] A soluble form of Klotho, produced by cleavage of the membrane-bound Klotho ectodomain, is released into the circulation and exerts both paracrine and endocrine functions independent of the *FGF23* signaling pathway.[5] Unlike the tissue-specific form, the soluble Klotho shows enzymatic activity with important implications in mineral homeostasis. By preventing endocytosis of tubular reabsorption of phosphate (TRP) V5, it enhances renal calcium reabsorption[6] and, through proteolysis

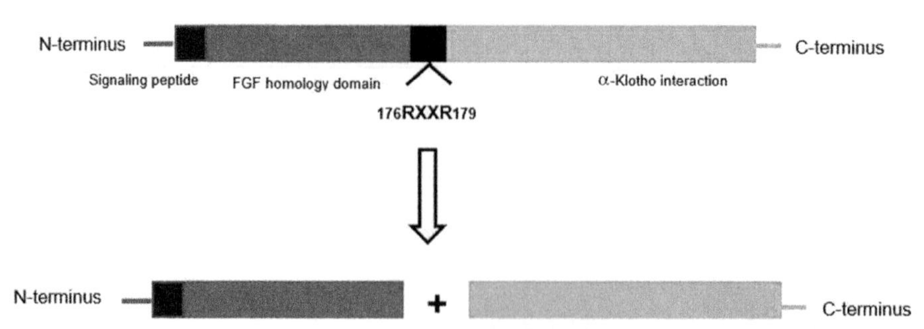

Fig. 1. Cleavage of the intact *FGF23* at the 176RXXR179 motif resulting in N-terminal and C-terminal inactive domains.

and internalization of sodium/phosphate cotransporter (NaPi) 2a, it inhibits phosphate reabsorption in the proximal renal tubule.[7]

Fibroblast Growth Factor 23 Functions

With the kidney as the main target, *FGF23* plays an essential role in phosphate homeostasis. **Fig. 2** summarizes the main functions of *FGF23*. Phosphate reabsorption in the kidney is highly dependent on sodium and involves the apical brush border NaPi 2a and NaPi 2c.[8] Approximately 80% of filtered phosphate is reabsorbed in the proximal tubule, 10% in the distal convoluted tubule, with the remaining 10% excreted in the urine. By interaction with the FGFR–α-Klotho coreceptor complex, *FGF23* directly inhibits transcription, translation, and apical translocation of the NaPi 2a, NaPi 2c transporters, thereby inhibiting renal phosphate reabsorption and promoting phosphaturia. *FGF23* also decreases $1,25(OH)_2D_3$ levels by directly suppressing 1-α-hydroxylase and increasing 24-α-hydroxylase activity. The overall effect is decreased

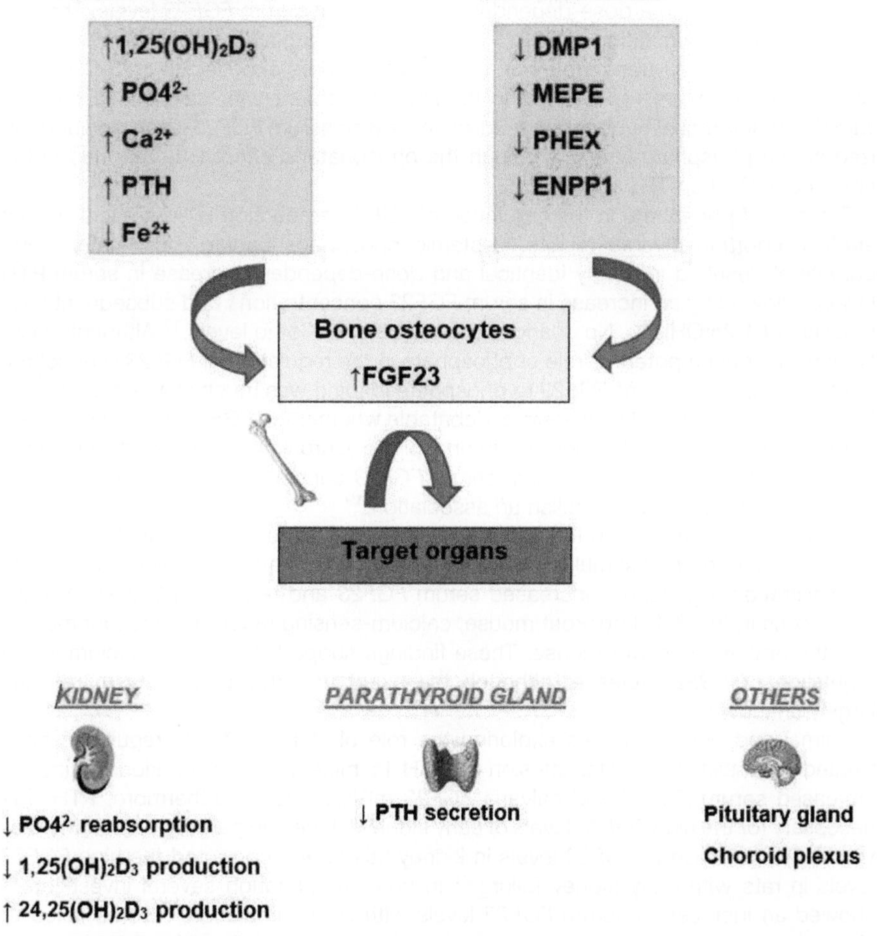

Fig. 2. Systemic and local regulators of *FGF23* production and main FGF actions at target tissues. Ca^{2+}, calcium; Fe^{2+}, iron; PTH, parathyroid hormone; $PO4^{2-}$, phosphate.

$1,25(OH)_2D_3$ production and increased $1,25(OH)_2D_3$ inactivation to the $24,25(OH)_2D_3$ form.[9] Data on *FGF23* action at the level of the parathyroid gland are more controversial, with studies reporting conflicting results. Although several investigators described *FGF23* as a negative regulator of PTH secretion,[10,11] others reported the opposite.[12] Because there is membrane-bound Klotho expression in the parathyroid gland, it has been suggested that *FGF23*-induced suppression of parathyroid hormone (PTH) secretion occurs in a Klotho-dependent manner. Recently, different mechanisms have been proposed. Using a parathyroid-specific Klotho knockout mouse, Olauson and colleagues[13] found a preserved PTH response to intravenous *FGF23*, suggesting that a Klotho-independent, calcineurin-mediated *FGF23* signaling pathway in parathyroid glands mediates the PTH suppression.

Regulators of Fibroblast Growth Factor 23 Production

The main regulators of *FGF23* production include $1,25(OH)_2D_3$, phosphate, calcium, PTH, and iron (see **Fig. 2**). Both animal and human data support the role of $1,25(OH)_2D_3$ in *FGF23* production, presumably via vitamin D receptors. Vitamin D null mice had very low *FGF23* levels[14] and administration of $1,25(OH)_2D_3$ in wild-type mice resulted in a dose-dependent stimulation of serum *FGF23* levels. The role of calcitriol in the regulation of *FGF23* secretion by osteoblasts was further supported by increased *FGF23* transcription in osteoblast cultures exposed to $1,25(OH)_2D_3$.[15] Similar findings were reproduced in humans. Treatment with calcitriol in patients with different forms of hypoparathyroidism increased serum *FGF23* levels and normalized serum phosphate levels, although the phosphaturic effect was reduced in the absence of PTH or PTH action.[16]

The role of phosphate in the regulation of *FGF23* production is controversial, with studies reporting diverse results. Systemic phosphate loading, both enteral and parenteral, resulted in nearly identical and dose-dependent increase in serum PTH levels, followed by an increase in serum *FGF23* concentrations and subsequent suppression of $1,25(OH)_2D_3$. No changes were seen in α-Klotho levels.[17] Although these findings suggest a potential role of phosphate in the regulation of *FGF23* production, the temporal response of *FGF23* to phosphate loading was much slower than the effect on PTH secretion. It is, therefore, debatable whether the *FGF23* response derived from the increase in PTH rather than in phosphate. Chronic phosphate administration was associated with an increase in serum *FGF23* concentration in some studies,[18] whereas others failed to establish an association.[19]

More recent data support the role of calcium in *FGF23* regulation, with hypercalcemia being an important stimulus for *FGF23* production. Intravenous calcium gluconate administration significantly increased serum *FGF23* and reduced $1,25(OH)_2D_3$ concentrations in the PTH knockout mouse, calcium-sensing receptor knockout mouse, and the double knockout mouse. These findings support the role of calcium in the regulation of *FGF23* release, although the exact underlying mechanism remains largely unknown.[20]

Animal and human studies exploring the role of PTH in *FGF23* regulation have yielded inconsistent results. Infusion of PTH to mice with normal kidney function increased serum *FGF23* and calvaria *FGF23* mRNA levels. Furthermore, PTH was necessary for the high *FGF23* levels of early kidney failure and parathyroidectomy prevented the increase in *FGF23* levels in kidney failure and corrected the high *FGF23* levels in rats with early kidney failure.[21] In humans, although several investigators showed an increase in serum *FGF23* levels with PTH stimulation,[22] some failed to show a connection,[23] whereas others reported opposite results with acute reduction of *FGF23* levels following PTH infusion.[24]

More recent data suggest an important role of iron in phosphate metabolism through alteration in *FGF23* levels. Inverse correlations between iron status and C-terminal but not intact *FGF23* have been described in patients with X-linked hypophosphatemic rickets (XLH)[25] and healthy individuals, whereas correlations with both C-terminal and intact *FGF23* were seen in patients with autosomal dominant hypophosphatemic rickets (ADHR).[26] Iron supplementation in children with anemia resulted in decrease of *FGF23* levels.[27]

DISORDERS ASSOCIATED WITH FIBROBLAST GROWTH FACTOR 23 EXCESS

Since its discovery in 2000, *FGF23* has been implicated in more than 12 human disorders. Disorders of *FGF23* excess and deficiency are summarized in **Table 1** and detailed later.

Table 1
Characteristics of inherited and acquired disorders involving fibroblast growth factor 23

Disease	Defect	Pathogenesis
Disorders associated with *FGF23* excess		
TIO	Mesenchymal tumors	↑ Production of *FGF23* and other phosphatonins
XLH	Inactivating *PHEX* mutations	↑ *FGF23* production from osteocytes
ADHR	Missense *FGF23* gene mutations	↑ *FGF23* resistance to cleavage and inactivation
ARHR1	Inactivating *DMP1* mutations	↑ *FGF23* production from immature osteocytes
ARHR2	Inactivating *ENPP1* mutations	↑ FGF23 production from bone
FD/MCAS	*GNAS* activating mutations	↑ *FGF23* production from fibrous dysplastic lesions
LNSS (ENS)	Excess *FGF23* production	↑ *FGF23* production from dysplastic bone lesions and nevi
OGD	FGFR1 activating mutations	↑ *FGF23* production from bone overgrowth
HR and HPT	Activating α-Klotho mutation	↑ α-Klotho and *FGF23*
Disorders associated with *FGF23* deficiency		
FTC (*GALNT3*, *FGF23*)	Inactivating mutations in *GALNT3*, *FGF23*	↑ C-terminal *FGF23* fragments and ↓ intact *FGF23*
FTC (α-Klotho)	Inactivating mutations in α-Klotho	↑ C-terminal and intact *FGF23*, *FGF23* resistance

Abbreviations: ADHR, autosomal dominant hypophosphatemic rickets; ARHR, autosomal recessive hypophosphatemic rickets; ENS, epidermal nevus syndrome; FD/MCAS, fibrous dysplasia/McCune-Albright syndrome; FTC, familial tumoral calcinosis; GNAS, guanine nucleotide binding protein, alpha stimulating; HPT, hyperparathyroidism; HR, hypophosphatemic rickets; LNSS, linear nevus sebaceous syndrome; OGD, osteoglophonic dysplasia; TIO, tumor-induced osteomalacia; XLH, X-linked hypophosphatemic rickets.

Tumor-Induced Osteomalacia

Tumor-induced osteomalacia (TIO) is a rare paraneoplastic disorder of renal phosphate wasting and impaired vitamin D synthesis, which results in hypophosphatemia, osteomalacia, fractures, and severe myopathy. First described by Robert McCance[28] in 1947, it was not until 1959 that a substance produced by the tumor was recognized as the disease mediator.[29] Although the exact prevalence of the disease is not known, more than 300 cases have been reported in the literature.[30]

Pathophysiology

TIO is usually caused by tumors of mesenchymal origin, also known as phosphaturic mesenchymal tumor mixed connective tissue variant (PMTMCT), and rarely by other tumor types such as osteosarcoma, giant cell tumor, pulmonary small cell carcinoma, or colon adenocarcinoma.[31–33] These mesenchymal tumors are small, slow growing, and produce *FGF23* and other phosphaturic factors known as phosphatonins. Although most PMTMCTs are benign, rare malignant forms have also been described.[33] *FGF23* is the predominant phosphaturic factor expressed by tumors, with a few other endocrine factors, including FGF7, MEPE and frizzled-related protein 4 (FRP4). Immunohistochemical staining has shown that approximately 70% of the tumors are positive for *FGF23*,[34] with many TIO tumors additionally expressing somatostatin receptors that make them detectable with somatostatin analogue imaging (octreotide scan).[35] Recent studies have identified a fibronectin 1 (FN1)–FGFR1 fusion gene expressed in PMTMCTs that may provide a possible mechanism for the tumorigenesis. About 42% of PMTMCTs express the FN1-FGFR1 fusion protein that is hypothesized to be secreted and to activate the FGFR1 expressed in these tumors in an autocrine fashion.[36,37]

Symptoms

Patients with TIO usually present with long-standing and progressive debilitating symptoms that typically go undiagnosed for years. Even after the syndrome is recognized it may take several years until the underlying tumor is identified, because most of the tumors are small and not easily detectable on physical examination or diagnostic imaging. Of the 308 TIO cases reviewed by Jiang and colleagues,[38] 40% were located in the skeleton and 55% in the soft tissues. Common complaints reported by patients are muscle weakness that eventually impairs ambulation; fatigue; bone pain; and multiple fractures, frequently of the vertebrae, ribs, and femur. In the rare instances when TIO occurs in children, it often presents with rachitic features, including muscle weakness, gait disturbance, growth retardation, and skeletal deformities. Often, patients are misdiagnosed with different musculoskeletal, rheumatologic, and even psychiatric disorders.[39] It is important that the correct laboratory evaluation is obtained for an accurate diagnosis.

Diagnostic tests/imaging study

Laboratory evaluation Several serum and urine measurements are required for a correct diagnosis, including fasting serum phosphorus, creatinine, calcium, intact PTH, $25(OH)D_3$, $1,25(OH)_2D_3$, alkaline phosphatase, with concurrent urine phosphorus and creatinine. The blood and urine are typically collected in the fasting state and the urine is the second morning-void sample. Hallmarks of the disorder are hypophosphatemia caused by phosphaturia as measured by either calculating the TRP or tubular maximum of phosphate corrected for glomerular filtration rate (TmP/GFR) (https://science.nichd.nih.gov/confluence/download/attachments/23920688/TRP%20TmPGFR%20Calculator.xls?version=1&modificationDate=1379358849000&api=v2) and low or inappropriately normal serum $1,25(OH)_2D_3$ level. Calcium and PTH are usually normal, although PTH may be modestly increased, reflecting secondary hyperparathyroidism caused by low $1,25(OH)_2D_3$ level.[40] Levels of serum electrolytes, creatinine, and $25(OH)D_3$ are usually normal and alkaline phosphatase is increased as a marker of osteoblast hyperactivity and increased bone remodeling. *FGF23* levels are typically increased.

Histomorphometry Histomorphometry of tetracycline-labeled iliac crest bone biopsies reveal findings of severe osteomalacia with increased osteoid surface and mineralization lag time.[40]

Imaging The small size, slow growth, and obscure location in bones and soft tissues make tumor localization extremely challenging, often requiring advanced imaging modalities. Plain skeletal radiographs show features of osteomalacia in adults and rickets in children with osteopenia, pseudofractures, and coarsened trabeculae. Technetium (Tc^{99}) bone scintigraphy shows diffuse skeletal uptake or localized uptake at the sites of fractures. Somatostatin receptors are expressed in many PMTMCT tumors[35] and scanning using radiolabeled somatostatin analogues, such as ^{111}In-pentetreotide scintigraphy (octreotide scan), has been successfully used.[38,41,42] Octreotide scanning typically detects tumors in half the cases. Similarly, whole-body MRI and F-18 fluorodeoxyglucose PET (FDG-PET/computed tomography) have been successfully used to localize tumors at rates similar to octreotide scanning.[43] Gallium-DOTATATE PET has recently emerged as a promising diagnostic tool, especially in patients with tumors undetectable by other techniques, performing even better than FDG-PET/CT or octreotide scan.[44] However, this imaging modality is not widely available. In rare circumstances, venous sampling for *FGF23* is necessary for tumor detection. Despite the advances in radiologic modalities, tumor localization remains unsuccessful in many patients. In this situation, close follow-up with periodic reimaging is necessary.

Differential diagnosis

Specific combinations of clinical and biochemical findings help in distinguishing TIO from other acquired or inherited disorders associated with hypophosphatemia and/or osteomalacia. Obtaining a detailed history is important because inherited disorders may run in families and show clinical features early in life. Acquired disorders presenting with hypophosphatemia and osteomalacia include vitamin D deficiency caused by insufficient nutritional intake or impaired conversion to active forms, nutritional calcium or phosphorus deficiency, use of bone mineralization inhibitors (such as bisphosphonates, fluoride, or aluminum), or Fanconi syndrome. Vitamin D deficiency is easily distinguishable from TIO by the presence of low serum calcium, low $25(OH)D_3$, and increased PTH concentrations. Serum phosphorus level tends to be low and urinary fractional phosphate excretion high because of decreased intestinal absorption and secondary hyperparathyroidism. Nutritional phosphate deficiency is associated with low urinary fractional phosphate excretion, low normal PTH level, increased $1,25(OH)_2D_3$ level, and urinary calcium excretion. Fanconi syndrome, a disorder of the proximal renal tubule leading to decreased phosphate reabsorption, can often present with laboratory findings similar to TIO. Glucosuria, aminoaciduria, and proximal renal tubular acidosis, as well as a history of medical conditions or use of medications associated with Fanconi syndrome, help differentiate it from TIO. Distinguishing TIO from the inherited forms of hypophosphatemic rickets with *FGF23* excess, such as XLH, ADHR, and autosomal recessive hypophosphatemic rickets (ARHR), can sometimes be challenging because the biochemical findings can be indistinguishable (**Table 2**). A negative family history, delayed age at onset, and more severe symptoms with rapid progression are features suggestive of TIO. Genetic testing of the *PHEX* (phosphate-regulating gene with homologies to endopeptidases on the X chromosome), *FGF23*, dentin matrix protein 1 (*DMP1*), and ectonucleotide pyrophosphatase/phosphodiesterase 1 (*ENPP1*) genes can distinguish TIO from these inherited forms of hypophosphatemic rickets and is commercially available.

Table 2
Biochemical and distinctive clinical features of disorders associated with fibroblast growth factor 23

Disease	Biochemical Findings				Distinctive Phenotypic Features
	$PO4^{2-}$	$1,25(OH)_2D$	*FGF23*	PTH	
Disorders Associated with *FGF23* Excess					
TIO	↓	N/↓	N/↑	N/↑	• More frequent in adults with slowly progressive symptoms • Bone pain, muscle weakness, recurrent fractures in adults • Growth retardation, skeletal deformities, bone pain in children
XLH	↓	N/↓	N/↑	N/↑	• Symptoms develop early in life with bowing of the legs, growth retardation, bone pain, recurrent dental abscesses, enthesopathy • Treatment indicated in children and symptomatic adults
ADHR	↓	N/↓	N/↑	N	• Incomplete/variable penetrance, variable age of onset and disease course; occasional loss of phosphate-wasting phenotype after puberty • Association between low iron and high *FGF23* levels
ARHR1	↓	N/↓	N/↑	N	• Present in early childhood with clinical and biochemical manifestations similar to XLH and ADHR; recessive inheritance
ARHR2	↓	N/↓	N/↑	N	• Symptoms develop in childhood • Linked recessive inheritance to generalized arterial calcification of infancy
FD/MCAS	↓	N/↓	N/↑	N	• Variable clinical presentation, waxing and waning course • Correlated with amount of dysplastic bone
LNSS (ENS)	↓	N/↓	N/↑	N	• Neurocutaneous and skeletal manifestations, hypophosphatemic rickets in some patients
OGD	↓	N/↓	N/↑	N	• Craniofacial deformity caused by dysplastic bone, dwarfism and hypophosphatemia in some patients
HR and HPT	↓	N/↓	N/↑	↑	• Rare form of hypophosphatemic rickets, inappropriately normal $1,25(OH)_2D_3$ and increased PTH levels

(*continued on next page*)

Table 2
(continued)

Disease	Biochemical Findings				Distinctive Phenotypic Features
	$PO4^{2-}$	$1,25(OH)_2D$	*FGF23*	PTH	
Disorders associated with *FGF23* deficiency					
FTC (*GALNT3, FGF23*)	↑	N/↑	↓**iFGF23** ↑cFGF23	N	• Ectopic calcifications in various tissues, including synovial joint spaces, soft tissues, eye, vasculature, and brain
FTC (α-Klotho)	↑	N/↑	↑**iFGF23** ↑cFGF23	N	• Ectopic calcifications in various tissues

Abbreviations: cFGF23, C-terminal FGF23; iFGF23, intact FGF23; N, normal.

Treatment

The definitive treatment of TIO is complete tumor resection, which results in clinical recovery, correction of biochemical abnormalities, and bone remineralization.[45] *FGF23* levels decrease rapidly (hours) after complete tumor resection followed by reversal of the biochemical abnormalities (days), but healing of osteomalacia can take months to a year. Because tumor resection is curative and recurrence is likely without complete resection, a wide surgical margin is important. In rare instances (<5%), the tumors metastasize to distant sites.[46] Radiofrequency ablation has been reported as a potential therapeutic option in these situations.[47]

Because of their obscure location, the tumors are not always identifiable and therefore are not amendable to surgical resection. In this scenario, medical therapy with phosphate supplementation in combination with calcitriol or alpha calcidiol becomes necessary in order to replace ongoing urinary phosphate loss and insufficient renal $1,25(OH)_2D_3$ production. Patients are usually treated with 1 to 4 g/d of phosphate divided into 3 to 4 doses and 1 to 3 μg/d of calcitriol.[40] The addition of calcitriol augments the intestinal phosphorus absorption and prevents the development of secondary hyperparathyroidism. The goal of the therapy is to improve symptoms, normalize alkaline phosphatase level, and maintain serum phosphorus level in the low normal range without inducing hypercalcemia, hypercalciuria, or secondary hyperparathyroidism. Serum measurements for calcium, phosphorus, PTH, renal function, and alkaline phosphatase as well as urinary calcium measurements should be frequently monitored (every 3–6 months), so complications related to the therapy such as nephrolithiasis, nephrocalcinosis, or renal insufficiency can be avoided.

Treatment with calcium-sensing receptor agonists has recently been used in 2 patients with TIO not tolerating phosphorus and calcitriol. Therapy with cinacalcet increased renal phosphate reabsorption and serum phosphorus, allowed the use of a more tolerable oral phosphate dose, and resulted in resolution of osteomalacia.[48]

Octreotide therapy was successfully used in 1 patient with TIO[49] but failed to show similar benefits in another patient.[50]

In 2009, Aono and colleagues[51] reported successful use of anti-*FGF23* antibodies in the *hyp* mouse, the murine homolog of XLH, with increased expression of the NaPi 2a cotransporter and 25-hydroxyvitamin-D-1α-hydroxylase and a suppressed expression of 24-hydroxylase in the kidney. Since then, the results of a phase I clinical trial evaluating a single injection of a humanized anti-*FGF23* antibody (KRN23) in adults with XLH have been published, that demonstrates increased renal phosphate reabsorption, increased serum phosphate, and increased $1,25(OH)_2D_3$ levels as well as a favorable safety profile.[52] Furthermore, monthly subcutaneous injections of anti-*FGF23* antibody in 28 adults with XLH for 12 months similarly increased serum phosphorous, 1,25$(OH)_2D_3$, and TmP/GFR levels and maintained serum phosphorus in the normal range in 58% to 85% of the patients.[53] A phase 2 clinical trial of (KRN23) use in prepubescent children, a phase 3 clinical trial in adults with XLH, and a phase 2 open-label trial of monthly KRN23 in adults with TIO and epidermal nevus syndrome are currently ongoing (ClinicalTrials.gov: NCT02163577, NCT02526160, NCT02304367).

The use of an FGFR inhibitor, NVP-BGJ398, in *Hyp* and *Dmp1*-null mice, normalized serum calcium and phosphate levels and enhanced bone growth and mineralization.[54] Furthermore, the finding of an FN1-FGFR1 genetic fusion in TIO tumors highlights the role of FGFR signaling in *FGF23* regulation. Treatment of a patient with widely metastatic TIO with FGFR1 rearrangement in tumor cells with NVP-BGJ398 resulted in disappearance of the pulmonary and hepatic metastasis, increase in serum phosphate level, and normalization of plasma *FGF23* level.[55]

More recently, *Cyp24*, which encodes the 24 hydroxylase gene, has been linked to the pathophysiology of *FGF23*-dependent renal phosphate wasting disorders and pharmacologic use of *Cyp24* inhibitors has been proposed as potential future therapy. Introduction of a null *Cyp24* allele into the *Hyp* and *FGF23* transgenic mice resulted in near-complete recovery of rachitic and osteomalacic bone abnormalities despite lack of changes in biochemical profiles, including the serum phosphorus.[56]

X-linked Hypophosphatemic Rickets

XLH is the most common genetic cause of hypophosphatemic rickets, with an estimated incidence of 1 per 20,000 live births.[57]

Pathophysiology

The gene responsible for this syndrome, *PHEX*, is located on chromosome Xp22.1 and shows the highest expression in bone cells such as osteocytes, osteoblasts, and odontoblasts in teeth.[58] Various inactivating mutations in *PHEX* result in increased bone-derived *FGF23* resulting in increased circulating *FGF23*, which is responsible for the biochemical phenotype. More recent data show that increased production of *FGF23*, rather than decreased degradation, is the underlying abnormality in XLH.[59] It is unclear how loss of *PHEX* function leads to increased *FGF23* production in bone. Excess *FGF23* impairs renal expression of NaPi 2a, NaPi 2c, and 1 α-hydroxylase activity, resulting in hypophosphatemia and decreased 1,25$(OH)_2D_3$ production. In the *Hyp* mouse model, hypophosphatemia decreased apoptosis of hypertrophic chondrocytes and impaired bone mineralization, which is responsible for the disorganized rachitic appearance in bones.[60]

Symptoms

The clinical findings of XLH are similar to TIO but some important distinctive features exist. Unlike patients with TIO, patients with XLH develop the symptoms early in life, usually within the first few years after birth. Although low serum phosphorus level is often present from birth, this can easily be missed if not specifically measured and compared with an age-specific and gender-specific normal range. Children are usually identified at the weight-bearing age when bowing leg deformities and departure from normal growth curve become noticeable. Enthesopathy (calcification of tendons and ligaments) is commonly seen in adults,[61] who often develop bone pain caused by the osteomalacia. Recurrent dental abscesses with loss of the permanent teeth in early adulthood is a common finding and dental issues continue into adulthood. Whether the dental abnormalities are caused by abnormal *PHEX* expression, high *FGF23* level, or resultant hypophosphatemia has been extensively debated in the literature.[60] Bone radiographs show evidence of rickets, especially at the growth plates around the knees in most children, and osteomalacia in adults. Cardiovascular disorders such as hypertension and left ventricular hypertrophy have been reported in many patients with XLH but whether they are direct manifestations of the disease or treatment complications remains largely unknown.[62]

Diagnostic tests/imaging studies

Early recognition of the disease can be challenging, especially in the absence of a family history. The biochemical findings are similar to TIO. In addition to hypophosphatemia and decreased tubular reabsorption of phosphate (TRP) and TmP/GFR levels, patients have decreased $1,25(OH)_2D_3$ production, increased alkaline phosphatase levels, and normal calcium and PTH levels.

The typical radiologic findings of rickets in children are widening and fraying of the metaphysis, whereas osteomalacia is usually seen in adults. The bones appear short with a coarse trabeculation in the axial skeleton.[63,64]

Genetic testing for the *PHEX* mutation can be useful to confirm the diagnosis and initiate therapy early in the disease course in order to prevent progression of rachitic changes in infants. About 60% to 70% of the time, *PHEX* gene mutations are identified in patients with the clinical diagnosis of XLH.

Differential diagnosis

The main differential diagnosis includes other forms of inherited hypophosphatemic rickets and rarely TIO when it presents in childhood. Because of the occurrence of symptoms early in life, other inherited disorders of phosphate metabolism need to be primarily excluded. The pattern of inheritance and age of onset can be helpful. Because XLH is an X-linked dominant disorder, there should be affected individuals in each generation, and this is also true of ADHR. If the disorder skips generations, then a recessive disorder such as ARHR should be considered. If there is evidence of father-to-son transmission, then ADHR should be considered because in X-linked inheritance father-to-son transmission is not observed. Delayed presentation in adolescence or early adulthood and even remission have been observed in ADHR.

Treatment

The goal of the therapy in XLH is highly dependent on the age of the patient. Early diagnosis in children and treatment initiation before walking begins may be beneficial. Quinlan and colleagues[65] showed that starting treatment early (before age 1 year) was associated with a better median height standard deviation score independent of gender or genotype. Variable responses to treatment have been reported by other investigators, with many of the treated children failing to achieve normal growth.[66] The goal of treatment in children is to correct or minimize rickets and maximize growth. Aiming for normal serum phosphate concentration should not be the primary therapeutic goal considering the potential higher complication rate. Administration of phosphate starting at 40 mg/kg/d in combination with calcitriol at 20 to 30 ng/kg/d is the preferred treatment, with further dose titration based on clinical, biochemical, and radiologic findings.[67] The use of phosphate alone is usually not adequate for treatment of rickets and has a significant risk of inducing iatrogenic hyperparathyroidism by increasing plasma phosphate level, decreasing plasma calcium and calcitriol concentrations, and further stimulating PTH production. With treatment, normal growth and improvement in leg deformities is frequently achieved, although the response is variable and some children still have a short stature and significant leg deformities requiring surgical interventions.

The role of therapy in adults is more controversial and is usually restricted to symptomatic patients, such as those experiencing bone pain, recurrent or nonunion fractures, preparing for orthopedic surgery, or with biochemical evidence of osteomalacia such as increased alkaline phosphatase level.[67] The minimal dose of medication able to achieve the treatment goal should be used in order to avoid complications, and close monitoring is required. Starting doses usually consist of calcitriol 0.5 μg in 2 divided doses and phosphate 250 mg thrice daily. Serum and urine calcium, creatinine, and PTH levels are monitored every 3 to 4 months while on therapy and adjusted to avoid complications of nephrocalcinosis, nephrolithiasis, and renal dysfunction. Imaging with renal ultrasonography at baseline and periodically is recommended. Conventional therapy has also been shown to improve dental manifestations, with mixed results for the effects on enthesopathy.[68,69]

The use of calcimimetics has been reported with favorable results. In a patient with XLH and long-term complications from conventional therapy with phosphate and calcitriol, including nephrolithiasis, renal dysfunction, secondary hyperparathyroidism, and hypertension, addition of cinacalcet resulted in blood pressure normalization, increase in serum phosphate level, and decrease in PTH and *FGF23* concentrations.[70]

Administration of a single dose of calcitonin resulted in a significant and sustained decrease in circulating levels of *FGF23* and an increase in serum levels of phosphorus in 7 patients with XLH, whereas no changes in these parameters were detected in the control group. There was a similar initial increase in $1,25(OH)_2D_3$ production in both groups, whereas no significant change in renal phosphate reabsorption (TmP/GFR) was seen.[71] Concomitant administration of phosphate and cinacalcet in 8 children with XLH resulted in suppression of PTH and serum calcium and increase in serum phosphate and TmP/GFR levels.[72] Although data look promising, larger studies are needed.

The use of hexa-D-arginine in the *Hyp* mouse model resulted in improvement in *FGF23* concentrations and rescued the *Hyp* phenotype by enhancing 7B2-subtilisin–like proprotein convertase 2 activity.[73]

Although growth hormone (GH) deficiency is not the underlying cause of growth retardation in patients with XLH, treatment with GH improved linear growth as well as serum phosphate and $1,25(OH)_2D_3$ levels in several studies. There were mixed results with respect to lower extremity deformity progression and concerns have been raised about potential exacerbation of secondary hyperparathyroidism and increased mortality in short children on high-dose long-term GH treatment.[74,75] Until more data are available, GH should be used with caution in patients with XLH with severe growth impairment.

As previously discussed, humanized anti-*FGF23* antibody (KRN23) use in adults with XLH showed promising results with respect to normalizing the biochemical manifestations in a phase 1/2 trial. Phase 2 and 3 clinical trials in children and adults with XLH are ongoing (ClinicalTrials.gov: NCT02163577 and NCT02526160).

Autosomal Dominant Hypophosphatemic Rickets

ADHR is a rare genetic disorder caused by mutations in the *FGF23* gene. Missense mutations in one of 2 arginine residues at positions 176 or 179 have been identified, resulting in *FGF23* resistance to cleavage by the subtilisinlike proprotein convertases and increased serum intact *FGF23* concentrations.[1,76]

The clinical and biochemical findings

The clinical and biochemical findings are similar to those of patients with XLH, but, because of its incomplete and variable penetrance, ADHR presents with variable age of onset and waxing and waning disease course. Patients with onset of the disease in early childhood present with phosphate wasting, radiologic rachitic findings, short stature, and lower extremity deformities. Some of these patients lose the renal phosphate wasting defect after puberty. When the disease first manifests in adulthood, the typical clinical findings are bone pain, muscle weakness, and pseudofractures, with most of the patients lacking lower extremity deformities or growth defects.[77] An interesting and more recent finding is the association between serum iron concentrations and ADHR phenotype, with low iron status increasing *FGF23* expression.[26] Iron supplementation in a patient with ADHR with iron deficiency anemia resulted in normalization of renal phosphate reabsorption, loss of ADHR phenotype, and withdrawal of medications.[78]

Treatment

Treatment of ADHR is similar to that of XLH, with phosphate and calcitriol supplementation as previously discussed. Considering the association between ADHR and iron deficiency anemia, patients with ADHR should be screened for iron deficiency followed by iron repletion as needed. Reduction and potential withdrawal of medications should be attempted once the iron status is normalized.

Autosomal Recessive Hypophosphatemic Rickets

Based on the underlying gene defect, ARHR has been divided into 2 main subtypes. ARHR1 is caused by inactivating mutations in the dentin matrix protein 1 (*DMP1*) gene, a matrix protein related to MEPE and member of the SIBLING (small integrin binding ligand N-linked glycoprotein) family. *DMP1* exerts important functions in osteocyte maturation and bone mineralization. Loss of *DMP1* function results in increased circulating *FGF23* levels caused by bone overproduction of *FGF23*, immature osteocytes, and impaired skeletal mineralization.[79,80] Inactivating mutations in *ENPP1* have been described in patients with ARHR2.[81] *ENPP1* is an important regulator of inorganic pyrophosphate required for bone mineralization and physiologic inhibition of calcification. Inactivating mutations in this gene have been linked to generalized arterial calcification of infancy.[82]

Patients with ARHR usually present in childhood with clinical and biochemical findings similar to XLH and ADHR. Treatment involves frequently administration of phosphate and calcitriol as described earlier.

OTHER DISORDERS ASSOCIATED WITH FIBROBLAST GROWTH FACTOR 23 EXCESS

Fibrous Dysplasia/McCune-Albright Syndrome

Fibrous dysplasia/McCune-Albright syndrome is caused by somatic activating mutations in the *GNAS* gene encoding a cyclic AMP pathway–associated G-protein, $G_s\alpha$. The clinical presentation ranges from incidentally discovered asymptomatic monostotic lesions to diffuse polyostotic disease associated with severe morbidity and occasionally death. It results from replacement of the medullary bone and bone marrow with fibrous tissue. Bianco and Robey[83] showed that in FD there is an arrest in the differentiation of the bone marrow stromal cells, which instead of progressing into the osteogenic lineage undergo proliferation and give rise to fibro-osseous masses of tissue. McCune-Albright syndrome is characterized by café-au-lait skin macules, fibrous dysplasia, and precocious puberty, although many other hyperfunctioning endocrine disorders can be present. Although the increased *FGF23* production in FD tissues results in renal phosphate wasting, hypophosphatemia and classic hypophosphatemic rickets are less common findings. Bhattacharyya and colleagues[84] showed that the underlying mechanism responsible for this phenotype is alterations in *FGF23* processing in FD tissue with increased cleavage of intact *FGF23* to its inactive fragments. The degree of *FGF23* overproduction correlates with the severity of fibrous dysplasia,[85] with a waxing and waning course of hypophosphatemia over a person's lifetime and potential resolution with advancing age.

Treatment often requires a multidisciplinary approach, targeted to the individual manifestations of the disease and focused on optimizing function and minimizing morbidity related to fractures and deformity. Treatment of frank hypophosphatemia is similar to that of other disorders of *FGF23* excess, with oral phosphate and calcitriol supplementation.

Linear Nevus Sebaceous Syndrome

Linear nevus sebaceous syndrome (LNSS), also known as epidermal nevus syndrome (ENS), is a rare disease associated with neurocutaneous and skeletal manifestations. Rarely, hypophosphatemic rickets has been described in association with epidermal nevi. Affected individuals present with typical skin lesions, various central nervous system abnormalities often resulting in mental retardation and seizures, as well as radiologic evidence of fibrous dysplasia. Increased circulating *FGF23* levels are thought to be responsible for the phosphate wasting and clinical rickets.[86] Treatment with phosphate and calcitriol is indicated with close monitoring for potential complications. There are mixed data with respect to the role of surgical removal of the skin lesions for correction of skeletal manifestations and normalization of serum phosphate.[87]

Osteoglophonic Dysplasia

Osteoglophonic dysplasia (OGD) is a very rare genetic disorder with autosomal dominant mode of inheritance, caused by an activating mutation in the FGFR1[88] and characterized by abnormal bone growth that leads to severe craniofacial abnormalities and dwarfism. Hypophosphatemia is present in some patients and is thought to be related to *FGF23* production by the abnormal bone because the extent of skeletal lesions has been correlated with *FGF23* levels and phosphate wasting severity.

Hypophosphatemic Rickets with Hyperparathyroidism

A rare form of renal phosphate wasting with hypophosphatemia, inappropriately normal $1,25(OH)_2D_3$ level, clinical and radiologic findings of rickets, and drastically increased PTH levels has been described.[12] A *de novo* translocation with a breakpoint adjacent to α-Klotho was reported, resulting in increased levels of plasma α-Klotho, a cofactor necessary for *FGF23* binding to and activation of its cognate receptor. An unexpected finding was the marked increase in *FGF23* level, implicating α-Klotho in the selective regulation of serum phosphate, *FGF23* expression, and regulation of parathyroid mass and function.

Chronic Kidney Disease

In patients with chronic kidney disease (CKD), serum *FGF23* level increases progressively as kidney function declines, reaching levels more than 200 times the normal limit in cases of advanced renal failure.[89] The increase in *FGF23* concentration precedes changes in serum phosphate, PTH, or $1,25\ (OH)_2\ D_3$ levels, although the exact explanation for these findings remains unknown. It has been suggested that the role of *FGF23* is to maintain a normal phosphate level with advancing CKD at the expense of worsening $1,25\ (OH)_2\ D_3$ deficiency and subsequent secondary hyperparathyroidism. Furthermore, treatment with calcitriol in patients with advanced CKD often exacerbates increases in *FGF23* levels. Epidemiologic studies have linked high *FGF23* level with increased mortality in patients with end-stage renal disease,[90] whereas other reports have shown associations between increased *FGF23* concentrations and endothelial dysfunction, arterial stiffness,[91] and left ventricular hypertrophy.[92]

DISORDERS ASSOCIATED WITH FIBROBLAST GROWTH FACTOR 23 DEFICIENCY

Familial Tumoral Calcinosis

Pathophysiology

Familial tumoral calcinosis (FTC) is a rare autosomal recessive metabolic disorder characterized by ectopic calcifications in soft tissues and the vasculature. Based on serum phosphate concentration, 2 disease categories have been described: normophosphatemic FTC, characterized by normal serum phosphate level; and hyperphosphatemic FTC, defined by increased phosphate concentrations. To date, 3 genetic mutations have been described in FTC, inactivating mutations *GALNT3*,[93] *FGF23*,[94] and α-Klotho.[95] Recall that *GALNT3* is an important enzyme for glycosylation of *FGF23* that protects the protein from cleavage and inactivation. Thus *GALNT3* deficiency leads to *FGF23* deficiency because of enhanced degradation. In contrast with ADHR, in which missense mutations in the *FGF23* gene disrupt the recognition site for *FGF23* proteolytic cleavage rendering *FGF23* resistant to inactivation, the mutations in *FGF23* in FTC are inactivating mutations that lead to *FGF23* deficiency. In the case of inactivating mutations in α-Klotho, this leads to *FGF23* resistance because α-Klotho is the coreceptor for *FGF23*. Therefore, patients with FTC with *GALNT3* and *FGF23* gene mutations have increased C-terminal *FGF23* and low intact *FGF23* levels, whereas increases in the intact and C-terminal *FGF23* fragments characterize patients with α-Klotho mutations.

Hyperostosis-hyperphosphatemia syndrome is a rare disorder caused by inactivating mutations in *GALNT3* with several clinical and metabolic features similar to FTC. It has, therefore, been suggested that the two syndromes may represent a spectrum of severity within the same disease.[96]

Symptoms

The clinical presentation of FTC is characterized by calcifications in various tissues, with common locations including synovial joint spaces, upper and lower extremities, and buttocks. Ectopic calcifications can also affect soft tissues and more rarely sites such as the eye, vasculature, and brain.[97] Some patients present with minimal or no symptoms, whereas others have debilitating pain requiring multiple surgical interventions. Severe inflammation with ulceration of the overlying skin and milky drainage can also be seen. Dental abnormalities include short bulbous roots, pulp stones, and partial obliteration of the pulp cavity.[98]

Diagnostic tests/imaging study

Biochemical abnormalities include hyperphosphatemia caused by renal phosphate retention and inappropriately normal or increased 1,25 $(OH)_2$ D_3 level with normal or mildly increased calcium and normal or suppressed PTH concentrations. Low intact *FGF23* levels with increased C-terminal *FGF23* fragments are seen in patients with *GALNT3* and *FGF23* gene mutations, whereas increase in both is found in patients with α-Klotho mutations.

Plain radiographs show the typical multilobulated and cystic calcifications in a periarticular location and computed tomography can be helpful in determining the extent and location of the lesions, especially when planning the surgical intervention.

Differential diagnosis
Differential diagnosis includes other disorders associated with abnormal calcifications, including calcinosis circumscripta, calcific tendonitis, osteosarcoma, myositis ossificans, tophaceous gout as well as connective tissue diseases. A thorough family history and typical biochemical findings are helpful in establishing the diagnosis.

Treatment
Treatment should be individualized to the symptoms of the patient, type of lesion, size, and location and includes medical therapy as well as surgical excision. Often repeat surgical interventions are needed because of the high recurrence rate of the lesions. The goal of medical therapy is to reduce the phosphate level and alter the biochemical profile toward a low–calcium-phosphate product. This goal can be achieved by reducing phosphate absorption through either dietary phosphate restriction or use of phosphate chelating agents such as oral aluminum hydroxide. Increasing urinary phosphate excretion by use of acetazolamide and calcitonin or blocking phosphate release from bone by bisphosphonates are alternative treatments.

SUMMARY

FGF23 is produced by osteocytes and exerts its action on the kidneys and parathyroid glands to maintain phosphate homeostasis and regulate vitamin D synthesis and metabolism, and is the first demonstration that circulating factors produced by the skeleton act in an endocrine fashion. *FGF23* excess results in hypophosphatemia secondary to reduced renal phosphate reabsorption and dysregulated vitamin D synthesis, which lead to bone demineralization and fractures. Causes of *FGF23* excess include ectopic production of *FGF23* (TIO), *FGF23* missense mutations that prevent *FGF23* protein degradation (ADHR), and overproduction of *FGF23* in bone through either overgrowth of dysplastic bone (FD, osteoglophonic dysplasia) or deficiency in local regulatory factors such as *PHEX* (XLH), *DMP1* (ARHR1), and *ENPP1* (ARHR2). *FGF23* deficiency results in hyperphosphatemia secondary to renal phosphate retention and increased $1,25(OH)_2D_3$ levels, which lead to ectopic calcification in various tissues. Mechanisms of *FGF23* deficiency include inactivating mutations in the *FGF23* gene, defective *FGF23* glycosylation caused by *GALNT3* mutations that render *FGF23* more susceptible to proteolytic cleavage and inactivation, and *FGF23* resistance caused by mutations in α-Klotho, the *FGF23* coreceptor. It is extraordinary that, in the 16 years since its discovery, at least 12 human disorders can be attributed to aberrations in the *FGF23* pathway. At present, novel therapies that target the *FGF23* pathway hold great promise for treating *FGF23*-mediated disease.

REFERENCES

1. Shimada T, Muto T, Urakawa I, et al. Mutant FGF-23 responsible for autosomal dominant hypophosphatemic rickets is resistant to proteolytic cleavage and causes hypophosphatemia in vivo. Endocrinology 2002;143(8):3179–82.
2. Kuro-o M, Matsumura Y, Aizawa H, et al. Mutation of the mouse klotho gene leads to a syndrome resembling ageing. Nature 1997;390(6655):45–51.
3. Shimada T, Kakitani M, Yamazaki Y, et al. Targeted ablation of Fgf23 demonstrates an essential physiological role of FGF23 in phosphate and vitamin D metabolism. J Clin Invest 2004;113(4):561–8.
4. Kurosu H, Ogawa Y, Miyoshi M, et al. Regulation of fibroblast growth factor-23 signaling by klotho. J Biol Chem 2006;281(10):6120–3.

5. Imura A, Iwano A, Tohyama O, et al. Secreted Klotho protein in sera and CSF: implication for post-translational cleavage in release of Klotho protein from cell membrane. FEBS Lett 2004;565(1–3):143–7.
6. Chang Q, Hoefs S, van der Kemp AW, et al. The beta-glucuronidase klotho hydrolyzes and activates the TRPV5 channel. Science 2005;310(5747):490–3.
7. Hu MC, Shi M, Zhang J, et al. Klotho: a novel phosphaturic substance acting as an autocrine enzyme in the renal proximal tubule. FASEB J 2010;24(9):3438–50.
8. Forster IC, Hernando N, Biber J, et al. Proximal tubular handling of phosphate: A molecular perspective. Kidney Int 2006;70(9):1548–59.
9. Shimada T, Hasegawa H, Yamazaki Y, et al. FGF-23 is a potent regulator of vitamin D metabolism and phosphate homeostasis. J Bone Miner Res 2004; 19(3):429–35.
10. Krajisnik T, Bjorklund P, Marsell R, et al. Fibroblast growth factor-23 regulates parathyroid hormone and 1alpha-hydroxylase expression in cultured bovine parathyroid cells. J Endocrinol 2007;195(1):125–31.
11. Ben-Dov IZ, Galitzer H, Lavi-Moshayoff V, et al. The parathyroid is a target organ for FGF23 in rats. J Clin Invest 2007;117(12):4003–8.
12. Brownstein CA, Adler F, Nelson-Williams C, et al. A translocation causing increased alpha-klotho level results in hypophosphatemic rickets and hyperparathyroidism. Proc Natl Acad Sci U S A 2008;105(9):3455–60.
13. Olauson H, Lindberg K, Amin R, et al. Parathyroid-specific deletion of Klotho unravels a novel calcineurin-dependent FGF23 signaling pathway that regulates PTH secretion. PLoS Genet 2013;9(12):e1003975.
14. Yu X, Sabbagh Y, Davis SI, et al. Genetic dissection of phosphate- and vitamin D-mediated regulation of circulating Fgf23 concentrations. Bone 2005;36(6): 971–7.
15. Liu S, Tang W, Zhou J, et al. Fibroblast growth factor 23 is a counter-regulatory phosphaturic hormone for vitamin D. J Am Soc Nephrol 2006;17(5):1305–15.
16. Collins MT, Lindsay JR, Jain A, et al. Fibroblast growth factor-23 is regulated by 1alpha,25-dihydroxyvitamin D. J Bone Miner Res 2005;20(11):1944–50.
17. Scanni R, vonRotz M, Jehle S, et al. The human response to acute enteral and parenteral phosphate loads. J Am Soc Nephrol 2014;25(12):2730–9.
18. Burnett SM, Gunawardene SC, Bringhurst FR, et al. Regulation of C-terminal and intact FGF-23 by dietary phosphate in men and women. J Bone Miner Res 2006; 21(8):1187–96.
19. Ito N, Fukumoto S, Takeuchi Y, et al. Effect of acute changes of serum phosphate on fibroblast growth factor (FGF)23 levels in humans. J Bone Miner Metab 2007; 25(6):419–22.
20. Quinn SJ, Thomsen AR, Pang JL, et al. Interactions between calcium and phosphorus in the regulation of the production of fibroblast growth factor 23 in vivo. Am J Physiol Endocrinol Metab 2013;304(3):E310–20.
21. Lavi-Moshayoff V, Wasserman G, Meir T, et al. PTH increases FGF23 gene expression and mediates the high-FGF23 levels of experimental kidney failure: a bone parathyroid feedback loop. Am J Physiol Renal Physiol 2010;299(4): F882–9.
22. Burnett-Bowie SM, Henao MP, Dere ME, et al. Effects of hPTH(1-34) infusion on circulating serum phosphate, 1,25-dihydroxyvitamin D, and FGF23 levels in healthy men. J Bone Miner Res 2009;24(10):1681–5.
23. Saji F, Shigematsu T, Sakaguchi T, et al. Fibroblast growth factor 23 production in bone is directly regulated by 1{alpha},25-dihydroxyvitamin D, but not PTH. Am J Physiol Renal Physiol 2010;299(5):F1212–7.

24. Gutierrez OM, Smith KT, Barchi-Chung A, et al. (1-34) Parathyroid hormone infusion acutely lowers fibroblast growth factor 23 concentrations in adult volunteers. Clin J Am Soc Nephrol 2012;7(1):139–45.
25. Imel EA, Gray AK, Padgett LR, et al. Iron and fibroblast growth factor 23 in X-linked hypophosphatemia. Bone 2014;60:87–92.
26. Imel EA, Peacock M, Gray AK, et al. Iron modifies plasma FGF23 differently in autosomal dominant hypophosphatemic rickets and healthy humans. J Clin Endocrinol Metab 2011;96(11):3541–9.
27. Braithwaite V, Prentice AM, Doherty C, et al. FGF23 is correlated with iron status but not with inflammation and decreases after iron supplementation: a supplementation study. Int J Pediatr Endocrinol 2012;2012(1):27.
28. McCance RA. Osteomalacia with Looser's nodes (Milkman's syndrome) due to a raised resistance to vitamin D acquired about the age of 15 years. Q J Med 1947; 16(1):33–46.
29. Prader A, Illig R, Uehlinger E, et al. Rickets following bone tumor. Helv Paediatr Acta 1959;14:554–65.
30. Dadoniene J, Miglinas M, Miltiniene D, et al. Tumour-induced osteomalacia: a literature review and a case report. World J Surg Oncol 2016;14(1):4.
31. Battoo AJ, Salih S, Unnikrishnan AG, et al. Oncogenic osteomalacia from nasal cavity giant cell tumor. Head Neck 2012;34(3):454–7.
32. Sauder A, Wiernek S, Dai X, et al. FGF23-associated tumor-induced osteomalacia in a patient with small cell carcinoma: a case report and regulatory mechanism study. Int J Surg Pathol 2016;24(2):116–20.
33. Leaf DE, Pereira RC, Bazari H, et al. Oncogenic osteomalacia due to FGF23-expressing colon adenocarcinoma. J Clin Endocrinol Metab 2013;98(3):887–91.
34. Folpe AL, Fanburg-Smith JC, Billings SD, et al. Most osteomalacia-associated mesenchymal tumors are a single histopathologic entity: an analysis of 32 cases and a comprehensive review of the literature. Am J Surg Pathol 2004;28(1):1–30.
35. Houang M, Clarkson A, Sioson L, et al. Phosphaturic mesenchymal tumors show positive staining for somatostatin receptor 2A (SSTR2A). Hum Pathol 2013; 44(12):2711–8.
36. Lee JC, Jeng YM, Su SY, et al. Identification of a novel FN1-FGFR1 genetic fusion as a frequent event in phosphaturic mesenchymal tumour. J Pathol 2015;235(4): 539–45.
37. Lee JC, Su SY, Changou CA, et al. Characterization of FN1-FGFR1 and novel FN1-FGF1 fusion genes in a large series of phosphaturic mesenchymal tumors. Mod Pathol 2016;2016:137.
38. Jiang Y, Xia WB, Xing XP, et al. Tumor-induced osteomalacia: an important cause of adult-onset hypophosphatemic osteomalacia in China: report of 39 cases and review of the literature. J Bone Miner Res 2012;27(9):1967–75.
39. Hautmann AH, Hautmann MG, Kolbl O, et al. Tumor-induced osteomalacia: an up-to-date review. Curr Rheumatol Rep 2015;17(6):512.
40. Jan de Beur SM. Tumor-induced osteomalacia. JAMA 2005;294(10):1260–7.
41. Jan de Beur SM, Streeten EA, Civelek AC, et al. Localisation of mesenchymal tumours by somatostatin receptor imaging. Lancet 2002;359(9308):761–3.
42. Jonsson KB, Zahradnik R, Larsson T, et al. Fibroblast growth factor 23 in oncogenic osteomalacia and X-linked hypophosphatemia. N Engl J Med 2003; 348(17):1656–63.
43. Chong WH, Yavuz S, Patel SM, et al. The importance of whole body imaging in tumor-induced osteomalacia. J Clin Endocrinol Metab 2011;96(12):3599–600.

44. Breer S, Brunkhorst T, Beil FT, et al. 68Ga DOTA-TATE PET/CT allows tumor localization in patients with tumor-induced osteomalacia but negative 111In-octreotide SPECT/CT. Bone 2014;64:222–7.
45. Shane E, Parisien M, Henderson JE, et al. Tumor-induced osteomalacia: clinical and basic studies. J Bone Miner Res 1997;12(9):1502–11.
46. Ogose A, Hotta T, Emura I, et al. Recurrent malignant variant of phosphaturic mesenchymal tumor with oncogenic osteomalacia. Skeletal Radiol 2001;30(2): 99–103.
47. Hesse E, Rosenthal H, Bastian L. Radiofrequency ablation of a tumor causing oncogenic osteomalacia. N Engl J Med 2007;357(4):422–4.
48. Geller JL, Khosravi A, Kelly MH, et al. Cinacalcet in the management of tumor-induced osteomalacia. J Bone Miner Res 2007;22(6):931–7.
49. Seufert J, Ebert K, Muller J, et al. Octreotide therapy for tumor-induced osteomalacia. N Engl J Med 2001;345(26):1883–8.
50. Paglia F, Dionisi S, Minisola S. Octreotide for tumor-induced osteomalacia. N Engl J Med 2002;346(22):1748–9 [author reply: 1748–9].
51. Aono Y, Yamazaki Y, Yasutake J, et al. Therapeutic effects of anti-FGF23 antibodies in hypophosphatemic rickets/osteomalacia. J Bone Miner Res 2009; 24(11):1879–88.
52. Carpenter TO, Imel EA, Ruppe MD, et al. Randomized trial of the anti-FGF23 antibody KRN23 in X-linked hypophosphatemia. J Clin Invest 2014;124(4):1587–97.
53. Imel EA, Zhang X, Ruppe MD, et al. Prolonged correction of serum phosphorus in adults with X-linked hypophosphatemia using monthly doses of KRN23. J Clin Endocrinol Metab 2015;100(7):2565–73.
54. Wohrle S, Henninger C, Bonny O, et al. Pharmacological inhibition of fibroblast growth factor (FGF) receptor signaling ameliorates FGF23-mediated hypophosphatemic rickets. J Bone Miner Res 2013;28(4):899–911.
55. Colling M. Striking response of tumor-induced osteomalacia to the FGFR inhibitor NVP-BGJ398. ASBMR 2015 Annual Meeting; 2015; Washington State Convention Center. Seattle (WA), October 19–22, 2015.
56. Bai X, Miao D, Xiao S, et al. CYP24 inhibition as a therapeutic target in FGF23-mediated renal phosphate wasting disorders. J Clin Invest 2016;126(2):667–80.
57. Alizadeh Naderi AS, Reilly RF. Hereditary disorders of renal phosphate wasting. Nat Rev Nephrol 2010;6(11):657–65.
58. Beck L, Soumounou Y, Martel J, et al. Pex/PEX tissue distribution and evidence for a deletion in the 3' region of the Pex gene in X-linked hypophosphatemic mice. J Clin Invest 1997;99(6):1200–9.
59. Liu S, Guo R, Simpson LG, et al. Regulation of fibroblastic growth factor 23 expression but not degradation by PHEX. J Biol Chem 2003;278(39):37419–26.
60. Lee JY, Imel EA. The changing face of hypophosphatemic disorders in the FGF-23 era. Pediatr Endocrinol Rev 2013;10(Suppl 2):367–79.
61. Polisson RP, Martinez S, Khoury M, et al. Calcification of entheses associated with X-linked hypophosphatemic osteomalacia. N Engl J Med 1985;313(1):1–6.
62. Nehgme R, Fahey JT, Smith C, et al. Cardiovascular abnormalities in patients with X-linked hypophosphatemia. J Clin Endocrinol Metab 1997;82(8):2450–4.
63. Mughal Z. Rickets in childhood. Semin Musculoskelet Radiol 2002;6(3):183–90.
64. Pavone V, Testa G, Gioitta Iachino S, et al. Hypophosphatemic rickets: etiology, clinical features and treatment. Eur J Orthop Surg Traumatol 2015;25(2):221–6.
65. Quinlan C, Guegan K, Offiah A, et al. Growth in PHEX-associated X-linked hypophosphatemic rickets: the importance of early treatment. Pediatr Nephrol 2012; 27(4):581–8.

66. Petersen DJ, Boniface AM, Schranck FW, et al. X-linked hypophosphatemic rickets: a study (with literature review) of linear growth response to calcitriol and phosphate therapy. J Bone Miner Res 1992;7(6):583–97.
67. Carpenter TO, Imel EA, Holm IA, et al. A clinician's guide to X-linked hypophosphatemia. J Bone Miner Res 2011;26(7):1381–8.
68. Connor J, Olear EA, Insogna KL, et al. Conventional therapy in adults with X-linked hypophosphatemia: effects on enthesopathy and dental disease. J Clin Endocrinol Metab 2015;100(10):3625–32.
69. Econs MJ. Conventional therapy in adults with XLH improves dental manifestations, but not enthesopathy. J Clin Endocrinol Metab 2015;100(10):3622–4.
70. Yavropoulou MP, Kotsa K, Gotzamani Psarrakou A, et al. Cinacalcet in hyperparathyroidism secondary to X-linked hypophosphatemic rickets: case report and brief literature review. Hormones (Athens) 2010;9(3):274–8.
71. Liu ES, Carpenter TO, Gundberg CM, et al. Calcitonin administration in X-linked hypophosphatemia. N Engl J Med 2011;364(17):1678–80.
72. Alon US, Levy-Olomucki R, Moore WV, et al. Calcimimetics as an adjuvant treatment for familial hypophosphatemic rickets. Clin J Am Soc Nephrol 2008;3(3): 658–64.
73. Yuan B, Feng JQ, Bowman S, et al. Hexa-D-arginine treatment increases 7B2*PC2 activity in hyp-mouse osteoblasts and rescues the HYP phenotype. J Bone Miner Res 2013;28(1):56–72.
74. Zivicnjak M, Schnabel D, Staude H, et al. Three-year growth hormone treatment in short children with X-linked hypophosphatemic rickets: effects on linear growth and body disproportion. J Clin Endocrinol Metab 2011;96(12):E2097–105.
75. Makitie O, Toiviainen-Salo S, Marttinen E, et al. Metabolic control and growth during exclusive growth hormone treatment in X-linked hypophosphatemic rickets. Horm Res 2008;69(4):212–20.
76. ADHR Consortium. Autosomal dominant hypophosphataemic rickets is associated with mutations in FGF23. Nat Genet 2000;26(3):345–8.
77. Econs MJ, McEnery PT. Autosomal dominant hypophosphatemic rickets/osteomalacia: clinical characterization of a novel renal phosphate-wasting disorder. J Clin Endocrinol Metab 1997;82(2):674–81.
78. Kapelari K, Kohle J, Kotzot D, et al. Iron supplementation associated with loss of phenotype in autosomal dominant hypophosphatemic rickets. J Clin Endocrinol Metab 2015;100(9):3388–92.
79. Lorenz-Depiereux B, Bastepe M, Benet-Pages A, et al. DMP1 mutations in autosomal recessive hypophosphatemia implicate a bone matrix protein in the regulation of phosphate homeostasis. Nat Genet 2006;38(11):1248–50.
80. Feng JQ, Ward LM, Liu S, et al. Loss of DMP1 causes rickets and osteomalacia and identifies a role for osteocytes in mineral metabolism. Nat Genet 2006;38(11): 1310–5.
81. Levy-Litan V, Hershkovitz E, Avizov L, et al. Autosomal-recessive hypophosphatemic rickets is associated with an inactivation mutation in the ENPP1 gene. Am J Hum Genet 2010;86(2):273–8.
82. Rutsch F, Ruf N, Vaingankar S, et al. Mutations in ENPP1 are associated with 'idiopathic' infantile arterial calcification. Nat Genet 2003;34(4):379–81.
83. Bianco P, Robey P. Diseases of bone and the stromal cell lineage. J Bone Miner Res 1999;14(3):336–41.
84. Bhattacharyya N, Wiench M, Dumitrescu C, et al. Mechanism of FGF23 processing in fibrous dysplasia. J Bone Miner Res 2012;27(5):1132–41.

85. Riminucci M, Collins MT, Fedarko NS, et al. FGF-23 in fibrous dysplasia of bone and its relationship to renal phosphate wasting. J Clin Invest 2003;112(5):683–92.
86. Heike CL, Cunningham ML, Steiner RD, et al. Skeletal changes in epidermal nevus syndrome: does focal bone disease harbor clues concerning pathogenesis? Am J Med Genet A 2005;139A(2):67–77.
87. Moreira AI, Ferreira G, Santos M, et al. Epidermal nevus syndrome associated with hypophosphatemic rickets. Dermatol Online J 2010;16(9):14.
88. White KE, Cabral JM, Davis SI, et al. Mutations that cause osteoglophonic dysplasia define novel roles for FGFR1 in bone elongation. Am J Hum Genet 2005;76(2):361–7.
89. Shigematsu T, Kazama JJ, Yamashita T, et al. Possible involvement of circulating fibroblast growth factor 23 in the development of secondary hyperparathyroidism associated with renal insufficiency. Am J Kidney Dis 2004;44(2):250–6.
90. Isakova T, Xie H, Yang W, et al. Fibroblast growth factor 23 and risks of mortality and end-stage renal disease in patients with chronic kidney disease. JAMA 2011; 305(23):2432–9.
91. Nakayama M, Kaizu Y, Nagata M, et al. Fibroblast growth factor 23 is associated with carotid artery calcification in chronic kidney disease patients not undergoing dialysis: a cross-sectional study. BMC Nephrol 2013;14(22):1–9.
92. Gutierrez OM, Januzzi JL, Isakova T, et al. Fibroblast growth factor 23 and left ventricular hypertrophy in chronic kidney disease. Circulation 2009;119(19): 2545–52.
93. Topaz O, Shurman DL, Bergman R, et al. Mutations in GALNT3, encoding a protein involved in O-linked glycosylation, cause familial tumoral calcinosis. Nat Genet 2004;36(6):579–81.
94. Benet-Pages A, Orlik P, Strom TM, et al. An FGF23 missense mutation causes familial tumoral calcinosis with hyperphosphatemia. Hum Mol Genet 2005;14(3): 385–90.
95. Ichikawa S, Imel EA, Kreiter ML, et al. A homozygous missense mutation in human KLOTHO causes severe tumoral calcinosis. J Musculoskelet Neuronal Interact 2007;7(4):318–9.
96. Frishberg Y, Topaz O, Bergman R, et al. Identification of a recurrent mutation in GALNT3 demonstrates that hyperostosis-hyperphosphatemia syndrome and familial tumoral calcinosis are allelic disorders. J Mol Med (Berl) 2005;83(1):33–8.
97. Folsom LJ, Imel EA. Hyperphosphatemic familial tumoral calcinosis: genetic models of deficient FGF23 action. Curr Osteoporos Rep 2015;13(2):78–87.
98. Burkes EJ Jr, Lyles KW, Dolan EA, et al. Dental lesions in tumoral calcinosis. J Oral Pathol Med 1991;20(5):222–7.

Bone–Fat Interaction

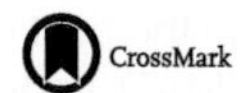

Elizabeth Rendina-Ruedy, PhD, Clifford J. Rosen, MD*

KEYWORDS

- Marrow adipose tissue • Marrow fat • Adiposity • Bone marrow

KEY POINTS

- In general, an inverse relationship exists between marrow fat and bone density.
- Multiple diseases associated with increased fracture risk also present with increased marrow adipose tissue.
- The composition of marrow adipose tissue differs between anatomic sites.
- The exact stem cell lineage and precise function of marrow adipocytes remains controversial.

INTRODUCTION

Osteoporosis and low bone mass (ie, osteopenia) are major public health concerns affecting a staggering 54 million in the United States.[1] Moreover, as the nation's demographic continues to shift toward an older population, these statistics are projected to continue to increase.[2] Approximately 2 million osteoporotic-related fracture occur each year, costing the nation $17 billion per year.[2] In addition to the financial burden, osteoporosis-related fractures often lead to multiple comorbidities (ie, hypertension, deficiency anemias, and fluid and electrolyte imbalance),[3] and patients frequently experience diminished quality of life owing to immobility, pain, and isolation.[4] Although therapeutic treatment options have aided significantly in the management of osteoporosis, some patients still experience undesirable, adverse side effects,[5–7] and therefore, continued development of refined options is necessary. As this quest continues, it is imperative to gain further insight in to the cellular and molecular responses occurring within the bone niche.

Bone is an incredibly dynamic tissue that undergoes continuous remodeling, involving bone-resorbing osteoclasts, bone-forming osteoblasts, and mechanical sensing osteocytes. Although much of bone biology has focused on these primary cell types, the bone marrow compartment also provides a unique environment in which communication between various cells can directly and indirectly impact the bone. One such cell population that has attracted much attention and scientific inquiry

Disclosure Statement: The authors have nothing to disclose.
Maine Medical Center Research Institute, 81 Research Drive, Scarborough, ME 04074, USA
* Corresponding author.
E-mail address: rosenc@mmc.org

Endocrinol Metab Clin N Am 46 (2017) 41–50
http://dx.doi.org/10.1016/j.ecl.2016.09.004
endo.theclinics.com

in the past decade are marrow adipocytes, often referred to as marrow adipose tissue (MAT) and/or yellow adipose tissue. These adipocytes can be found interspersed throughout the marrow compartment. Recently, 2 "types" of MAT, constitutive MAT and regulated MAT, have been described based on their (1) cellular morphology, (2) region specificity, and (3) fatty acid composition.[8] Both in human and mouse tissues, constitutive MAT is described as containing large adipocytes localized at the distal tibia, and is primarily composed of unsaturated lipids.[8] Conversely, regulated MAT is found mainly in the proximal tibia, interspersed with active hematopoiesis, and composed of saturated lipids.[8] Although our understanding of MAT has advanced significantly in the past decade, many questions remain. It is therefore the aim of this review is to provide the most current opinions relative to MAT and bone, while providing a brief overview of clinical scenarios in which MAT is altered.

CURRENT CONTROVERSIES AND FUNDAMENTAL QUESTIONS

Lineage of Bone Marrow Adipocytes

Unlike peripheral adipocytes or white adipose tissue, which are primarily derived from mesenchymal stem cells through vascular infiltration,[9,10] the definitive lineage of marrow adipocytes remains largely unknown and controversial. For example, although these cells have classic adipocyte functions and pathology by their hallmark ability to store lipids, bone marrow adipocytes express the osteoprogenitor marker osterix, encoded by the *Sp7* gene.[11] Given the expression of *Sp7*, one theory is that the development of marrow adipocytes results from a shift in allocation of mesenchymal stem cells from the osteoblast lineage toward the adipocyte lineage, subsequently decreasing bone formation.[12–14] Another possibility is that the marrow adipocyte could arise from bone lining cells, poorly characterized flat fibroblastic cells that express some markers of the osteogenic lineage (eg, *Sp7*).

In addition to demonstrating features characteristic of white adipose tissue and *Sp7*, marrow adipocytes also exhibit some brown adipose tissue transcriptional markers and target genes (ie, *Prdm16, FoxC2, Pgc1*α*, Dio2,* β*3AR*, and *Ucp1*).[15] Some literature also describes fibroblast adventitial reticular cells of the venous sinusoids accumulating lipids to "convert" to adipocytes. Under these circumstances, marrow adipocytes are presumed to primarily function as space fillers in the marrow cavity for inactive or reduced numbers of hematopoietic cells,[16,17] Another, more recent discovery completely shifts the idea that bone marrow adipocytes exclusively develop from mesenchymal stem cell pools and suggests they may arise from hematopoietic stem cells. These data demonstrate that hematopoietic stem cells have the ability to hone to nontissue resident fat depots, differentiate to adipocytes, and undergo de novo generation.[9,18] Moreover, the identification of differential bone marrow adipose depots (ie, constitutive MAT and regulated MAT) has given rise to the possibility that adipocytes within the marrow space are a heterogeneous population, derived from multiple sources. Nonetheless, the controversy surrounding the origin of bone marrow adipocytes underscores the complexity of these unique cells and further investigation is warranted.

Bone Marrow Adipocyte Function

Aside from the lineage tracing of marrow adipocytes, the next fundamental question that arises is that of MAT function. Our understanding of marrow adipocytes now extends well beyond their historical role as passive, "space-filling" support for the hematopoietic microenvironment. Although marrow adipocytes have a defined function as regulators of hematopoietic activity,[19] evidence also suggests MAT impacts systemic metabolism as well as bone turnover. Given their adipose pathology and biology, bone marrow adipocytes store fatty acids and, therefore, can impact global metabolism either by clearance of circulating fats and/or by their mobilization. Additionally, the recent identification of MAT as an endocrine organ capable of producing hormones such as adiponectin and leptin strongly suggests that bone marrow adipocytes regulate systemic metabolism.[20,21] Although the impact of marrow adipocytes on bone seems to be complex, evidence also indicates that an inverse relationship exists between MAT and skeletal mass (**Table 1**). As described in the previous section, one theory could involve the "see-saw" effect between osteoblasts and adipocytes; however, it is likely more complicated than proposed. The predominant localization of marrow adipocytes to the trabecular compartment of bone suggests their direct interaction facilitates bone turnover.[8] Although many questions remain, clinical scenarios in which MAT is altered has allowed investigators to gain further insight into how this novel organ impacts bone and fracture risk.

CLINICAL SCENARIOS OF ALTERED MARROW ADIPOSE TISSUE AND THEIR BONE PHENOTYPE

Anorexia Nervosa

Anorexia nervosa is a prevalent psychiatric disorder characterized by extreme self-imposed starvation as well as the subsequent weight loss and depletion of energy stores. A striking health consequence of anorexia nervosa is an approximately 7-fold increase in fracture risk, which is predominantly owing to significant bone loss and decreased bone turnover.[22–24] Another, somewhat paradoxic feature of anorexia nervosa is that, despite the lack of peripheral fat, the bone medullary space experiences a dramatic but reversible increase in MAT.[25,26] Histologic and pathologic

Table 1
Relationship between marrow adiposity, bone mineral density, and fracture risk in various clinical conditions

	Marrow Adiposity	Bone Mineral Density	Fracture Risk	References
Anorexia nervosa	↑	↓	↑	Misra & Klibanski,[22] 2006; Vestergaard et al,[23] 2002; Bredella et al,[25] 2009
Type 1 diabetes mellitus	*Inconclusive*	↓	↑	Kemink et al,[35] 2000; Slade et al,[42] 2012; Nicodemus and Folsom,[47] 2001
Type 2 diabetes mellitus	*Inconclusive*	No change or ↑	↑	Patsch et al,[55] 2013; Gorman et al,[77] 2011; Schwartz et al,[78] 2011
Aging	↑	↓	↑	National Osteoporosis Foundation,[1] 2002;Schellinger et al,[57] 2011; Schwartz et al,[79] 2013
Gonadal deficiency	↑	↓	↑	Li et al,[61] 2014; Limonard et al,[62] 2015
Unloading	↑	↓	↑	LeBlanc et al,[66] 2007; Trudel et al,[68] 2009

Abbreviations: ↓, decreased; ↑, increased.

evaluation of the bone marrow cavity is characterized by hypoplasia accompanied by the accumulation of adipocytes and a pink gelatinous material.[27] This gelatinous material tends to surround adipocytes and is thought to be a result of fat atrophy during severe starvation. The progression of these changes within the marrow space seems to primarily depend on body weight loss or weight gain with treatment.[28] As a cautionary note, serous changes occurring in the bone marrow of patients with anorexia nervosa can often mask stress fracture during routine MRI.[29] Anorexia nervosa patients also experience decreases in serum leptin,[30,31] insulin-like growth factor-1 (IGF1)[31] as well as increases in adiponectin[20] and preadipocyte factor-1 (Pref1).[32] Whether the relationship of these various biomarkers is associated directly with MAT and their precise mechanisms of action remain to be further elucidated in patients with anorexia nervosa; however, they all have documented effects on bone metabolism. Furthermore, some of the bone loss and the excess marrow adiposity is reversible, when eating resumes normally and weight is restored.

Type 1 Diabetes Mellitus

Type 1 diabetes mellitus (T1DM) is another condition in which patients experience dramatic bone loss and increased risk of fracture[33–35]; however, the MAT phenotype seems to be slightly more ambiguous. Mouse models of T1DM (ie, streptozotocin induced) have been characterized as an appropriate model based on their (1) ablation of β-cells and subsequent attenuation of insulin production, (2) decreased body weight, (3) hyperglycemia, and (4) significant bone loss.[36] Additionally, these animal models have consistently demonstrated an increase in marrow adiposity.[36–40] Despite these observations in animal models, assessment of MAT in patients with T1DM has yielded less impressive results. For example, patients with T1DM and severe sensory polyneuropathy revealed a slight shift in T1 waves of routine MRI, indicative of marrow fat, in the tibia compared with matched controls.[41] However, the authors noted that although this signaling shift was significant it was not overtly abnormal.[41] Somewhat consistent with this finding, Slade and colleagues[42] reported no differences in marrow adiposity from any site tested (eg, vertebrae, femur epiphysis, femur metaphysis, and tibia metaphysis) between control and T1DM patients. An unexpected and key finding to this study was that serum lipids (eg, cholesterol, cholesterol/high-density lipoprotein ratio, low-density lipoprotein, and triglycerides) demonstrated a strong relationship with marrow adiposity, not duration of T1DM or hemoglobin A_{1C}.[42] Taken together, these studies reveal that further clinical studies are warranted to fully understand whether MAT is altered clinically during T1DM.

Obesity and Type 2 Diabetes Mellitus

One of the most striking health consequences related to the prevalence of obesity (body mass index $\geq$30 kg/m^2 in adults) has been the staggering increase in cases of type 2 diabetes mellitus (T2DM), and although not all type 2 diabetics are overweight or obese, the majority of the cases occur in this population.[43] Understanding the bone phenotype in obese individuals and patients with T2DM has been extremely complex and outside of the scope of the current review; however, the current stance within the field is that type 2 diabetics experience an increased risk of fracture, independent of bone mineral density (BMD).[44–52] In one study, it seems that visceral fat in otherwise healthy women correlated with vertebral marrow adiposity; however, bone density was not reported.[53] In addition to marrow visceral fat, bone marrow fat content was also shown to be associated with intramyocellular and intrahepatic lipids, as well as serum cholesterol and triglycerides, both of which are increased in obesity.[54] A logical explanation of increased MAT in obesity would be that cells within the marrow compartment are exposed to or come in contact with more fatty acids and, therefore, readily accumulate and store these substrates. Given the intimate relationship between obesity and T2DM, similar changes in MAT have also been documented. Interestingly, one study noted that although total lipids were not different between type 2 diabetics and control subjects, patients with T2DM had higher saturated fat in the marrow compartment.[55] Moreover, T2DM patients with previous fracture had the highest saturated fatty acids and lowest unsaturated fatty acids.[55] These data suggest that bone marrow fat composition may serve as a novel tool to assess fracture risk within patients with T2DM. It is also interesting to note that weight loss from Roux-en-Y gastric bypass surgery reduces MAT after 6 months only in diabetic patients and not the nondiabetic group.[56] Although the implications of obesity and T2DM on bone health remains somewhat controversial, these data further implicate the role of MAT as a regulator of systemic metabolism.

Aging and Gonadal Deficiency

Age-related changes in bone (ie, decreased BMD, increased risk of fracture) are often thought of as the most classic alterations occurring in the skeleton. Aside from affecting an enormous portion of the population, age-related and gonadal deficiency osteoporosis have a strong historical presence in the bone literature. In 2000, Schellinger and colleagues[57] used proton MR to determine that fat content within the vertebra (L2) increased with age, and, interestingly, men had higher fat content than women. These results were corroborated independently shortly thereafter.[58] In addition to the age-associated increase in bone marrow adipocytes and decrease in BMD, bone formation rates have also been inversely correlated with MAT.[59] These data provide evidence that, as the adipocyte portion increased within the bone marrow cavity, osteoblast activity decreased. Moreover, the composition of marrow fat in age-related osteoporosis seems to be preferentially composed of unsaturated fatty acids.[60]

As aging progresses in women, gonadal deficiency or menopause is a natural physiologic consequence. As such, the inverse relationship between BMD and MAT also exists in postmenopausal women.[61] The changes in marrow adiposity are most evident in the axial skeleton and it has been reported that the increase in MAT can occur quickly after withdrawal of estrogen or decrease rapidly in response to exogenous estrogen.[62] Furthermore, the fatty acid composition of MAT in postmenopausal women also follows a similar profile demonstrating lower saturated fatty acids and increased monounsaturated fatty acids, particularly in participants with previous fracture.[63] This is particularly interesting given the opposite observation in T2DM. It is also important to note that the treatment of postmenopausal osteoporosis with the bisphosphonates risendronate and zoledronate not only significantly reduces the risk of fracture, but can also decrease MAT.[64,65] Collectively, these data clearly demonstrate that an inverse relationship exists between bone density and MAT in age-related and postmenopausal osteoporosis.

Disuse and Unloading of the Skeleton

Mechanical loading of the skeleton is crucial to overall bone health and quality. This is demonstrated in the severe loss of bone experienced by astronauts and cosmonauts during spaceflight as well as in bedridden patients.[66] Likewise, loading of the skeleton by gravity and weight-bearing exercises has shown to increase BMD and decrease fracture risk.[67] Although clinical data remain relatively scarce owing to the uniqueness and vulnerability of the primary populations affected by disuse, Trudel and colleagues,[68] demonstrated that 60 days of bedrest increased fat accumulation in vertebral bone marrow. The authors go on to describe that the elevated MAT remained even after 1 year of recovery (reambulation or normal physical activity).[68] It should also be noted this increase in bone marrow adiposity has been documented in rodent models of disuse (ie, hindlimb suspension)[69] and during microgravity/spaceflight. Additionally, when mechanical stress or loading is introduced to bone in the form of exercise, it seems to decrease MAT while increasing BMD.[70,71] Although more research is needed to elucidate fully how mechanical stress, or the lack thereof, affects MAT, the decrease of BMD seems to be accompanied by an increase in marrow adiposity.

Other Clinical Scenarios

The most extensively studied clinical diseases and conditions that alterations in MAT have been studied are outlined; however, other unique scenarios in the clinic exist in which changes in MAT have been documented. For example, bone loss and increased fracture risk is associated with alcoholism. It has also been demonstrated in rodent models that alcohol consumption dramatically increases vertebral fat accumulation.[72] Treatment options for various conditions and disease states can also impact marrow adiposity and bone. One such example of this is from radiation exposure used to treat various cancers. Exposure of the bone marrow compartment to radiation is sometimes targeted, as in Hodgkin's lymphoma, but can also occur secondary owing to the proximity of the targeted area, as in many pelvic cancers. Nonetheless, radiation treatment causes direct damage to red and white blood cells often eradicating blood-related cancers; however, the repopulation of the marrow compartment is accomplished by adipocyte replacement.[73–75] Perhaps consequent to this massive expansion of MAT, the risk of fracture to the irradiated area is often 3 times that of nonirradiated populations.[76] Although this is by no means an all-inclusive list of clinical scenarios in which MAT is altered, it is imperative to continue to collect these data to gain further insight into how this novel tissue can impact multiple disease states. The advent of techniques such as MR spectroscopy in larger clinical trials is likely to provide greater insight into the pathophysiology of MAT.

FUTURE CONSIDERATIONS AND SUMMARY

MAT is an active dynamic depot that contributes to overall metabolic homeostasis. Understanding both its function and origin will go a long way in terms of determining how marrow adipocytes sense energy needs in the organism and how these cells respond to environmental and nutrient stress. Importantly, defining if these adipocytes are unique in their fatty acid transport and in their adipokine secretion should help to clarify the role of MAT in bone acquisition and maintenance.

REFERENCES

1. National Osteoporosis Foundation (NOF). America's bone health: the state of osteoporosis and low bone mass in our nation. 2002.
2. The Surgeon General. Bone health and osteoporosis: a Report of the Surgeon General. 2004.
3. Nikkel LE, Fox EJ, Black KP, et al. Impact of comorbidities on hospitalization costs following hip fracture. J Bone Joint Surg Am 2012;94(1):9–17.
4. Cummings SR, Melton LJ. Epidemiology and outcomes of osteoporotic fractures. Lancet 2002;359(9319):1761–7.
5. Purcell PM, Boyd IW. Bisphosphonates and osteonecrosis of the jaw. Med J Aust 2005;182(8):417–8.

6. Rizzoli R, Reginster JY, Boonen S, et al. Adverse reactions and drug-drug interactions in the management of women with postmenopausal osteoporosis. Calcif Tissue Int 2011;89(2):91–104.
7. Schilcher J, Koeppen V, Aspenberg P, et al. Risk of atypical femoral fracture during and after bisphosphonate use. N Engl J Med 2014;371(10):974–6.
8. Scheller EL, Doucette CR, Learman BS, et al. Region-specific variation in the properties of skeletal adipocytes reveals regulated and constitutive marrow adipose tissues. Nat Commun 2015;6:7808.
9. Gavin KM, Gutman JA, Kohrt WM, et al. De novo generation of adipocytes from circulating progenitor cells in mouse and human adipose tissue. FASEB J 2016; 30(3):1096–108.
10. Majka SM, Barak Y, Klemm DJ. Concise review: adipocyte origins: weighing the possibilities. Stem Cells 2011;29(7):1034–40.
11. Liu Y, Strecker S, Wang L, et al. Osterix-cre labeled progenitor cells contribute to the formation and maintenance of the bone marrow stroma. PLoS One 2013;8(8): e71318.
12. Song L, Liu M, Ono N, et al. Loss of wnt/beta-catenin signaling causes cell fate shift of preosteoblasts from osteoblasts to adipocytes. J Bone Miner Res 2012; 27(11):2344–58.
13. Velletri T, Xie N, Wang Y, et al. P53 functional abnormality in mesenchymal stem cells promotes osteosarcoma development. Cell Death Dis 2016;7:e2015.
14. Takada I, Suzawa M, Matsumoto K, et al. Suppression of PPAR transactivation switches cell fate of bone marrow stem cells from adipocytes into osteoblasts. Ann N Y Acad Sci 2007;1116:182–95.
15. Krings A, Rahman S, Huang S, et al. Bone marrow fat has brown adipose tissue characteristics, which are attenuated with aging and diabetes. Bone 2012;50(2): 546–52.
16. Bianco P, Costantini M, Dearden LC, et al. Alkaline phosphatase positive precursors of adipocytes in the human bone marrow. Br J Haematol 1988;68(4):401–3.
17. Bianco P, Riminucci M, Kuznetsov S, et al. Multipotential cells in the bone marrow stroma: regulation in the context of organ physiology. Crit Rev Eukaryot Gene Expr 1999;9(2):159–73.
18. Majka SM, Miller HL, Sullivan T, et al. Adipose lineage specification of bone marrow-derived myeloid cells. Adipocyte 2012;1(4):215–29.
19. Naveiras O, Nardi V, Wenzel PL, et al. Bone-marrow adipocytes as negative regulators of the haematopoietic microenvironment. Nature 2009;460(7252):259–63.
20. Cawthorn WP, Scheller EL, Learman BS, et al. Bone marrow adipose tissue is an endocrine organ that contributes to increased circulating adiponectin during caloric restriction. Cell Metab 2014;20(2):368–75.
21. Dib LH, Ortega MT, Fleming SD, et al. Bone marrow leptin signaling mediates obesity-associated adipose tissue inflammation in male mice. Endocrinology 2014;155(1):40–6.
22. Misra M, Klibanski A. Anorexia nervosa and osteoporosis. Rev Endocr Metab Disord 2006;7(1–2):91–9.
23. Vestergaard P, Emborg C, Stoving RK, et al. Fractures in patients with anorexia nervosa, bulimia nervosa, and other eating disorders–a nationwide register study. Int J Eat Disord 2002;32(3):301–8.
24. Fazeli PK, Klibanski A. Bone metabolism in anorexia nervosa. Curr Osteoporos Rep 2014;12(1):82–9.
25. Bredella MA, Fazeli PK, Miller KK, et al. Increased bone marrow fat in anorexia nervosa. J Clin Endocrinol Metab 2009;94(6):2129–36.

26. Ecklund K, Vajapeyam S, Feldman HA, et al. Bone marrow changes in adolescent girls with anorexia nervosa. J Bone Miner Res 2010;25(2):298–304.
27. Cornbleet PJ, Moir RC, Wolf PL. A histochemical study of bone marrow hypoplasia in anorexia nervosa. Virchows Arch A Pathol Anat Histol 1977;374(3):239–47.
28. Abella E, Feliu E, Granada I, et al. Bone marrow changes in anorexia nervosa are correlated with the amount of weight loss and not with other clinical findings. Am J Clin Pathol 2002;118(4):582–8.
29. Tins B, Cassar-Pullicino V. Marrow changes in anorexia nervosa masking the presence of stress fractures on MR imaging. Skeletal Radiol 2006;35(11):857–60.
30. Cawthorn WP, Scheller EL, Parlee SD, et al. Expansion of bone marrow adipose tissue during caloric restriction is associated with increased circulating glucocorticoids and not with hypoleptinemia. Endocrinology 2016;157(2):508–21.
31. Devlin MJ, Cloutier AM, Thomas NA, et al. Caloric restriction leads to high marrow adiposity and low bone mass in growing mice. J Bone Miner Res 2010;25(9): 2078–88.
32. Fazeli PK, Bredella MA, Freedman L, et al. Marrow fat and preadipocyte factor-1 levels decrease with recovery in women with anorexia nervosa. J Bone Miner Res 2012;27(9):1864–71.
33. Hui SL, Epstein S, Johnston CC Jr. A prospective study of bone mass in patients with type I diabetes. J Clin Endocrinol Metab 1985;60(1):74–80.
34. Piepkorn B, Kann P, Forst T, et al. Bone mineral density and bone metabolism in diabetes mellitus. Horm Metab Res 1997;29(11):584–91.
35. Kemink SA, Hermus AR, Swinkels LM, et al. Osteopenia in insulin-dependent diabetes mellitus; prevalence and aspects of pathophysiology. J Endocrinol Invest 2000;23(5):295–303.
36. Botolin S, McCabe LR. Bone loss and increased bone adiposity in spontaneous and pharmacologically induced diabetic mice. Endocrinology 2007;148(1): 198–205.
37. Botolin S, Faugere MC, Malluche H, et al. Increased bone adiposity and peroxisomal proliferator-activated receptor-gamma2 expression in type I diabetic mice. Endocrinology 2005;146(8):3622–31.
38. Botolin S, McCabe LR. Inhibition of PPARgamma prevents type I diabetic bone marrow adiposity but not bone loss. J Cell Physiol 2006;209(3):967–76.
39. Motyl KJ, McCabe LR. Leptin treatment prevents type I diabetic marrow adiposity but not bone loss in mice. J Cell Physiol 2009;218(2):376–84.
40. Motyl KJ, Raetz M, Tekalur SA, et al. CCAAT/enhancer binding protein beta-deficiency enhances type 1 diabetic bone phenotype by increasing marrow adiposity and bone resorption. Am J Physiol Regul Integr Comp Physiol 2011; 300(5):R1250–60.
41. Poll LW, Chantelau EA. Routine MRI findings of the asymptomatic foot in diabetic patients with unilateral Charcot foot. Diabetol Metab Syndr 2010;2:25.
42. Slade JM, Coe LM, Meyer RA, et al. Human bone marrow adiposity is linked with serum lipid levels not T1-diabetes. J Diabetes Complications 2012;26(1):1–9.
43. Clinical guidelines on the identification, evaluation, and treatment of overweight and obesity in adults- The evidence report. National Institutes of Health. Obes Res 1998;6(Suppl 2):51S–209S.
44. Valerio G, Galle F, Mancusi C, et al. Prevalence of overweight in children with bone fractures: a case control study. BMC Pediatr 2012;12:166.
45. Schwartz AV, Sellmeyer DE, Ensrud KE, et al. Older women with diabetes have an increased risk of fracture: a prospective study. J Clin Endocrinol Metab 2001; 86(1):32–8.

46. van Daele PL, Stolk RP, Burger H, et al. Bone density in non-insulin-dependent diabetes mellitus. The Rotterdam Study. Ann Intern Med 1995;122(6):409–14.
47. Nicodemus KK, Folsom AR. Type 1 and type 2 diabetes and incident hip fractures in postmenopausal women. Diabetes Care 2001;24(7):1192–7.
48. de Liefde II, van der Klift M, de Laet CE, et al. Bone mineral density and fracture risk in type-2 diabetes mellitus: the Rotterdam Study. Osteoporos Int 2005;16(12): 1713–20.
49. Janghorbani M, Feskanich D, Willett WC, et al. Prospective study of diabetes and risk of hip fracture: the Nurses' Health Study. Diabetes Care 2006;29(7):1573–8.
50. Farr JN, Drake MT, Amin S, et al. In Vivo assessment of bone quality in postmenopausal women with type 2 diabetes. J Bone Miner Res 2014;29:787–95.
51. Cole ZA, Harvey NC, Kim M, et al. Increased fat mass is associated with increased bone size but reduced volumetric density in pre pubertal children. Bone 2012;50(2):562–7.
52. Goulding A, Taylor RW, Jones IE, et al. Overweight and obese children have low bone mass and area for their weight. Int J Obes Relat Metab Disord 2000;24(5): 627–32.
53. Bredella MA, Torriani M, Ghomi RH, et al. Vertebral bone marrow fat is positively associated with visceral fat and inversely associated with IGF-1 in obese women. Obesity (Silver Spring) 2011;19(1):49–53.
54. Bredella MA, Gill CM, Gerweck AV, et al. Ectopic and serum lipid levels are positively associated with bone marrow fat in obesity. Radiology 2013;269(2):534–41.
55. Patsch JM, Li X, Baum T, et al. Bone marrow fat composition as a novel imaging biomarker in postmenopausal women with prevalent fragility fractures. J Bone Miner Res 2013;28(8):1721–8.
56. Schafer AL, Li X, Schwartz AV, et al. Changes in vertebral bone marrow fat and bone mass after gastric bypass surgery: a pilot study. Bone 2015;74:140–5.
57. Schellinger D, Lin CS, Fertikh D, et al. Normal lumbar vertebrae: anatomic, age, and sex variance in subjects at proton MR spectroscopy–initial experience. Radiology 2000;215(3):910–6.
58. Kugel H, Jung C, Schulte O, et al. Age- and sex-specific differences in the 1H-spectrum of vertebral bone marrow. J Magn Reson Imaging 2001;13(2):263–8.
59. Verma S, Rajaratnam JH, Denton J, et al. Adipocytic proportion of bone marrow is inversely related to bone formation in osteoporosis. J Clin Pathol 2002;55(9): 693–8.
60. Yeung DK, Griffith JF, Antonio GE, et al. Osteoporosis is associated with increased marrow fat content and decreased marrow fat unsaturation: a proton MR spectroscopy study. J Magn Reson Imaging 2005;22(2):279–85.
61. Li GW, Xu Z, Chen QW, et al. Quantitative evaluation of vertebral marrow adipose tissue in postmenopausal female using MRI chemical shift-based water-fat separation. Clin Radiol 2014;69(3):254–62.
62. Limonard EJ, Veldhuis-Vlug AG, van DL, et al. Short-Term Effect of Estrogen on Human Bone Marrow Fat. J Bone Miner Res 2015;30(11):2058–66.
63. Miranda M, Pino AM, Fuenzalida K, et al. Characterization of fatty acid composition in bone marrow fluid from postmenopausal women: modification after hip fracture. J Cell Biochem 2016;117:2370–6.
64. Duque G, Li W, Adams M, et al. Effects of risedronate on bone marrow adipocytes in postmenopausal women. Osteoporos Int 2011;22(5):1547–53.
65. Yang Y, Luo X, Yan F, et al. Effect of zoledronic acid on vertebral marrow adiposity in postmenopausal osteoporosis assessed by MR spectroscopy. Skeletal Radiol 2015;44(10):1499–505.

66. LeBlanc AD, Spector ER, Evans HJ, et al. Skeletal responses to space flight and the bed rest analog: a review. J Musculoskelet Neuronal Interact 2007;7(1):33–47.
67. Kodama Y, Umemura Y, Nagasawa S, et al. Exercise and mechanical loading increase periosteal bone formation and whole bone strength in C57BL/6J mice but not in C3H/Hej mice. Calcif Tissue Int 2000;66(4):298–306.
68. Trudel G, Payne M, Madler B, et al. Bone marrow fat accumulation after 60 days of bed rest persisted 1 year after activities were resumed along with hemopoietic stimulation: the Women International Space Simulation for Exploration study. J Appl Physiol (1985) 2009;107(2):540–8.
69. Hamrick MW, Shi X, Zhang W, et al. Loss of myostatin (GDF8) function increases osteogenic differentiation of bone marrow-derived mesenchymal stem cells but the osteogenic effect is ablated with unloading. Bone 2007;40(6):1544–53.
70. Rantalainen T, Nikander R, Heinonen A, et al. Differential effects of exercise on tibial shaft marrow density in young female athletes. J Clin Endocrinol Metab 2013;98(5):2037–44.
71. Styner M, Thompson WR, Galior K, et al. Bone marrow fat accumulation accelerated by high fat diet is suppressed by exercise. Bone 2014;64:39–46.
72. Maddalozzo GF, Turner RT, Edwards CH, et al. Alcohol alters whole body composition, inhibits bone formation, and increases bone marrow adiposity in rats. Osteoporos Int 2009;20(9):1529–38.
73. Ramsey RG, Zacharias CE. MR imaging of the spine after radiation therapy: easily recognizable effects. AJR Am J Roentgenol 1985;144(6):1131–5.
74. Casamassima F, Ruggiero C, Caramella D, et al. Hematopoietic bone marrow recovery after radiation therapy: MRI evaluation. Blood 1989;73(6):1677–81.
75. Cao X, Wu X, Frassica D, et al. Irradiation induces bone injury by damaging bone marrow microenvironment for stem cells. Proc Natl Acad Sci U S A 2011;108(4): 1609–14.
76. Baxter NN, Habermann EB, Tepper JE, et al. Risk of pelvic fractures in older women following pelvic irradiation. JAMA 2005;294(20):2587–93.
77. Gorman E, Chudyk AM, Madden KM, et al. Bone health and type 2 diabetes mellitus: a systematic review. Physiother Can 2011;63(1):8–20.
78. Schwartz AV, Vittinghoff E, Bauer DC, et al. Association of BMD and FRAX score with risk of fracture in older adults with type 2 diabetes. JAMA 2011;305(21): 2184–92.
79. Schwartz AV, Sigurdsson S, Hue TF, et al. Vertebral bone marrow fat associated with lower trabecular BMD and prevalent vertebral fracture in older adults. J Clin Endocrinol Metab 2013;98(6):2294–300.

Endothelin Signaling in Bone

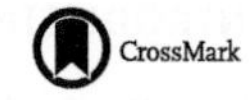

Jasmin Kristianto, PhD[a], Michael G. Johnson, PhD[b], Rafia Afzal, MBBS[c], Robert D. Blank, MD, PhD[a,d,*]

KEYWORDS

- WNT Signaling • Endothelin 1 signaling • Osteogenesis • Mechanotransduction
- Micro-RNA

KEY POINTS

- The endothelin system includes 3 small peptide hormones that are secreted as inactive precursors, a pair of G-protein–coupled receptors, and a pair of membrane-bound, extracellular converting enzymes.
- Endothelin 1/endothelin receptor A signaling is essential for the development of the craniofacial skeleton. Knockouts of the *Edn1*, *Ednra*, and *Ece1* genes have lethal phenotypes.
- Endothelin signaling is osteogenic in the setting of prostate and breast cancer.
- Genetic evidence points to allelic variation of *Ece1* as a mediator of bone biomechanical performance.
- In vitro experiments indicate that ET signaling derepresses WNT signaling, and thus may function upstream of WNT in mediating mechanical homeostasis of skeletal mass.

Grant Support: This work was supported in part by VA 1I21 RX1440 and American Heart Association grant 15GRNT25700126 to R.D. Blank.
Disclosure: Dr R.D. Blank is an investigator in a clinical trial sponsored by Novo Nordisk, a consultant for Bristol-Myers Squibb, and a contributor to UpToDate and receives royalties for this work. Drs J. Kristianto, M.G. Johnson, and R. Afzal have nothing to disclose.
This work was supported in part by SPiRe Award #1I21 RX1440 from the United States Department of Veterans Affairs Rehabilitation Research and Development Service to R.D. Blank. In addition, this material is the result of work supported with resources and the use of facilities at the Geriatrics Research, Education, and Clinical Center at the William S. Middleton Veterans Hospital in Madison, WI. The opinions expressed herein are those of the authors, and do not represent the views of the US government.
[a] Divisions of Endocrinology, Metabolism, and Clinical Nutrition, Department of Medicine, Medical College of Wisconsin, 9200 West Wisconsin Avenue, Milwaukee, WI 53226, USA; [b] Department of Medicine, University of Wisconsin, 600 Highland Avenue, Madison, WI 53792, USA; [c] Department of Anesthesiology, Aga Khan University Hospital, Stadium Road, Karachi 74800, Pakistan; [d] Medical Service, Clement J. Zablocki VAMC, 5000 West National Avenue, Milwaukee, WI 53295, USA
* Corresponding author. 9200 West Wisconsin Avenue, Milwaukee, WI 53226.
E-mail address: roblank@mcw.edu

Endocrinol Metab Clin N Am 46 (2017) 51–62
http://dx.doi.org/10.1016/j.ecl.2016.09.014
0889-8529/17/Published by Elsevier Inc.

INTRODUCTION

Endothelin 1 (ET1; **Table 1** for gene and protein abbreviations) signaling has been recognized as a driver of osteoblastic metastasis for more than a decade and recent work points to its having a broader role in bone biology. This review first outlines the ET signaling pathway and ET metabolism. It next summarizes the role of ET1 signaling in craniofacial development. Then, it discusses observations relating ET signaling to osteoblastic and other osteosclerotic processes in cancer. Finally, it describes recent work in our laboratory that points to endothelin signaling as the role of an upstream mediator of WNT signaling, promoting bone matrix synthesis and mineralization. It concludes with a statement of some remaining gaps in knowledge and proposals for future research. These are informed by insights gained from study of ET signaling in the development and physiology of the cardiovascular system.

OVERVIEW OF THE ENDOTHELIN SIGNALING PATHWAY

The ET system includes 3 small peptide hormones,[1–3] ET1, ET2, and ET3; 2 G-protein–coupled receptors,[4,5] EDNRA and EDNRB; and 2 specific converting enzymes,[6,7] ECE1 and ECE2. The ETs are synthesized as prepropeptides that are first processed to biologically inactive, 37 to 41 amino acid propeptides, commonly known as "big ETs," by furinlike proteases before secretion.[8,9] After secretion, the big ETs must be converted to their active forms by proteolytic cleavage in the extracellular space. ECE1 and ECE2, which have different pH optima (neutral pH optimal for ECE1, acidic pH optimal for ECE2), catalyze ET activation by cleaving the big ETs to 21 amino acid active ETs. In addition, big ETs can be converted by a variety of other proteases (**Figs. 1** and **2**).[10–12]

The ET system was discovered in arteries, and it has since been shown that various elements of the system are expressed in a wide variety of tissues, but expression is not ubiquitous. Immortalized osteoblasts in culture express ET1, EDNRA, and ECE1, thus having the capacity for autocrine ET signaling within the lineage.[13] Conversely, ET2, ET3, EDNRB, and ECE2 are either not detected or expressed at very low levels in these cells.[13]

ENDOTHELIN 1 SIGNALING IN DEVELOPMENT

Knockout mice lacking either ET1 or EDNRA have very similar, lethal phenotypes that result from malformations of the craniofacial bones.[14,15] Mice die shortly after birth due to asphyxia, which can be overcome by tracheostomy. They have hypoplastic mandibles, homeotic transformation of the mandible to a maxillary morphology.[16,17]

Table 1
Gene and protein abbreviations

	Protein	Human Gene	Mouse Gene
Endothelin 1	ET1	*EDN1*	*Edn1*
Endothelin 2	ET2	*EDN2*	*Edn2*
Endothelin 3	ET3	*EDN3*	*Edn3*
Endothelin A-type receptor	EDNRA	*EDNRA*	*Ednra*
Endothelin B-type receptor	EDNRA	*EDNRB*	*Ednrb*
Endothelin converting enzyme 1	ECE1	*ECE1*	*Ece1*
Endothelin converting enzyme 2	ECE2	*ECE2*	*Ece2*

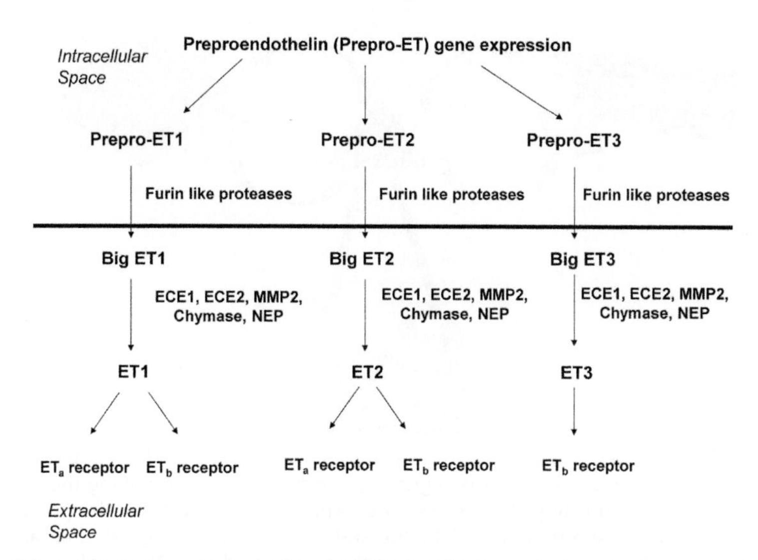

Fig. 1. Schematic representation of endothelin synthesis, secretion, and receptor binding. The horizontal line represents the cell membrane, with events above the line occurring intracellularly and those below the line occurring extracellularly. Both the ET receptors and the ECEs are membrane bound, but their ligand binding/catalytic sites are extracellular. ET_a represents the A-type endothelin receptor, encoded by *EDNRA* in humans and *Ednra* in mice. ET_b represents the B-type endothelin receptor, encoded by *EDNRB* in humans and *Ednrb* in mice. All 3 endothelins are initially synthesized as prepropeptides, encoded by *EDN1*, *EDN2*, and *EDN3* in humans and *Edn1*, *Edn2*, and *Edn3* in mice. They are processed to the respective big ETs by furin-like proteases before secretion. The big ETs are further processed to the mature, biologically active ETs by the ECEs or other extracellular proteases. B-type receptors in endothelial cells promote NO synthesis, cell survival, and ET clearance. Both A-type and B-type receptors promote smooth muscle cell contraction and collagen synthesis by fibroblasts.

There are multiple defects in other facial and basilar skull bones, and the hyoid bones. Together, these defects obstruct the airway, leading to the observed lethality. Identical craniofacial defects are observed in ECE1 knockout mice.[18]

In addition to the craniofacial abnormalities, ET1 and EDNRA knockout mice share defects of the cardiac outflow tract and great vessels.[15,19] These defects are not fully penetrant, and include tubular hypoplasia of the aortic arch, absent right subclavian artery, and perimembranous ventricular septal defect. In ECE1 knockout mice, these defects are both more severe and more penetrant than in the ET1 and EDNRA knockouts.[18] **Box 1** provides further information about ET signaling in cardiovascular physiology.

The common element linking the craniofacial and cardiovascular anomalies is that the affected structures are derived from the neural crest. Cranial and cardiac neural crest cells migrate early in development and express EDNRA.[15] It is worth noting that knockouts of ET3 and EDNRB, which are also lethal, affect a different population of neural crest derivatives. Phenotypes of these mutations include colonic aganglionosis (Hirschsprung disease) and white spotting.[20,21] As in the case of EDNRA/ET1, EDNRB/ET3 knockouts have very similar phenotypes. ECE1 knockout animals have all the defects characteristic of both the EDNRA/ET1 and EDNRB/ET3 knockouts.[18]

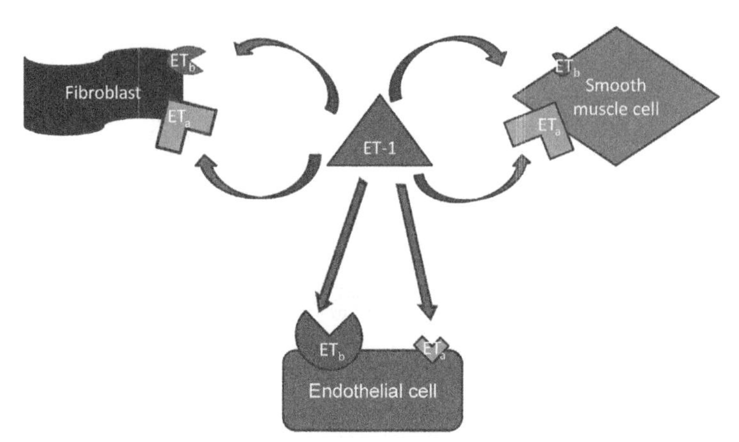

Fig. 2. Schematic representation of autocrine and paracrine ET1 signaling. In blood vessels, the balance of autocrine and paracrine signaling is important in determining the biological response to ET signaling. Big ET1 is secreted by endothelial cells. It can be processed to mature ET1 by membrane-bound ECE1 by the endothelial cells and signal in an autocrine fashion via either A-type or B-type receptors on the endothelial cells. These cells express predominantly B-type receptor, thus favoring vasodilatory responses. Alternatively, mature ET1 (21 amino acids) or big ET1 (38 amino acids) can diffuse in the extracellular space. Big ET1 can be activated by other tissue proteases and can signal via ET receptors located on smooth muscle cells, fibroblasts, or other cells present in the vessel wall or perivascular space. Activation of these cell types by ET1 promotes vasoconstriction and thickening/stiffening of the media. The activity of ECE1 can alter the balance of autocrine versus paracrine ET1 signaling.

ENDOTHELIN SIGNALING IN OSTEOBLASTIC METASTASIS

ET signaling occurs in both mammary and prostate glands, and when it is expressed in neoplasms arising from those tissues, it promotes osteoblastic metastasis.[22–26] Osteoblastic metastasis is common in prostate cancer and uncommon in breast cancer. In both cases, lesions feature synthesis of sclerotic, woven bone that is mechanically deficient. We recently found that ET1 is highly expressed in the setting of osteosclerosis associated with myelofibrosis,[27] with similar features to those encountered in breast and prostate cancer. Promotion of osteogenesis by ET1 signaling is mediated at least in part by modulation of WNT signaling. In cultured mouse calvarial osteoblasts, ET1 reduces transcription and secretion of DKK1, and concomitantly increases bone formation.[28] In men with metastatic prostate cancer, EDNRA blockade suppressed progression of bone disease as measured by bone turnover markers.[29]

Human breast cancer cells can convert big ET1 to active ET1,[24,30] suggesting the potential role of ET1 in bone metastasis in breast cancer. EDNRA blockade reduced osteoblastic lesions in mice inoculated with ZR-75-1 human breast cancer cells.[24] Collectively, these results show that ET1 action via EDNRA mediate bone formation in both breast and prostate cancer. The bone cells, in turn, secrete factors that can support proliferation of the tumor cells, such as IGF1, resulting in a vicious cycle of concurrent bone and tumor growth supported by reciprocal paracrine signaling between tumor cells and osteoblasts.

ENDOTHELIN SIGNALING IN BONE PHYSIOLOGY

In the course of pursuing our long-standing interest in the genetic basis of bone biomechanical performance, we identified *Ece1* as a candidate gene for a

Box 1
Physiologic endothelin signaling in the cardiovascular system

The endothelin (ET) system was first discovered in the vasculature and its biology is best understood in that setting. ET signaling via EDNRB on endothelial cells causes vasodilation and clearance of ETs from the circulation.[48–50] In contrast, signaling via both EDNRA and EDNRB in smooth muscle cells has potent vasoconstrictive effects.[1,51] Endothelial cells are the primary source of ET1 and have a high density of EDNRB, so autocrine signaling favors vasodilation and hypotensive responses, whereas paracrine signaling leads to hypertensive responses. In experiments we performed using the same mice in which we identified *Ece1* as a candidate gene for bone biomechanical performance, we found that mice harboring a high-expressing *Ece1* allele had larger femoral and arterial cross-sections, greater arterial compliance, and lower blood pressure than mice harboring a low-expressing *Ece1* allele.[52]

Shear stress plays a critical role in vascular remodeling, both in developmental[53] and physiologic[54–56] settings. NO is known to play a central role in mediating vascular remodeling in pregnancy and its induction by shear stress is well established.[57–59] In this setting, NO is produced by NOS3 and the *Nos3* gene is induced by EDNRB activation in endothelial cells.[49] Insufficient EDNRB function exacerbates inward hypotrophic vascular remodeling by low flow.[60] Taken together, these findings suggest that ET signaling via EDNRB could contribute to outward remodeling in response to high shear stress.

Although osteoblasts and endothelial cells express all the genes necessary for autocrine ET1 signaling, in blood vessels there is a necessary balance between autocrine and paracrine ET1 signaling. Paracrine signaling contributes to the greater thickness and higher smooth muscle content of arterial versus venous walls. Even though arterial and venous identities are established before the onset of circulation,[61] mechanical signals reinforce and amplify those differences.[53] It is presently unknown whether specific mechanical environments lead to differential endothelial cell expression of *Edn1* and of *Ece1*. Should this prove to be the case, differential regulation of these genes by distinct mechanical environments could provide a mechanism by which wall stress and shear stress might lead to distinct adaptive responses.

pleiotropic quantitative trait locus (QTL) for bone size, shape, and strength.[31–35] The QTL increases the cross-sectional size and ellipticity of the femoral diaphysis, leading to an increase in the whole bone strength as measured by 3-point bending. This constellation of phenotypes suggested that the primary process affected by the QTL was bone modeling in response to mechanical loading (**Box 2**). Other investigators had determined that our QTL lies within a genomic region that contributes to load-induced bone modeling,[36] leading us to hypothesize that both sets of phenotypes were mediated by the same genes. It is worth noting that the mouse QTL corresponds to a confirmed human bone mineral density (BMD) QTL.[37]

In subsequent experiments, we found that murine osteoblasts grown in tissue culture engage in autocrine ET1 signaling via EDNRA[13] (Johnson and colleagues, unpublished data, 2014-2016). They express *Edn1*, *Ednra*, and *Ece1*, but not *Ednrb*. These cells recapitulate maturation of the osteoblast lineage when placed in medium supplemented with vitamin C and phosphate, forming mineralized nodules after 2 weeks in mineralization medium. Supplementation of the medium with big ET1 increases mineralization, which is blocked by pharmacologic inhibition of either ECE1 or EDNRA, treatment with sclerostin (SOST), or by transfection of small interfering RNA targeting *Ece1* message. In addition to promoting mineralization, ET1 treatment reduces secretion of SOST and DKK1, in spite of increasing transcription of their mRNAs. These

Box 2
The skeletal mechanostat and the WNT pathway

The ability of bone to alter its size and shape in response to its habitual mechanical environment is well established. Overloading leads to an increase in long bone cross-sectional size, as was demonstrated in elite racquet sport athletes.[62] Conversely, underloading, as occurs in spaceflight, prolonged bed rest, or spinal cord injury, leads to loss of skeletal mass.[63–65] The notion that bone mass is physiologically regulated has been formalized in the mechanostat model of bone modeling.[66,67] Briefly stated, the model holds that bone modeling (change in diameter and/or cross-sectional geometry) occurs to maintain mechanical strain (fractional change in length) within a narrow physiologic range. Once such physiologic equilibrium is reached, bone size and shape remain stable unless disturbed.

Widely accepted experimental interventions to allow study of defined skeletal loading conditions in experimental animals have been developed. Ulnar and tibial loading coupled with dynamic histomorphometry allow the in vivo modeling response to loading to be measured, using the contralateral, unloaded limb as a control.[12] Tail suspension[68] and sciatic neurectomy[69] both allow study of in vivo unloading. These powerful investigative tools have been used in genetically engineered mice to identify critical molecules mediating mechanotransduction.

The canonical WNT signaling pathway is one of the principal mechanisms by which bone responds to its mechanical environment. Recognition of its central role in bone biology emerged from the recognition that inactivating and activating mutations of *LRP5*, a WNT coreceptor, caused 2 rare Mendelian conditions, the osteoporosis pseudoglioma syndrome and hereditary high bone mass, respectively.[70–72] Mendelian high bone mass disorders, sclerosteosis and Van Buchem disease, arise as a consequence of mutations in *SOST*, the gene encoding the WNT antagonist sclerostin.[73,74] Overexpression of the WNT inhibitor DKK1 drives bone resorption in multiple myeloma.[75]

Although human disease provided the first clues that WNT signaling is critical in bone physiology, mechanistic understanding of bone mass regulation has been achieved through study of mouse models. Experiments featuring ulnar loading demonstrated that loss of function *Lrp5* (mouse homolog of *LRP5*) mutations lead to decreased load-induced modeling,[76,77] whereas mutations that mimic human high bone mass variants display increased modeling in response to mechanical loading.[77–79] These modeling responses demonstrate that disruption of the WNT pathway affects physiology as well as development.

SOST is a WNT inhibitor and is produced constitutively by mature osteocytes, but its expression is decreased in the presence of mechanical loading.[47] Mice in which *Sost* (the mouse gene encoding SOST) has been knocked out display increased bone mass, mimicking the human sclerosteosis phenotype.[80,81]

Furthermore, SNPs within or near genes involved in the WNT pathway are associated with mass and fractures in humans.[37,82–85] In the case of *LRP5*, there is evidence from the Framingham cohort that the association with BMD is exercise dependent.[86] Anti-SOST antibodies are presently being tested as possible drugs to increase bone mass and prevent fracture.[87,88]

divergent effects on transcription and protein secretion are mediated in part by miR 126-3p, which is increased by approximately 120-fold via ET signaling, which targets *Sost* message. The effects of ET1 signaling on mineralization and SOST secretion are mimicked by transfection of a miR 126-3p expressing lentivirus, whereas the effects of ET1 signaling blockade are mimicked by transfection of a lentivirus expressing a miR 126-3p antagonist.

MiR 126-3p is a critical molecule in angiogenesis.[38] MiR 126-3p ablated mice have a high rate of embryonic lethality with impaired blood vessel formation, whereas the surviving mice are deficient in the angiogenic response to experimental ischemia.[39] Important endothelial cell targets of miR-126-3p include, but are not limited to, mRNAs encoding a pair of vascular endothelial growth factor inhibitors, *Pik3r2* and *Spred1*. It is interesting to note that both in osteoblasts and in endothelial cells, miR 126-3p acts by releasing repression of critical signaling pathways.

FUTURE CONSIDERATIONS

Current understanding of ET biology is very uneven. The developmental roles of ET signaling are relatively well characterized, as is ET signaling within arterial walls. It is also clear that ET drives osteoblastic metastasis in breast and prostate cancer, but little is known regarding the role of ET signaling in the normal function of each of these glands, or of the contribution of ET signaling to normal bone physiology. Greater understanding of the ET signaling pathway's role in the normal biology of tissues outside the vasculature is therefore of great importance.

It is important to recall that ET1 signaling is essential in development,[14,15,18,19] and that the phenotypes resulting from knockout of *Edn1*, *Ednra*, and *Ece1* overlap some of those arising from mutants affecting WNT signaling. Ablation of *Ece1*, unlike that of either *Edn1* or *Ednra*, leads to significant mid-gestational in utero lethality due to heart failure, reflecting a greater severity of cardiac outflow tract abnormalities.[18] In the chick, ET1 signaling mediates essential mechanotransductive signals in Purkinje system development.[40–43]

However, the situation is more complex. WNT signaling has an unequivocal trophic impact on cells already committed to the osteoblast lineage; indeed, canonical WNT signaling has been shown by some investigators to inhibit commitment of mesenchymal stem cells to the osteoblast lineage.[44,45] In addition, mice constitutively expressing β-catenin in late stage osteoblasts and osteocytes have *both* increased bone volume and osteomalacia.[46] These findings demonstrate that normal bone mineralization requires downregulation of canonical WNT signaling at late stages of osteoblast maturation, even while elaboration of bone matrix by less mature cells is promoted.

Downregulation of SOST, leading to derepression of the WNT pathway has been demonstrated in an *in vivo* experimental mechanical loading protocol.[47] It is unknown at this point whether ET signaling mediates the SOST response in this setting, thus functioning upstream of the WNT pathway in mediating mechanotransduction in bone. Our laboratory's findings that ET1 signaling reduces SOST expression via miR-126-3p provide a mechanistic basis for pursuing this line of investigation[13] (Johnson and colleagues, unpublished data, 2014-2016). Other investigators have identified DKK1 as another WNT-related target of ET1 signaling in cancer,[28] further supporting the idea that ET signaling is upstream of the WNT pathway in bone.

More broadly, little attention has been devoted to identifying common mechanisms of mechanotransduction in bones and arteries. Both are tubular organs whose function requires adaptation to highly variable mechanical environments. Bone and vascular biology might both benefit by further work in this area.

Finally, osteoblastic metastases arise in other tumors in addition to prostate and breast cancer. It is worth studying other tumor types to determine whether they share ET1 signaling as the underlying mechanism.

REFERENCES

1. Yanagisawa M, Kurihara H, Kimura S, et al. A novel potent vasoconstrictor peptide produced by vascular endothelial cells. Nature 1988;332(6163):411–5.
2. Yanagisawa M, Inoue A, Ishikawa T, et al. Primary structure, synthesis, and biological activity of rat endothelin, an endothelium-derived vasoconstrictor peptide. Proc Natl Acad Sci U S A 1988;85(18):6964–7.

3. Inoue A, Yanagisawa M, Kimura S, et al. The human endothelin family: three structurally and pharmacologically distinct isopeptides predicted by three separate genes. Proc Natl Acad Sci U S A 1989;86(8):2863–7.
4. Arai H, Hori S, Aramori I, et al. Cloning and expression of a cDNA encoding an endothelin receptor. Nature 1990;348(6303):730–2.
5. Sakurai T, Yanagisawa M, Takuwa Y, et al. Cloning of a cDNA encoding a non-isopeptide-selective subtype of the endothelin receptor. Nature 1990; 348(6303):732–5.
6. Xu D, Emoto N, Giaid A, et al. ECE-1: a membrane-bound metalloprotease that catalyzes the proteolytic activation of big endothelin-1. Cell 1994;78(3):473–85.
7. Emoto N, Yanagisawa M. Endothelin-converting enzyme-2 is a membrane-bound, phosphoramidon-sensitive metalloprotease with acidic pH optimum. J Biol Chem 1995;270(25):15262–8.
8. Denault JB, Claing A, D'Orleans-Juste P, et al. Processing of proendothelin-1 by human furin convertase. FEBS Lett 1995;362(3):276–80.
9. Inoue A, Yanagisawa M, Takuwa Y, et al. The human preproendothelin-1 gene. Complete nucleotide sequence and regulation of expression. J Biol Chem 1989;264(25):14954–9.
10. Fernandez-Patron C, Radomski MW, Davidge ST. Vascular matrix metalloproteinase-2 cleaves big endothelin-1 yielding a novel vasoconstrictor. Circ Res 1999;85(10):906–11.
11. Wypij DM, Nichols JS, Novak PJ, et al. Role of mast cell chymase in the extracellular processing of big-endothelin-1 to endothelin-1 in the perfused rat lung. Biochem Pharmacol 1992;43(4):845–53.
12. Abassi ZA, Tate JE, Golomb E, et al. Role of neutral endopeptidase in the metabolism of endothelin. Hypertension 1992;20(1):89–95.
13. Johnson MG, Kristianto J, Yuan B, et al. Big endothelin changes the cellular miRNA environment in TMOb osteoblasts and increases mineralization. Connect Tissue Res 2014;55(Suppl 1):113–6.
14. Kurihara Y, Kurihara H, Suzuki H, et al. Elevated blood pressure and craniofacial abnormalities in mice deficient in endothelin-1. Nature 1994;368(6473):703–10.
15. Clouthier DE, Hosoda K, Richardson JA, et al. Cranial and cardiac neural crest defects in endothelin-A receptor-deficient mice. Development 1998;125(5): 813–24.
16. Ozeki H, Kurihara Y, Tonami K, et al. Endothelin-1 regulates the dorsoventral branchial arch patterning in mice. Mech Dev 2004;121(4):387–95.
17. Ruest LB, Clouthier DE. Elucidating timing and function of endothelin-A receptor signaling during craniofacial development using neural crest cell-specific gene deletion and receptor antagonism. Dev Biol 2009;328(1):94–108.
18. Yanagisawa H, Yanagisawa M, Kapur RP, et al. Dual genetic pathways of endothelin-mediated intercellular signaling revealed by targeted disruption of endothelin converting enzyme-1 gene. Development 1998;125(5):825–36.
19. Kurihara Y, Kurihara H, Oda H, et al. Aortic arch malformations and ventricular septal defect in mice deficient in endothelin-1. J Clin Invest 1995;96(1):293–300.
20. Baynash AG, Hosoda K, Giaid A, et al. Interaction of endothelin-3 with endothelin-B receptor is essential for development of epidermal melanocytes and enteric neurons. Cell 1994;79(7):1277–85.
21. Hosoda K, Hammer RE, Richardson JA, et al. Targeted and natural (piebald-lethal) mutations of endothelin-B receptor gene produce megacolon associated with spotted coat color in mice. Cell 1994;79(7):1267–76.

22. Nelson JB, Hedican SP, George DJ, et al. Identification of endothelin-1 in the pathophysiology of metastatic adenocarcinoma of the prostate. Nat Med 1995; 1(9):944–9.
23. Berruti A, Dogliotti L, Gorzegno G, et al. Differential patterns of bone turnover in relation to bone pain and disease extent in bone in cancer patients with skeletal metastases. Clin Chem 1999;45(8 Pt 1):1240–7.
24. Yin JJ, Mohammad KS, Kakonen SM, et al. A causal role for endothelin-1 in the pathogenesis of osteoblastic bone metastases. Proc Natl Acad Sci U S A 2003;100(19):10954–9.
25. Mohammad KS, Guise TA. Mechanisms of osteoblastic metastases: role of endothelin-1. Clin Orthop Relat Res 2003;415(Suppl):S67–74.
26. Guise TA, Yin JJ, Mohammad KS. Role of endothelin-1 in osteoblastic bone metastases. Cancer 2003;97(3 Suppl):779–84.
27. Yachoui R, Kristianto J, Sitwala K, et al. Role of endothelin-1 in a syndrome of myelofibrosis and osteosclerosis. J Clin Endocrinol Metab 2015;100(11):3971–4.
28. Clines GA, Mohammad KS, Bao Y, et al. Dickkopf homolog 1 mediates endothelin-1-stimulated new bone formation. Mol Endocrinol 2007;21(2):486–98.
29. Nelson JB, Nabulsi AA, Vogelzang NJ, et al. Suppression of prostate cancer induced bone remodeling by the endothelin receptor A antagonist atrasentan. J Urol 2003;169(3):1143–9.
30. Patel KV, Sheth HG, Schrey MP. Stimulation or endothelin-1 secretion by human breast cancer cells through protein kinase A activation: a possible novel paracrine loop involving breast fibroblast-derived prostaglandin E2. Mol Cell Endocrinol 1997;126(2):143–51.
31. Saless N, Litscher SJ, Vanderby R, et al. Linkage mapping of principal components for femoral biomechanical performance in a reciprocal HCB-8 x HCB-23 intercross. Bone 2011;48(3):647–53.
32. Saless N, Litscher SJ, Houlihan MJ, et al. Comprehensive skeletal phenotyping and linkage mapping in an intercross of recombinant congenic mouse strains HcB-8 and HcB-23. Cells Tissues Organs 2011;194(2–4):244–8.
33. Saless N, Lopez Franco GE, Litscher S, et al. Linkage mapping of femoral material properties in a reciprocal intercross of HcB-8 and HcB-23 recombinant mouse strains. Bone 2010;46(5):1251–9.
34. Saless N, Litscher SJ, Lopez Franco GE, et al. Quantitative trait loci for biomechanical performance and femoral geometry in an intercross of recombinant congenic mice: restriction of the Bmd7 candidate interval. FASEB J 2009;23(7): 2142–54.
35. Kristianto J, Litscher SJ, Johnson MG, et al. Congenic strains confirm the pleiotropic effect of chromosome 4 QTL on mouse femoral geometry and biomechanical performance. PLoS One 2016;11(2):e0148571.
36. Robling AG, Li J, Shultz KL, et al. Evidence for a skeletal mechanosensitivity gene on mouse chromosome 4. FASEB J 2003;17(2):324–6.
37. Rivadeneira F, Styrkarsdottir U, Estrada K, et al. Twenty bone-mineral-density loci identified by large-scale meta-analysis of genome-wide association studies. Nat Genet 2009;41(11):1199–206.
38. Fish JE, Santoro MM, Morton SU, et al. miR-126 regulates angiogenic signaling and vascular integrity. Dev Cell 2008;15(2):272–84.
39. Wang S, Aurora AB, Johnson BA, et al. The endothelial-specific microRNA miR-126 governs vascular integrity and angiogenesis. Dev Cell 2008;15(2):261–71.

40. Gourdie RG, Wei Y, Kim D, et al. Endothelin-induced conversion of embryonic heart muscle cells into impulse-conducting Purkinje fibers. Proc Natl Acad Sci U S A 1998;95(12):6815–8.
41. Hall CE, Hurtado R, Hewett KW, et al. Hemodynamic-dependent patterning of endothelin converting enzyme 1 expression and differentiation of impulse-conducting Purkinje fibers in the embryonic heart. Development 2004;131(3):581–92.
42. Sedmera D, Harris BS, Grant E, et al. Cardiac expression patterns of endothelin-converting enzyme (ECE): implications for conduction system development. Dev Dyn 2008;237(6):1746–53.
43. Takebayashi-Suzuki K, Yanagisawa M, Gourdie RG, et al. In vivo induction of cardiac Purkinje fiber differentiation by coexpression of preproendothelin-1 and endothelin converting enzyme-1. Development 2000;127(16):3523–32.
44. Boland GM, Perkins G, Hall DJ, et al. Wnt 3a promotes proliferation and suppresses osteogenic differentiation of adult human mesenchymal stem cells. J Cell Biochem 2004;93(6):1210–30.
45. Liu G, Vijayakumar S, Grumolato L, et al. Canonical Wnts function as potent regulators of osteogenesis by human mesenchymal stem cells. J Cell Biol 2009;185(1):67–75.
46. Chen S, Feng J, Bao Q, et al. Adverse effects of osteocytic constitutive activation of ss-Catenin on bone strength and bone growth. J Bone Miner Res 2015;30(7):1184–94.
47. Robling AG, Niziolek PJ, Baldridge LA, et al. Mechanical stimulation of bone in vivo reduces osteocyte expression of Sost/sclerostin. J Biol Chem 2008;283(9):5866–75.
48. Masaki T, Kimura S, Yanagisawa M, et al. Molecular and cellular mechanism of endothelin regulation. Implications for vascular function. Circulation 1991;84(4):1457–68.
49. Tsukahara H, Ende H, Magazine HI, et al. Molecular and functional characterization of the non-isopeptide-selective ETB receptor in endothelial cells. Receptor coupling to nitric oxide synthase. J Biol Chem 1994;269(34):21778–85.
50. Frangos JA, Eskin SG, McIntire LV, et al. Flow effects on prostacyclin production by cultured human endothelial cells. Science 1985;227(4693):1477–9.
51. Sumner MJ, Cannon TR, Mundin JW, et al. Endothelin ETA and ETB receptors mediate vascular smooth muscle contraction. Br J Pharmacol 1992;107(3):858–60.
52. Wang Z, Kristianto J, Yen Ooi C, et al. Blood pressure, artery size, and artery compliance parallel bone size and strength in mice with differing ece1 expression. J Biomech Eng 2013;135(6):61003–9.
53. Lucitti JL, Jones EA, Huang C, et al. Vascular remodeling of the mouse yolk sac requires hemodynamic force. Development 2007;134(18):3317–26.
54. Langille BL, O'Donnell F. Reductions in arterial diameter produced by chronic decreases in blood flow are endothelium-dependent. Science 1986;231(4736):405–7.
55. Tuttle JL, Nachreiner RD, Bhuller AS, et al. Shear level influences resistance artery remodeling: wall dimensions, cell density, and eNOS expression. Am J Physiol Heart Circ Physiol 2001;281(3):H1380–9.
56. Rudic RD, Shesely EG, Maeda N, et al. Direct evidence for the importance of endothelium-derived nitric oxide in vascular remodeling. J Clin Invest 1998;101(4):731–6.

57. Li Y, Zheng J, Bird IM, et al. Effects of pulsatile shear stress on nitric oxide production and endothelial cell nitric oxide synthase expression by ovine fetoplacental artery endothelial cells. Biol Reprod 2003;69(3):1053–9.
58. Li Y, Zheng J, Bird IM, et al. Effects of pulsatile shear stress on signaling mechanisms controlling nitric oxide production, endothelial nitric oxide synthase phosphorylation, and expression in ovine fetoplacental artery endothelial cells. Endothelium 2005;12(1–2):21–39.
59. Sladek SM, Magness RR, Conrad KP. Nitric oxide and pregnancy. Am J Physiol 1997;272(2 Pt 2):R441–63.
60. Murakoshi N, Miyauchi T, Kakinuma Y, et al. Vascular endothelin-B receptor system in vivo plays a favorable inhibitory role in vascular remodeling after injury revealed by endothelin-B receptor-knockout mice. Circulation 2002;106(15): 1991–8.
61. Wang HU, Chen ZF, Anderson DJ. Molecular distinction and angiogenic interaction between embryonic arteries and veins revealed by ephrin-B2 and its receptor Eph-B4. Cell 1998;93(5):741–53.
62. Jones HH, Priest JD, Hayes WC, et al. Humeral hypertrophy in response to exercise. J Bone Joint Surg Am 1977;59(2):204–8.
63. Lang T, LeBlanc A, Evans H, et al. Cortical and trabecular bone mineral loss from the spine and hip in long-duration spaceflight. J Bone Miner Res 2004;19(6): 1006–12.
64. Donaldson CL, Hulley SB, Vogel JM, et al. Effect of prolonged bed rest on bone mineral. Metabolism 1970;19(12):1071–84.
65. Griffiths HJ, Zimmerman RE. The use of photon densitometry to evaluate bone mineral in a group of patients with spinal cord injury. Paraplegia 1973;10(4): 279–84.
66. Frost HM. The Utah paradigm of skeletal physiology: an overview of its insights for bone, cartilage and collagenous tissue organs. J Bone Miner Metab 2000; 18(6):305–16.
67. Frost HM. From Wolff's law to the Utah paradigm: insights about bone physiology and its clinical applications. Anat Rec 2001;262(4):398–419.
68. Morey-Holton ER, Globus RK. Hindlimb unloading of growing rats: a model for predicting skeletal changes during space flight. Bone 1998;22(5 Suppl):83S–8S.
69. Hert J, Sklenska A, Liskova M. Reaction of bone to mechanical stimuli. 5. Effect of intermittent stress on the rabbit tibia after resection of the peripheral nerves. Folia Morphol (Praha) 1971;19(4):378–87.
70. Boyden LM, Mao J, Belsky J, et al. High bone density due to a mutation in LDL-receptor-related protein 5. N Engl J Med 2002;346(20):1513–21.
71. Gong Y, Slee RB, Fukai N, et al. LDL receptor-related protein 5 (LRP5) affects bone accrual and eye development. Cell 2001;107(4):513–23.
72. Little RD, Carulli JP, Del Mastro RG, et al. A mutation in the LDL receptor-related protein 5 gene results in the autosomal dominant high-bone-mass trait. Am J Hum Genet 2002;70(1):11–9.
73. Brunkow ME, Gardner JC, Van Ness J, et al. Bone dysplasia sclerosteosis results from loss of the SOST gene product, a novel cystine knot-containing protein. Am J Hum Genet 2001;68(3):577–89.
74. Balemans W, Patel N, Ebeling M, et al. Identification of a 52 kb deletion downstream of the SOST gene in patients with van Buchem disease. J Med Genet 2002;39(2):91–7.

75. Tian E, Zhan F, Walker R, et al. The role of the Wnt-signaling antagonist DKK1 in the development of osteolytic lesions in multiple myeloma. N Engl J Med 2003; 349(26):2483–94.
76. Sawakami K, Robling AG, Ai M, et al. The Wnt co-receptor LRP5 is essential for skeletal mechanotransduction but not for the anabolic bone response to parathyroid hormone treatment. J Biol Chem 2006;281(33):23698–711.
77. Cui Y, Niziolek PJ, MacDonald BT, et al. Lrp5 functions in bone to regulate bone mass. Nat Med 2011;17(6):684–91.
78. Akhter MP, Wells DJ, Short SJ, et al. Bone biomechanical properties in LRP5 mutant mice. Bone 2004;35(1):162–9.
79. Robinson JA, Chatterjee-Kishore M, Yaworsky PJ, et al. Wnt/beta-catenin signaling is a normal physiological response to mechanical loading in bone. J Biol Chem 2006;281(42):31720–8.
80. Li X, Ominsky MS, Niu QT, et al. Targeted deletion of the sclerostin gene in mice results in increased bone formation and bone strength. J Bone Miner Res 2008; 23(6):860–9.
81. Balemans W, Ebeling M, Patel N, et al. Increased bone density in sclerosteosis is due to the deficiency of a novel secreted protein (SOST). Hum Mol Genet 2001; 10(5):537–43.
82. Sims AM, Shephard N, Carter K, et al. Genetic analyses in a sample of individuals with high or low BMD shows association with multiple Wnt pathway genes. J Bone Miner Res 2008;23(4):499–506.
83. Richards JB, Rivadeneira F, Inouye M, et al. Bone mineral density, osteoporosis, and osteoporotic fractures: a genome-wide association study. Lancet 2008; 371(9623):1505–12.
84. Uitterlinden AG, Arp PP, Paeper BW, et al. Polymorphisms in the sclerosteosis/van Buchem disease gene (SOST) region are associated with bone-mineral density in elderly whites. Am J Hum Genet 2004;75(6):1032–45.
85. Estrada K, Styrkarsdottir U, Evangelou E, et al. Genome-wide meta-analysis identifies 56 bone mineral density loci and reveals 14 loci associated with risk of fracture. Nat Genet 2012;44(5):491–501.
86. Kiel DP, Ferrari SL, Cupples LA, et al. Genetic variation at the low-density lipoprotein receptor-related protein 5 (LRP5) locus modulates Wnt signaling and the relationship of physical activity with bone mineral density in men. Bone 2007;40(3): 587–96.
87. McClung MR, Grauer A. Romosozumab in postmenopausal women with osteopenia. N Engl J Med 2014;370(17):1664–5.
88. Recker RR, Benson CT, Matsumoto T, et al. A randomized, double-blind phase 2 clinical trial of blosozumab, a sclerostin antibody, in postmenopausal women with low bone mineral density. J Bone Miner Res 2015;30(2):216–24.

Diabetes and Bone Disease

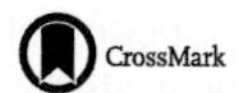

G. Isanne Schacter, MD, FRCPC[a], William D. Leslie, MD, MSc, FRCPC[b,*]

KEYWORDS

- Diabetes • Bone • Osteoporosis • Fracture • Bone mineral density
- Dual-energy x-ray absorptiometry

KEY POINTS

- Both TYPES 1 and 2 diabetes are associated with an increased risk of fracture.
- The pathophysiology of the increased fracture risk differs between types 1 and 2 diabetes.
- Several modalities, including bone mineral density, are available to stratify risk, but may not accurately capture the increased risk of fracture.
- First-line management is with bisphosphonates, although their efficacy in diabetes-induced osteoporosis is uncertain.
- Treatment-related suppression in bone turnover has not been shown to influence glucose metabolism or precipitate diabetes.

INTRODUCTION

The World Health Organization estimated that diabetes mellitus occurs in more than 415 million people worldwide, and that this number could double by 2040, because the incidences of both TYPE 1 (T1D) and TYPE 2 (T2D) diabetes are increasing.[1] T1D accounts for less than 10% of all patients with diabetes, and recent studies have shown that the global incidence is increasing by approximately 2% to 3% per year.[2,3] T2D currently affects 25% of older adults in the United States (including diagnosed and undiagnosed cases),[4] with worldwide estimates suggesting that it affects more than 15% of adults greater than age 55 years.[1]

The major complications of diabetes are well-known, namely, microvascular complications such as nephropathy, retinopathy, and neuropathy, as well as the macrovascular complications including cardiovascular disease. More recently, epidemiologic data have shown that other tissues and organs may be adversely impacted by diabetes. The skeletal system seems to be an additional target of diabetes-mediated damage, leading to the subsequent development of diabetes-

The authors have nothing to disclose.
[a] Department of Medicine, University of Manitoba, GF-335, 820 Sherbrook Street, Winnipeg, Manitoba R3A 1R9, Canada; [b] Department of Medicine, University of Manitoba, C5121, 409 Tache Avenue, Winnipeg, Manitoba R2H 2A6, Canada
* Corresponding author.
E-mail address: bleslie@sbgh.mb.ca

Endocrinol Metab Clin N Am 46 (2017) 63–85
http://dx.doi.org/10.1016/j.ecl.2016.09.010

induced osteoporosis. A conceptual framework for this increase in fracture burden is illustrated in **Fig. 1**.

Osteoporosis and diabetes are increasingly prevalent diseases, in part owing to aging populations worldwide.[1,5] At the age of 50, the lifetime risk of hip fracture is approximately 17.5% for women, and 6% for men in the United States,[6] with an even higher lifetime risk for vertebral fracture.[7] Nine percent of adults aged 50 and over have osteoporosis, as defined by a low bone mineral density (BMD) at either the femoral neck or the lumbar spine.[8] The total number of hip fractures in 1990 was estimated to be 1.26 million, and is projected to double twice, to 2.6 million hip fractures annually by 2025 and 4.5 million by 2050.[9]

EPIDEMIOLOGY

It has long been well-established that T1D is associated with an increased risk of both osteoporosis and osteopenia.[10–14] A metaanalysis demonstrated reduced BMD.[15] In addition, there is an increased risk of fracture in patients with T1D, more so than in those with T2D.[15] In a study of more than 33,000 Swedish adults (ages 25–60 years old), the strongest risk factor for hip fracture in both women and men was diabetes (relative risk [RR], 3.89; 95% confidence interval [CI], 1.69–8.93 [*P* = .001] for women; RR, 6.13; 95% CI 3.19–11.8 [*P* = .001] for men).[16] The increase in fracture risk, which is particularly marked at the hip, is much greater than what would be expected on the basis of the BMD decrement, implying that there are other factors independent of BMD that contribute to this increased fracture risk.[15,17]

Both T2D and low-trauma fracture become more common with advancing age. T2D is associated with both greater weight and higher BMD,[18] which was historically assumed to be protective against fracture. However, a paradoxic increased risk of fracture has been observed in many[19–23] but not all studies.[24,25] A metaanalysis by Janghorbani and colleagues[26] described an increased risk for all nonvertebral fractures (adjusted RR, 1.2; 95% CI, 1.01–1.5). An updated metaanalysis by Dytfeld and

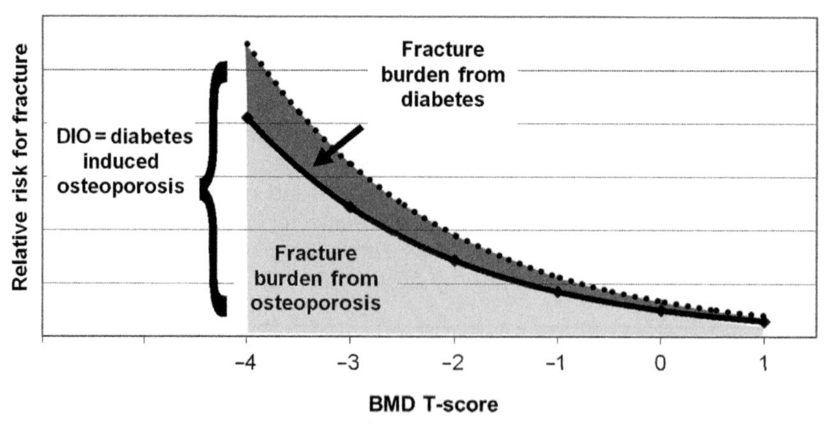

Fig. 1. Conceptual framework for diabetes and fractures. The light gray region below the solid line indicates the fracture burden attributable to osteoporosis; the dark gray region between the dotted and solid lines indicates the additional fracture burden attributable to diabetes. BMD, bone mineral density. (*Reprinted from* Schacter GI, Leslie WD. DXA based measurements in diabetes: can they predict fracture risk? Calcif Tissue Int 2016. [Epub ahead of print]; with permission.)

Michalak[27] assessed 15 observational studies including 263,000 individuals with diabetes and 502,000 controls. T2D was associated with a higher risk for hip fracture (odds ratio [OR], 1.296; 95% CI, 1.069–1.571), although there was significant heterogeneity and vertebral fracture risk was not significantly greater (OR, 1.134; 95% CI, 0.936–1.374). The Health, Aging and Body Composition study showed an increase in fracture risk in T2D even after adjustment for age, calcaneal BMD, body mass index (BMI), and other covariates.[28] Strotmeyer and colleagues[29] concluded that diabetes was associated with higher hip, whole body and volumetric spine BMD, independent of body composition and fasting insulin.

RISK FACTORS

As outlined in **Table 1**, clinical risk factors associated with lower BMD in T1D include male gender,[30–33] longer duration of disease,[14] younger age at diagnosis,[34] lower endogenous insulin and/or C-peptide levels,[35] lower BMI,[30,36] and potentially the comorbidities and/or autoimmunity associated with the chronic disease.[37] Other studies have cited chronic poor glycemic control[38] or the presence of microvascular complications,[39] including retinopathy,[40] neuropathy,[41,42] and nephropathy.[43]

Risk factors for fractures in T1D include longer duration of disease,[44] microvascular complications[45] (specifically retinopathy[44] and nephropathy[46]), and potentially long-term glycemic control or decreased vitamin D levels.[47,48] This increased fracture risk is amplified by the increase in risk of falls, contributed to by increased rates of hypoglycemia, visual defects, peripheral neuropathy, or disability.[21,49,50]

Risk factors for fractures in T2D include older age,[51] lower BMD, lower BMI, and falls.[26,29,52] As in T1D, diabetes duration[19,20,22,23,28,53] and diabetes complications[46,54] are also associated with greater risk.

Antidiabetic medications may contribute to increased risk of fracture in diabetes. In general, there is a lack of definitive clinical evidence regarding the skeletal effects of antidiabetic medications, because fracture is rarely the primary outcome of interest. In addition, although medications may produce changes in BMD, this cannot be assumed to have a predictable effect on fracture risk.[55] Furthermore, dual-energy x-ray absorptiometry (DXA), the most widely used method for quantitative skeletal assessment, does not reflect non-BMD changes in skeletal integrity (such as cortical

Table 1
Risk factors for fracture in diabetes

Type 1 diabetes	• Long-term glycemic control • Decreased vitamin D levels
Type 2 diabetes	• General population risk factors • Older age • Lower bone mineral density • Lower body mass index • FRAX score and risk factors • Lower trabecular bone score
Both TYPES 1 and 2 diabetes	• Longer duration of diabetes • Presence of complications (specifically retinopathy and nephropathy) • Increased fall risk • Hypoglycemia • Visual defects • Peripheral neuropathy • Disability

porosity). There are no randomized trials of insulin therapy with fracture or BMD outcomes, and observational trials have been mixed. Thiazolidinediones in particular are associated with adverse effects on the skeleton, likely via activation of peroxisome proliferator activated receptor-Υ promotion of adipogenesis at the expense of osteoblastogenesis, thus inhibiting bone formation and inducing bone loss.[56,57] In addition, recent studies involving the newest agents, sodium–glucose cotransporter 2 inhibitors, have revealed a decrease in total hip BMD of up to 1.2% after 2 years of use, although no changes at other sites were found.[58] Canagliflozin has also been found to be associated with a higher fracture incidence within 12 weeks of initiation of therapy, primarily affecting distal extremities. These effects are thought to be attributable to the weight loss often accompanying sodium–glucose cotransporter 2 inhibitor use. Metformin[59] and sulfonylureas[60] do not seem to affect fracture risk, and dipeptidyl peptidase 4 inhibitors may in fact decrease risk, although the mechanism for this is uncertain.[61]

Some studies implicate insulin use as a risk for fracture, but it is difficult to distinguish its use from potential surrogacy for duration and severity of diabetes.[20] A recent study from Pscherer and colleagues[62] suggests a lower risk for fracture with glargine use as compared with NPH (neutral protamine Hagedorn insulin).

PATHOPHYSIOLOGY

Although patients with T1D and T2D are at increased risk for fractures, the pathophysiology differs.[21,29,63,64] T1D is associated with decreased BMD. In comparison, in T2D, BMD is frequently increased or normal. Both are commonly stated to show relatively reduced bone formation, osteoblast dysfunction, and low bone turnover. A metaanalysis comparing biochemical bone turnover among diabetes patients and controls identified 22 relevant papers.[65] Significant (but relatively small) reductions were seen among diabetes patients for osteocalcin (−1.15 ng/mL [range, −1.78 to −0.52]) and C-terminal cross-linked telopeptide (−0.14 ng/mL [range, −0.22 to −0.05]), with a borderline reduction in N-terminal cross-linked telopeptide. Other markers (including bone-specific alkaline phosphatase, collagen type 1C propeptide, and deoxypyridinoline) did not differ and all markers displayed very high heterogeneity. There were insufficient studies that stratified according the diabetes type to compare T1D and T2D directly. The observed reductions, even when significant, were modest with considerable overlap between the diabetes and control groups. Some large trials even failed to detect any difference between subjects with and without diabetes.[66]

Ultimately, the pathophysiology of diabetes-induced osteoporosis is likely multifactorial in nature. Diabetes and hyperglycemia are associated with hyperglycemia, hyperlipidemia, decreased insulin signaling, decreased insulinlike growth factor 1, reactive oxygen species production,[67–71] and inflammation. All of these factors could potentially contribute to suppressed osteoblast activity. Potential factors degrading bone quality include chronic hyperglycemia,[72] microarchitectural bone defects,[18] and skeletal advanced glycation end products (AGEs),[73] which accrue irreversibly from the nonenzymatic addition of sugar moieties to the amine groups of proteins.[74–76] The dysregulated accumulation of AGEs in bone likely has a negative impact on the integrity of skeletal tissues,[77] especially type 1 collagen, as the AGEs can change the structural and functional properties of proteins. As such, their levels correlate with diabetes complication severity. AGEs increase collagen cross-linking, which contributes to decreased bone strength and increased brittleness.[78] Owing to low bone turnover, long-lived proteins accumulate AGEs, and these levels are especially high in those with diabetes.[79] There are several molecularly well-defined AGEs that are specific to nonenzymatic glycation, such as pentosidine.[80,81] With aging and diabetes, increased glucose levels enhance bone matrix glycation while impairing collagen turnover and matrix renewal. The end result is impaired bone formation leading to more fragile bones containing higher levels of AGEs per gram of collagen. The collagen modifications stiffen bone matrix and modify the material properties of bone, leading to brittleness and mechanical failure under physiologic levels of stress.[80]

Hyperglycemia increases oxidative stress through 2 mechanisms: (1) the mitochondria become overloaded with glucose and (2) AGEs and polyol signaling.[82] The oxidative stress in turn negatively affects osteoblast maturation,[83] and may trigger increased osteoblast apoptosis.[84]

A primary derangement in T1D is decreased bone formation secondary to decreased osteoblast activity.[39,44,85] Studies have suggested a potential connection to serum osteocalcin,[38,86–88] which is expressed in the late stages of osteoblast maturation, and is carboxylated at 3 residues to increase affinity to the bone matrix.[89] In mice, it has been shown that the undercarboxylated form of osteocalcin stimulates insulin secretion, insulin signaling sensitivity, and glucose hemostasis.[89] A similar effect has been sought in humans with support from 2 recent metaanalyses.[90,91] Lower serum osteocalcin levels have been found in both patients with T1D or T2D as compared with subjects without diabetes.[70,92,93] Osteocalcin is correlated negatively with glycosylated hemoglobin levels in patients with T1D.[92]

Given that diabetes is marked by reduced bone turnover and osteoblast activity, a role for altered Wnt signaling has been suggested.[94,95] Increased levels of sclerostin (an osteocyte product that antagonizes the Wnt signaling pathway) would inhibit bone formation.[94] The end result is uncoupling in bone formation and resorption.

Last, both obesity and diabetes itself can increase bone marrow inflammation, resulting in inflammatory cytokines that impair osteoblast activity.[96] Inflammation in the bone marrow favors an increase in osteoclast number and activity, leading to increased bone loss.[97] Increased levels of inflammatory cytokines have been found in subjects with both T1D[98] and T2D.[99]

RISK ASSESSMENT

General Background

Osteoporosis and fracture risk are assessed traditionally with BMD measured by DXA. Osteoporosis is defined as a BMD that is 2.5 or more standard deviations (SD) below the young adult mean population (T-score ≤ -2.5), with the proposed reference standard relying on BMD measured at the femoral neck with DXA and a uniform reference database (National Health and Nutrition Examination Survey III for white women aged 20–29 years).[100] The risk of fracture increases 1.4- to 2.6-fold for each SD decrease in BMD.[101,102]

Although BMD is the most commonly reported measurement from DXA, other DXA-derived parameters for evaluating fracture risk are available. These include skeletal geometry, trabecular bone score (TBS), vertebral fracture assessment (VFA), and body composition. Additionally, fracture prediction tools such as the World Health Organization fracture risk assessment tool (FRAX; available: www.shef.ac.uk/FRAX/index.aspx), the Garvan fracture risk calculator (available: www.garvan.org.au/bone-fracture-risk), and the QFracture score (available: www.qfracture.org) have all been derived to aid with fracture risk prediction in the general population, although only the QFracture score has specific inputs for T1D and T2D.[103]

Available measurements of hip geometry include hip structural analysis (HSA), hip axis length, and neck shaft angle.[104] TBS, a texture parameter derived from pixel–gray level variations in the spine DXA image, can be used to enhance fracture risk predictions independent of BMD.[105] TBS has now been implemented as an adjustment to the FRAX score, and was validated in a multicohort metaanalysis.[106] VFA by DXA visualizes the thoracic and lumber spine to detect vertebral fractures,[107] because the presence of morphometric vertebral fractures increases the risk of both vertebral and nonvertebral fractures, independent of BMD.[108]

Reduced appendicular muscle mass and function, known as sarcopenia, commonly occurs in later life and is of interest as a potential risk factor for fracture.[109–112] DXA is a well-validated technique for analyzing body composition, muscle, and fat mass.[113] DXA can also estimate visceral adipose tissue (VAT), a metabolically active pathogenic fat depot that is implicated in insulin resistance and T2D. VAT is also been shown to be a risk factor for fracture.[114,115]

Type 1 diabetes

Bone mineral density Reduced bone density in patients with T1D as compared with normal controls has been demonstrated in a metaanalysis, where a significant reduction in BMD *Z*-score (comparison of the subject's BMD with the age- and sex-matched controls) was seen at both the hip (mean, −0.37) and lumbar spine (mean, −0.22).[15] However, the decrease in BMD reported in subjects with T1D only partially explains the observed 6.4- to 6.9-fold higher hip fracture risk (expected approximately 1.42) compared with individuals without diabetes.[15,26] To date, no studies have been sufficiently powered to adequately examine the ability of BMD to predict fractures in T1D.

Skeletal geometry Only 2 small studies[32,34] have assessed geometric properties of bone strength in adults with T1D. Maser and colleagues[34] studied 60 adults with T1D to look at the association of age of onset of diabetes, with BMD as well as estimates of bone strength. Earlier age at onset of T1D was associated significantly with lower measures of bone strength. Miazgowski and colleagues[32] compared BMD, hip axis length, cross-sectional area and cross-sectional moment of inertia in 36 men with T1D. Hip BMD and geometry were not significantly different than that of age-, weight-, and height-matched controls.

There have been no studies of hip geometry in patients with T1D with fracture as the outcome, thereby precluding a determination of whether bone geometry contributes to excess fracture risk.

Trabecular bone score There are sparse data on spine TBS in T1D. Neumann and colleagues[116] conducted a cross-sectional study of subjects with and without diabetes (gender-, age- and BMI-matched) subjects. This study revealed a borderline reduction in mean TBS for T1D patients versus controls (1.357 $\pm$ 0.129 vs 1.389 $\pm$ 0.085, respectively; P = .075). T1D patients with prevalent fractures had significantly decreased TBS as compared with T1D patients without fractures (1.309 $\pm$ 0.125 vs 1.370 $\pm$ 0.127; P = .04). TBS and hemoglobin A1c were associated independently with prevalent fractures. A TBS cutoff of less than 1.42 captured prevalent fractures with 91.7% sensitivity and 43.2% specificity. Only TBS and total hip BMD discriminated between diabetic patients with and without fractures (area under the curve [AUC], 0.63 [95% CI, 0.51–0.74; P = .048] and AUC, 0.64 [95% CI, 0.51–0.78; P = .032], respectively). The combination of lumbar spine TBS and total hip BMD increased the AUC to 0.68 (95% CI, 0.55–0.81; P = .007), suggesting potential additive value of TBS and BMD.

Vertebral fracture assessment Evidence for the use of VFA for fracture risk prediction in T1D is limited. One small cross-sectional study assessed 82 patients with T1D and

82 controls.[17] The patients with T1D had a higher prevalence of vertebral fractures than the controls (24.4 vs 6.1%; $P = .002$), and were mostly asymptomatic. However, prospective studies are needed to determine whether vertebral fractures detected on VFA predict clinical fractures in T1D.

Body composition There are no adult studies that examine the role of body composition in fracture risk in T1D. Abd El Dayem and colleagues[117] studied 47 children (mean age, 13 years) with T1D and 30 age- and sex-matched controls. Both lean body mass and lean fat ratio were found to be lower in patients with T1D. Total fat mass, abdominal fat percentage, soft tissue fat mass percentage, and fat/lean ratio were all higher in T1D patients as compared with the controls. It is uncertain whether either absolute or relative reduction in lean mass contributes to the excess fracture risk in adults with T1D.

Fracture prediction tools The World Health Organization fracture risk assessment tool (FRAX) is based on easily assessed risk factors identified in metaanalyses of population-based prospective cohorts.[118] FRAX has been adapted to more than 60 countries and widely adopted into numerous international clinical guidelines for osteoporosis management. T1D is not presented as a primary entry variable in the FRAX algorithm, but is considered one of the potential causes of secondary osteoporosis, and as such is given the same weight as rheumatoid arthritis (the prototype for all causes of secondary osteoporosis). Importantly, coding secondary osteoporosis only increases fracture probability when BMD is not included in the FRAX calculation.[119] Including secondary osteoporosis or BMD in the FRAX calculation may partially account for the excess risk for major osteoporotic fractures (clinical spine, forearm, hip, or shoulder fracture) in T1D, but would not account for the very high RR for hip fractures. No studies have directly assessed the performance of FRAX (with or without BMD) for predicting fracture risk in T1D.

Type 2 diabetes

Bone mineral density The reported effect of T2D on BMD is inconsistent across individual studies. Metaanalyses provide robust evidence for normal or even high BMD at both the hip and the spine in T2D,[15,18] although there is paradoxically increased fracture risk.[15,26] Vestergaard and colleagues[15] reported an increased age-adjusted RR for hip fracture of 1.38 (95% CI, 1.25–1.53) in patients with T2D, as compared with healthy controls, and the metaanalysis by Janghorbani and colleagues[26] found an even stronger effect of T2D on hip fracture risk (summary RR, 1.7; 95% CI, 1.3–2.2). This contrasts with an expected RR 0.7 (ie, 30% lower risk) based on the degree of BMD elevation in T2D. This highlights the difficulty in relying on BMD alone to assess fracture risk in T2D.

Pooled results from 3 large prospective observational studies found that the fracture risk for any given femoral neck BMD T-score and age was increased in patients with T2D when compared with normal controls.[120] The mean difference in femoral neck T-score when comparing subjects with and without diabetes at the same hip fracture risk was approximately 0.5 SD (0.59 [95% CI, 0.31–0.87] in women and 0.38 [95% CI, 0.09–0.66] in men). Although there was a systematically higher fracture risk attributable to T2D, the age-adjusted hazard ratios (HRs) per SD decrease in BMD predicted hip fracture and nonspine fracture equally well in those with and without diabetes.

Leslie and colleagues[52] conducted an observational registry-based study of more than 62,000 individuals (10% with diabetes; mean age, 66.5 years), with 4218 sustaining 1 or more incident major osteoporotic fractures (hip, spine, humerus, or forearm). An additional 1108 subjects sustained incident hip fractures during the follow-up period. Femoral neck BMD was significantly greater in those with diabetes ($P<.001$). The adjusted HR per SD decrease in femoral neck T-score in individuals without diabetes (1.68; 95% CI 1.61–1.75) was similar to those with diabetes (1.60; 95% CI, 1.44–1.79; P for interaction = .456). For major osteoporotic fracture prediction, each SD decrease in femoral neck T-score strongly predicted hip fracture in those without diabetes (HR, 2.17; 95% CI, 1.98–2.38) as well as in those with diabetes (2.15; 95% CI, 1.75–2.6; P for interaction = 0.956).

In summary, a lower BMD is strongly predictive of fractures in T2D, similar to the general population. However, the excess fracture risk in T2D is not captured by BMD, which is paradoxically higher, even after adjustment for greater BMI. Although BMD can stratify fracture risk within the T2D population, it does not account for differences between the T2D and general population. Conceptually, diabetes-induced osteoporosis represents the combined fracture burden attributable to low BMD and conventional osteoporosis with the additional fracture burden attributable to diabetes (see **Fig. 1**).

Skeletal geometry There are few studies evaluating hip structure in T2D and no studies have evaluated fracture as an outcome. Garg and colleagues[121] studied almost 6000 postmenopausal women from the WHI-OS (Women's Health Initiative Observational Study), among whom 427 had T2D. BMD and many of the HSA-derived measures were higher in the women with T2D, but these differences disappeared after adjustment for other variables (including total lean body weight). Cross-sectional area and BMD normalized to lean body mass were both lower in T2D women receiving insulin as compared with controls, or compared with women with T2D not receiving insulin. Moseley and colleagues[122] conducted a small cross-sectional study of 134 men and women with non–insulin-requiring T2D. They found that lean mass (but not fat mass) was positively correlated with BMD and HSA-derived measurements (cross-sectional area, SM, and buckling ratio).

Hamilton and colleagues[123] studied more than 3600 women (157 of whom with T2D) enrolled in the CaMos (Canadian Multicenter Osteoporosis Study) with hip geometry and HSA data. Using engineering beam theory, stresses were found to be 4.5% higher in women with T2D as compared with those without (11.03 $\pm$ 0.18 MPa vs 10.56 $\pm$ 0.04 MPa; $P = .0093$), indicating weaker geometry and an impaired skeletal load response in those with T2D.

Ishii and colleagues[124] analyzed more than 1800 women (81 with T2D) enrolled in the SWAN (Study of Women's Health Across the Nation) trial. They found that even though women with T2D had a greater BMD at the femoral neck than the controls, they had lower composite indices of strength relative to load (−0.20 SD [95% CI, -0.38 to −0.03 SD] for compression; -0.19 SD [95% CI, -0.38 to −0.003 SD] for bending; and −0.19 SD [95% CI, -0.37 to −0.02 SD] for impact). Finally, Akeroyd and colleagues[125] studied more than 1100 men (12.5% with T2D) and found no association between T2D and HSA-based geometry measurements of strength. The clinical usefulness of skeletal strength measurements derived from DXA for fracture prediction in T2D is unproven.

Trabecular bone score Leslie and colleagues[126] performed a retrospective cohort study of almost 30,000 women (approximately 2300 with diabetes) using BMD results from a large clinical registry for the province of Manitoba, Canada. They found that diabetes was associated with higher BMD at all sites, whereas lumbar spine TBS was lower in both unadjusted and covariate-adjusted models (all $P<.001$). Lumbar spine TBS was an equally strong and BMD-independent predictor of fracture in women with diabetes (adjusted HR, 1.27; 95% CI, 1.10–1.46) and women without diabetes

(HR, 1.31; 95% CI, 1.24–1.38). Fracture risk stratification from lumbar spine TBS (AUC, 0.63; 95% CI, 0.61–0.64) was similar to lumbar spine BMD (AUC, 0.64; 95% CI, 0.63–0.65). Lumbar spine TBS partially explained the effect of diabetes on fracture risk in the prediction model, but the opposite effect was seen when BMD measurements were added where the effect of diabetes was paradoxically increased. Combining lumbar spine TBS with BMD may incrementally improve fracture prediction in those with diabetes, as it has for the general population.

In summary, TBS predicts major osteoporotic fractures in postmenopausal women with and without diabetes. TBS scores in T2D are lower, and this partially accounts for the excess fracture risk in T2D.

Vertebral fracture assessment There are no published studies assessing VFA in T2D and as such its ability to predict incident fractures and capture excess fracture risk is untested. VFA image quality is degraded in obese patients, which may affect test performance in T2D. It is clinically important to detect vertebral fractures in T2D; a previous study by Leslie and colleagues[19] showed that prior vertebral fracture predicts future major osteoporotic fracture and hip fracture in women with and without diabetes.

Body composition It is well-known that body composition and fat distribution (namely, abdominal adiposity) are strongly associated with metabolic morbidities, including T2D, and may have a causal role in their development.[117,127,128] Intraabdominal fat is closely linked to the metabolic syndrome and its complications, including T2D.[129,130] A study by Rothney and colleagues[131] demonstrated the strong positive associated between VAT and T2D. In this cross-sectional analysis of more than 900 subjects, sex-specific, age-adjusted multivariable regression analysis revealed that DXA VAT was significantly associated with increased odds of cardiometabolic indicators, including impaired fasting glucose and T2D ($P<.001$). After adjustment for BMI and waist circumference, the OR per SD increase in VAT for T2D was 2.07 (95% CI, 0.73–5.87) for women and 2.25 (95% CI, 1.21–4.19) for men.

In a study by Akeroyd and colleagues, [125] it was concluded that men with T2D have lower muscle mass and strength, but a similar BMD when compared with nondiabetic controls. The authors concluded that the differences in nonskeletal factors could explain at least in part the greater incidence of falls and fractures in the patients with T2D.[125] However, there are no studies available that examined whether either body composition or VAT is a predictor of fracture in T2D or whether sarcopenic obesity can identify bone fragility and fracture risk in T2D.

Fracture prediction tools Several studies have evaluated the predictive performance of FRAX in patients with T2D and have show that, for a given FRAX probability, there is an increased risk of fracture in subjects with diabetes as compared with those without diabetes.[51,120] In the study by Schwartz and colleagues, [120] 3 prospective observational studies of older community-dwelling adults (comprising >9500 women and 7400 men) were combined. For a given FRAX probability, both women and men with T2D had a higher observed fracture risk. Despite the globally higher fracture risk attributable to T2D, FRAX was found to predict hip and nonspine fracture equally well in those with and without diabetes (all P for interaction >0.10).

A more recent study of more than 3500 older patients with diagnosed diabetes (predominantly T2D) from a large clinical cohort in Manitoba, Canada, found diabetes to be a risk factor for subsequent major osteoporotic fracture (MOF) (adjusted HR, 1.61; 95% CI, 1.42–1.83) or hip fracture (adjusted HR, 6.27; 95% CI, 3.62–10.87 aged < 65 years; 2.22; 95% CI, 1.71–2.90 aged $\geq$ 65 years).[51] FRAX was able to stratify fracture risk in those with diabetes (AUC for MOF, 0.67; 95% CI, 0.63–0.70; AUC for hip fracture, 0.77; 95% CI, 0.72–0.81), only slightly less well than in those without diabetes, but FRAX again underestimated MOF and hip fracture risk in those with diabetes, even after accounting for mortality differences.

A related analysis from the same Manitoba database of 62,000 individuals aged 40 years and older (10% with diabetes) showed that diabetes and the FRAX risk factors were associated independently with MOFs and hip fractures.[52] Diabetes did not significantly modify the effect of individual FRAX risk factors for major osteoporotic fractures: a 10-year increase in age in those without diabetes (HR, 1.43) versus those with diabetes (HR, 1.39; *P* for interaction = .781), rheumatoid arthritis (1.43 vs 1.74; *P* for interaction = .325), and prior fracture (1.62 vs 1.72; *P* for interaction = .588) when adjusted for BMD. When BMD was excluded, an increase in BMI of 5 kg/m^2 was similarly protective against major osteoporotic fracture in those without diabetes (HR, 0.83) and those with diabetes (HR, 0.79; *P* for interaction = .0276).

In summary, the individual FRAX risk factors (including BMD) remain important in patients with T2D, and FRAX provides fracture discrimination in the diabetes population similar to that seen in the general population. However, the absolute fracture risk is underestimated, possibly owing to alterations in material strength and greater risk for falls.

The lack of significant interactions between diabetes status and FRAX risk factors or FRAX scores for predicting MOF implies the potential for a simple recalibration of the FRAX tool to accommodate the unmeasured effect of T2D. Several methods have been proposed to capture the effect of T2D despite its absence as an input variable in FRAX. One such method is to use rheumatoid arthritis in the calculation as a proxy for T2D, because the effect seems to be very similar to that of T2D,[103] whereas other options are to use the recently validated TBS adjustment for FRAX[105,106] or lower the femoral neck T-score by 0.5 SD.[120]

The Garvan fracture risk calculator was constructed using information on women and men from the Australian Dubbo Osteoporosis Epidemiology Study (DOES).[132,133] The 5- and 10-year fracture probability nomograms were constructed using inputs of age, sex, femoral neck BMD (or weight), history of prior fractures after age 50 years (none to $\geq$3), and falls in the previous 12 months (none to $\geq$3). Diabetes is not an input, and no studies have evaluated the Garvan calculator in subjects with T1D or T2D. The appropriateness of using a 0.5 SD lower femoral neck T-score input has not been specifically tested in this calculator.[120] Because the Garvan calculator includes falls, it may capture some of the diabetes-associated risk.

The QFracture score was derived from a cohort including more than 1 million women and more than 1 million men age 30 to 85 years with 24,350 incident osteoporotic fractures in women (9302 hip fractures) and 7934 osteoporotic fractures in men (5424 hip fractures).[134] It provides outputs for any osteoporotic fracture (hip, wrist, or spine) and hip fracture over a user-selected follow-up period from 1 to 10 years. This algorithm includes T1D or T2D as a direct input, but does not allow for the use of BMD in the risk estimation. Furthermore, the QFracture tool was developed for use in the UK and its applicability to other regions including North America is unknown.

A comparison of inputs, outputs, and potential T2D adjustments from the 3 fracture risk calculators and the effect on estimated fracture risk in a hypothetical case is demonstrated in **Table 2**.

MANAGEMENT

Nonpharmacologic management should not be overlooked. The Institute of Medicine recommends 700 to 1300 mg/d of calcium intake (preferably from food sources)

Table 2
Comparison of inputs, outputs, and potential T2D adjustments

Fracture Prediction Tool	Risk Factor Inputs	Osteoporotic Fracture 10 y (%)	Hip Fracture 10 y (%)	Potential Adjustments for Diabetes	Osteoporotic Fracture 10 y (%)	Hip Fracture 10 y (%)
FRAX	• Age and sex • Height and weight • Prior fracture • Glucocorticoid use • Secondary OP (includes T1D) • RA • Parental hip fracture • Smoking • Alcohol ≥3 U/d • Femoral neck BMD (optional)	15 (major = hip, clinical spine, distal forearm, proximal humerus)	2.5	RA input as proxy for diabetes TBS Decrease femoral neck T-score by 0.5 SD	20 23 19	3.6 4.6 4.3
Garvan	• Age and sex • Prior fracture (0, 1, 2, ≥3) • Falls last 12 mo (0, 1, 2, ≥3) • Femoral neck BMD or weight	48 (any = all fragility fractures except digits)	21	None available	—	—
QFracture	• Age, sex, and 10 ethnicities • Height and weight • Diabetes (T1D, T2D) • 20 other risk factors (but not BMD)	6.2 (major = hip, wrist, shoulder or spine)	2.3	T1D input T2D input	11.6 7.8	10.3 3.6

From 3 fracture risk calculators and the effect on estimated fracture risk in a hypothetical case (65-year-old female with T2D, body mass index 30.5 kg/m^2, prior fractures distal radius and humerus, one recent fall, hip T-score −2.1, TBS at the 10th percentile = 1.160).

Abbreviations: BMD, bone mineral density; OP, osteoporosis; RA, rheumatoid arthritis; SD, standard deviation; T1D, type 1 diabetes; T2D, type 2 diabetes.

depending on life-stage group at least 1 year of age, and 600 IU/d of vitamin D for those aged 1 to 70 years of age, and 800 IU/d for ages 71 and older.[135] These recommendations are applicable to the diabetes population. Despite the positive effects on fracture risk, recent studies have raised concerns about the possible adverse effects of calcium with regard to cardiovascular outcomes and death.[136–139] This topic remains controversial, and beyond the scope of this review.

Subjects with T1D have been found to have significantly lower 25-hydroxyvitamin D levels.[65] Individuals with T2D may require a larger daily dose of vitamin D, which is fat soluble, owing to obesity. The safe upper level of intake for vitamin D in adults is 4000 IU/d intake, although the practice of giving such high doses remains controversial.[135] The importance of falls prevention, particularly in the frail or elderly patient with diabetes, cannot be overemphasized.[21,26,29,30,49]

Antiresorptive agents, usually a bisphosphonate, are currently first-line therapy for the majority of patients initiating treatment for osteoporosis because they decrease osteoclast activity and slow bone turnover, allowing for a modest gain in BMD with stabilization in skeletal microstructure leading to reduced fracture risk.[140] Additional options are raloxifene, a selective estrogen receptor modulator, and denosumab, an antibody directed against RANK ligand. However, if bone is already deficient in osteoblast function then it might be questioned whether antiresorptive agents would be less effective. Indeed, there is some evidence that high bone turnover in comparison with low bone turnover at baseline significantly predicts greater response to bisphosphonate treatment.[141] However, bisphosphonates are the treatment of choice for glucocorticoid-induced osteoporosis, which is also characterized by an osteoblast defect. It makes sense to select an agent with demonstrated efficacy for hip fracture prevention given the particularly high risk for hip fractures in T1D and T2D.

There is very little information available from comparative studies on the effectiveness of traditional osteoporosis treatment in diabetes-induced osteoporosis in general, and in T1D specifically. This has been compounded by the fact that diabetes is often an exclusion criteria for enrollment in clinical trials, as a secondary cause of osteoporosis. Animal studies involving an intermittent parenteral parathyroid hormone analogue (teriparatide) have shown increased osteoblast survival and a subsequent decrease in diabetes associated bone loss.[142] This measure might support use of an osteoanabolic agent, especially if markers confirm low bone turnover, or if BMD is very low, although this approach has never been tested specifically in patients with diabetes. However, this needs to be weighed against the significant increase in cortical porosity seen with teriparatide monotherapy that is not seen with denosumab, alone or in combination with teriparatide.[143]

There have been a few trials evaluating response to antiresorptives in predominantly T2D populations. Keegan and colleagues[66] used the data collected in the FIT (Fracture Intervention Trial) involving 6450 women aged 54 to 81 years with low femoral neck BMD who were randomly assigned to either placebo or alendronate for 7 years. In the patients with diabetes, after 3 years of treatment with alendronate, there was an increase in BMD at all sites, including 6.6% at the lumbar spine and 2.4% at the hip. This was similar to the gains seen in subjects without diabetes, and contrasted with subjects with diabetes in the placebo group, who lost more BMD at the total hip as compared with those subjects without diabetes. Women with and without diabetes also experienced similar decreases in markers of bone turnover. The authors concluded that antiresorptive therapy was just as effective in patients with T2D as in those without diabetes, but the study was underpowered to compare fracture outcomes. Iwamoto and colleagues[144] studied 151 postmenopausal osteoporotic women (16 with T2D) who had been treated with alendronate for more than 3 years.

Bone markers were similar in women both with and without diabetes by the end of the follow-up period.

Johnell and colleagues[145] examined for interactions between 30 baseline risk factors and the effectiveness of raloxifene in the randomized MORE (Multiple Outcomes of Raloxifene Evaluation) trial. Of interest, raloxifene showed greater efficacy for vertebral fracture prevention in patients with T2D compared with those without diabetes ($P = .04$). In hemodialysis patients, raloxifene similarly suppressed bone turnover markers and improved quantitative heel ultrasound in postmenopausal women with and without T2D.[146]

Of potential relevance in T2D is the potential for differential treatment responses according to baseline factors. The FIT was conducted in postmenopausal women without prior vertebral fractures, and demonstrated an interaction between femoral neck BMD and prevention of clinical fractures during 4 years of treatment with alendronate versus placebo: active treatment significantly reduced the risk of clinical fractures among women with osteoporosis but not among women with higher BMD.[147] A similar subgroup analysis was performed by McClung and associates[148] for the FREEDOM (Fracture REduction Evaluation of Denosumab in Osteoporosis Every 6 Months) trial evaluating fracture outcomes in 7808 women randomly assigned to receive denosumab or placebo for 3 years: active treatment significantly reduced the risk of nonvertebral fractures among women with osteoporotic femoral neck T-scores (but not for T-scores > -2.5) and in those BMI of less than 25 kg/m^2 (but not in the those with BMI between 25 and 30 or > 30 kg/m^2).[148] In contrast, no interactions were seen for prevention of vertebral fractures. These observations may be relevant for individuals with T2D given their greater likelihood of having an high BMI and nonosteoporotic BMD.

Vestergaard and colleagues[149] investigated whether further decreasing bone turnover by use of antiresorptives would be detrimental to subjects with diabetes given their low baseline bone turnover. Using nationwide Danish registry data from 1996 to 2006, 103,562 patients with diabetes and 310,683 age- and gender-matched controls were studied. The authors found that there was an increased risk of hip, spine, and forearm fractures in subjects with diabetes, which they attributed to a higher baseline risk in patients being treated for osteoporosis. However, there was no difference observed in antifracture efficacy between subjects with and without diabetes, nor between those with T1D and T2D. The authors concluded that the low turnover state did not affect the action of antiresorptive medications in diabetic subjects. Most important, there was no suggestion that further reduction of bone turnover by antiresorptive drugs resulted in an increase in fracture risk.

CURRENT CONTROVERSIES

The optimal duration of therapy is uncertain and a subject of increasing importance given reports regarding serious complications, potentially related to the cumulative intake of some drugs.[150–153] The prolonged skeletal retention of bisphosphonates (but not other agents) introduces the potential for a temporary interruption in therapy ("drug holiday") after 3 to 5 years of therapy in selected individuals.[154] A rare side effect of osteoporosis treatment, osteonecrosis of the jaw, may be more common in patients with diabetes who are receiving bisphosphonates or denosumab.[150–152] Kajizono and colleagues[150] reported that diabetes was strongly associated with osteonecrosis of the jaw (OR, 6.7; 95% CI, 1.435–31.277; $P = .016$). Whether diabetes is a risk factor for atypical femoral fractures, potential complications of long-term antiresorptive therapy (initially bisphosphonates and more recently denosumab), is uncertain, because the data are conflicting.[155,156] Although diabetes was originally a minor criterion for the atypical femoral fractures case definition proposed by the American Society of Bone and Mineral Research, this was dropped from the most recent Task Force report.[153]

Schwartz and colleagues[157] set out to determine if treatment-related suppression in bone turnover played a significant role in glucose metabolism. Undercarboxylated osteocalcin is normally a hormone that promotes insulin sensitivity and secretion demonstrated in rodent models. If it played a similar role in humans, antiresorptive agents that decreased circulating undercarboxylated osteocalcin may subsequently increase insulin resistance and subsequent development of diabetes. Schwartz and colleagues performed a post hoc analysis of 3 trials: the FIT trial (involving >6000 subjects treated with alendronate for 4 years), the HORIZON-PFT (HORIZON Pivotal Fracture Trial) trial (involving >7000 subjects treated with zolendronate for 3 years), and the FREEDOM trial (involving >7000 subjects treated with denosumab for 3 years).[157] Serum fasting blood glucose levels were collected regularly in all 3 trials. There was no clinically significant change in fasting blood glucose levels in any of the trials (-0.47 g/dL in FIT, 0.20 mg/dL in HORIZON-PFT, and 0.90 mg/dL in FREEDOM; all $P>.6$). When analyses of the 3 trials were combined, new incidence of diabetes was found in 203 women in the active treatment groups, versus 225 in the placebo groups, which was not clinically significant. The pooled RR of developing diabetes was 0.90 (95% CI, 0.74–1.10). The authors concluded that there was no demonstrable role of decreased bone turnover on the regulation of insulin and glucose metabolism in humans, despite contrary experimental data from rodent models.

Additional studies have reported lower or similar risk for T2D. Vestergaard and colleagues[158] found that the incident risk of developing T2D was reduced with the use of bisphosphonates. Chan and colleagues[159] conducted a retrospective cohort study including osteoporotic patients without diabetes from a population-based cohort of 1,000,000 subjects. Approximately 1000 subjects were exposed to alendronate and were compared with nonexposed controls. The nonexposed group had a significantly higher rate of development of diabetes (OR, 1.21; 95% CI, 1.03–1.41). Toulis and colleagues[160] performed a retrospective open cohort study of 36,000 individuals without diabetes at baseline. The risk of incident diabetes was much lower in those exposed to bisphosphonates (adjusted incidence rate ratio 0.52; 95% CI, 0.48–0.56; $P<.0001$). Most recently, Yang and colleagues[161] reported no effect in 33,640 women. During a mean of 4.2 years of follow-up, 3.7% of new antiresorptive therapy users and 4.2% of nonusers acquired a new diagnosis of diabetes (adjusted hazards ratio 1.01; 95% CI, 0.87–1.15). Importantly, no study to date has shown a convincing increased risk for developing diabetes in humans initiating osteoporosis treatment.

FUTURE CONSIDERATIONS/SUMMARY

Diabetes-induced osteoporosis in both T1D and T2D is characterized by an increase in fracture risk. As the prevalence of diabetes (especially T2D) continues to increase, one would expect that increased skeletal complications will follow, which may be exacerbated by some of the medications used to control hyperglycemia.

Several fracture risk assessment tools are available to help stratify fracture risk, but these only partially capture the risk in T1D, and slightly underestimate the risk in T2D. Although BMD from DXA and FRAX are still useful clinically and stratify fracture risk in those with diabetes, recent enhancements can help to better identify patients at increased risk of fracture. Incorporating this additional information into risk prediction may help to identify subjects with diabetes who are at high risk for fracture and in whom treatment for osteoporosis is most likely to be beneficial.

REFERENCES

1. Internal Diabetes Federation. Available at: http://www.idf.org/diabetesatlas. Accessed September 23, 2016.
2. Egro FM. Why is type 1 diabetes increasing? J Mol Endocrinol 2013;51(1):R1–13.
3. Atkinson MA, Eisenbarth GS, Michels AW. Type 1 diabetes. Lancet 2014; 383(9911):69–82.
4. Prevalence of diabetes and impaired fasting glucose in adults–United States, 1999-2000. MMWR Morb Mortal Wkly Rep 2003;52(35):833–7.
5. Cole ZA, Dennison EM, Cooper C. Osteoporosis epidemiology update. Curr Rheumatol Rep 2008;10(2):92–6.
6. Melton LJ 3rd, Chrischilles EA, Cooper C, et al. How many women have osteoporosis? JBMR Anniversary Classic. JBMR, Volume 7, Number 9, 1992. J Bone Miner Res 2005;20(5):886–92.
7. Schousboe JT. Epidemiology of vertebral fractures. J Clin Densitom 2016;19(1): 8–22.
8. Looker AC, Borrud LG, Dawson-Hughes B, et al. Osteoporosis or low bone mass at the femur neck or lumbar spine in older adults: United States, 2005-2008. NCHS Data Brief 2012;(93):1–8.
9. Gullberg B, Johnell O, Kanis JA. World-wide projections for hip fracture. Osteoporos Int 1997;7(5):407–13.
10. Mathiassen B, Nielsen S, Johansen JS, et al. Long-term bone loss in insulin-dependent diabetic patients with microvascular complications. J Diabetic Complications 1990;4(4):145–9.
11. Hui SL, Epstein S, Johnston CC Jr. A prospective study of bone mass in patients with type I diabetes. J Clin Endocrinol Metab 1985;60(1):74–80.
12. Bouillon R. Diabetic bone disease. Calcified Tissue Int 1991;49(3):155–60.
13. McNair P, Christiansen C, Christensen MS, et al. Development of bone mineral loss in insulin-treated diabetes: a 1 1/2 years follow-up study in sixty patients. Eur J Clin Invest 1981;11(1):55–9.
14. Miazgowski T, Czekalski S. A 2-year follow-up study on bone mineral density and markers of bone turnover in patients with long-standing insulin-dependent diabetes mellitus. Osteoporos Int 1998;8(5):399–403.
15. Vestergaard P. Discrepancies in bone mineral density and fracture risk in patients with type 1 and type 2 diabetes–a meta-analysis. Osteoporos Int 2007; 18(4):427–44.
16. Holmberg AH, Johnell O, Nilsson PM, et al. Risk factors for hip fractures in a middle-aged population: a study of 33,000 men and women. Osteoporos Int 2005;16(12):2185–94.
17. Zhukouskaya VV, Eller-Vainicher C, Vadzianava VV, et al. Prevalence of morphometric vertebral fractures in patients with type 1 diabetes. Diabetes care 2013; 36(6):1635–40.
18. Armas LA, Akhter MP, Drincic A, et al. Trabecular bone histomorphometry in humans with Type 1 Diabetes Mellitus. Bone 2012;50(1):91–6.
19. Leslie WD, Lix LM, Prior HJ, et al. Biphasic fracture risk in diabetes: a population-based study. Bone 2007;40(6):1595–601.
20. Melton LJ 3rd, Leibson CL, Achenbach SJ, et al. Fracture risk in type 2 diabetes: update of a population-based study. J Bone Mineral Res 2008;23(8):1334–42.
21. Bonds DE, Larson JC, Schwartz AV, et al. Risk of fracture in women with type 2 diabetes: the Women's Health Initiative Observational Study. J Clin Endocrinol Metab 2006;91(9):3404–10.

22. Hothersall EJ, Livingstone SJ, Looker HC, et al. Contemporary risk of hip fracture in type 1 and type 2 diabetes: a national registry study from Scotland. J Bone Mineral Res 2014;29(5):1054–60.
23. Lipscombe LL, Jamal SA, Booth GL, et al. The risk of hip fractures in older individuals with diabetes: a population-based study. Diabetes Care 2007;30(4): 835–41.
24. Dobnig H, Piswanger-Solkner JC, Roth M, et al. Type 2 diabetes mellitus in nursing home patients: effects on bone turnover, bone mass, and fracture risk. J Clin Endocrinol Metab 2006;91(9):3355–63.
25. Martinez-Laguna D, Tebe C, Javaid MK, et al. Incident type 2 diabetes and hip fracture risk: a population-based matched cohort study. Osteoporos Int 2015; 26(2):827–33.
26. Janghorbani M, Van Dam RM, Willett WC, et al. Systematic review of type 1 and type 2 diabetes mellitus and risk of fracture. Am J Epidemiol 2007;166(5): 495–505.
27. Dytfeld J, Michalak M. Type 2 diabetes and risk of low-energy fractures in postmenopausal women: meta-analysis of observational studies. Aging Clin Exp Res 2016. [Epub ahead of print].
28. Schwartz AV, Sellmeyer DE, Ensrud KE, et al. Older women with diabetes have an increased risk of fracture: a prospective study. J Clin Endocrinol Metab 2001; 86(1):32–8.
29. Strotmeyer ES, Cauley JA, Schwartz AV, et al. Diabetes is associated independently of body composition with BMD and bone volume in older white and black men and women: The Health, Aging, and Body Composition Study. J Bone Miner Res 2004;19(7):1084–91.
30. Hamilton EJ, Rakic V, Davis WA, et al. Prevalence and predictors of osteopenia and osteoporosis in adults with Type 1 diabetes. Diabetic Med 2009;26(1): 45–52.
31. Hadjidakis DJ, Raptis AE, Sfakianakis M, et al. Bone mineral density of both genders in Type 1 diabetes according to bone composition. J Diabetes Complications 2006;20(5):302–7.
32. Miazgowski T, Pynka S, Noworyta-Zietara M, et al. Bone mineral density and hip structural analysis in type 1 diabetic men. Eur J Endocrinology/European Fed Endocr Societies 2007;156(1):123–7.
33. Hamilton EJ, Rakic V, Davis WA, et al. A five-year prospective study of bone mineral density in men and women with diabetes: the Fremantle Diabetes Study. Acta Diabetol 2012;49(2):153–8.
34. Maser RE, Kolm P, Modlesky CM, et al. Hip strength in adults with type 1 diabetes is associated with age at onset of diabetes. J Clin Densitom 2012; 15(1):78–85.
35. Lopez-Ibarra PJ, Pastor MM, Escobar-Jimenez F, et al. Bone mineral density at time of clinical diagnosis of adult-onset type 1 diabetes mellitus. Endocr Pract 2001;7(5):346–51.
36. Eller-Vainicher C, Zhukouskaya VV, Tolkachev YV, et al. Low bone mineral density and its predictors in type 1 diabetic patients evaluated by the classic statistics and artificial neural network analysis. Diabetes care 2011;34(10):2186–91.
37. Lombardi F, Franzese A, Iafusco D, et al. Bone involvement in clusters of autoimmune diseases: just a complication? Bone 2010;46(2):551–5.
38. Danielson KK, Elliott ME, LeCaire T, et al. Poor glycemic control is associated with low BMD detected in premenopausal women with type 1 diabetes. Osteoporos Int 2009;20(6):923–33.

39. Munoz-Torres M, Jodar E, Escobar-Jimenez F, et al. Bone mineral density measured by dual X-ray absorptiometry in Spanish patients with insulin-dependent diabetes mellitus. Calcified Tissue Int 1996;58(5):316–9.
40. Campos Pastor MM, Lopez-Ibarra PJ, Escobar-Jimenez F, et al. Intensive insulin therapy and bone mineral density in type 1 diabetes mellitus: a prospective study. Osteoporos Int 2000;11(5):455–9.
41. Rix M, Andreassen H, Eskildsen P. Impact of peripheral neuropathy on bone density in patients with type 1 diabetes. Diabetes Care 1999;22(5):827–31.
42. Forst T, Pfutzner A, Kann P, et al. Peripheral osteopenia in adult patients with insulin-dependent diabetes mellitus. Diabetic Med 1995;12(10):874–9.
43. Smets YF, de Fijter JW, Ringers J, et al. Long-term follow-up study on bone mineral density and fractures after simultaneous pancreas-kidney transplantation. Kidney Int 2004;66(5):2070–6.
44. Ivers RQ, Cumming RG, Mitchell P, et al. Diabetes and risk of fracture: The Blue Mountains Eye Study. Diabetes Care 2001;24(7):1198–203.
45. Miao J, Brismar K, Nyren O, et al. Elevated hip fracture risk in type 1 diabetic patients: a population-based cohort study in Sweden. Diabetes Care 2005; 28(12):2850–5.
46. Vestergaard P, Rejnmark L, Mosekilde L. Diabetes and its complications and their relationship with risk of fractures in type 1 and 2 diabetes. Calcif Tissue Int 2009;84(1):45–55.
47. Christodoulou S, Goula T, Ververidis A, et al. Vitamin D and bone disease. Biomed Res Int 2013;2013:396541.
48. Lips P, Hosking D, Lippuner K, et al. The prevalence of vitamin D inadequacy amongst women with osteoporosis: an international epidemiological investigation. J Intern Med 2006;260(3):245–54.
49. Maurer MS, Burcham J, Cheng H. Diabetes mellitus is associated with an increased risk of falls in elderly residents of a long-term care facility. J Gerontol A Biol Sci Med Sci 2005;60(9):1157–62.
50. Schwartz AV, Hillier TA, Sellmeyer DE, et al. Older women with diabetes have a higher risk of falls: a prospective study. Diabetes Care 2002;25(10):1749–54.
51. Giangregorio LM, Leslie WD, Lix LM, et al. FRAX underestimates fracture risk in patients with diabetes. J Bone Miner Res 2012;27(2):301–8.
52. Leslie WD, Morin SN, Lix LM, et al. Does diabetes modify the effect of FRAX risk factors for predicting major osteoporotic and hip fracture? Osteoporos Int 2014; 25(12):2817–24.
53. Janghorbani M, Feskanich D, Willett WC, et al. Prospective study of diabetes and risk of hip fracture: the Nurses' Health Study. Diabetes care 2006;29(7): 1573–8.
54. Nickolas TL, Leonard MB, Shane E. Chronic kidney disease and bone fracture: a growing concern. Kidney Int 2008;74(6):721–31.
55. Silverman SL, Cummings SR, Watts NB. Recommendations for the clinical evaluation of agents for treatment of osteoporosis: consensus of an expert panel representing the American Society for Bone and Mineral Research (ASBMR), the International Society for Clinical Densitometry (ISCD), and the National Osteoporosis Foundation (NOF). J Bone Mineral Res 2008;23(1):159–65.
56. Yki-Jarvinen H. Thiazolidinediones. New Engl J Med 2004;351(11):1106–18.
57. Grey A. Skeletal consequences of thiazolidinedione therapy. Osteoporos Int 2008;19(2):129–37.

58. Alba M, Xie J, Fung A, et al. The effects of canagliflozin, a sodium glucose co-transporter 2 inhibitor, on mineral metabolism and bone in patients with type 2 diabetes mellitus. Curr Med Res Opin 2016;32(8):1375–85.
59. Vestergaard P, Rejnmark L, Mosekilde L. Relative fracture risk in patients with diabetes mellitus, and the impact of insulin and oral antidiabetic medication on relative fracture risk. Diabetologia 2005;48(7):1292–9.
60. Lapane KL, Yang S, Brown MJ, et al. Sulfonylureas and risk of falls and fractures: a systematic review. Drugs Aging 2013;30(7):527–47.
61. Monami M, Dicembrini I, Antenore A, et al. Dipeptidyl peptidase-4 inhibitors and bone fractures: a meta-analysis of randomized clinical trials. Diabetes Care 2011;34(11):2474–6.
62. Pscherer S, Kostev K, Dippel FW, et al. Fracture risk in patients with type 2 diabetes under different antidiabetic treatment regimens: a retrospective database analysis in primary care. Diabetes Metab Syndr Obes 2016;9:17–23.
63. Hanley DA, Brown JP, Tenenhouse A, et al. Associations among disease conditions, bone mineral density, and prevalent vertebral deformities in men and women 50 years of age and older: cross-sectional results from the Canadian Multicentre Osteoporosis Study. J bone Mineral Res 2003;18(4):784–90.
64. Petit MA, Paudel ML, Taylor BC, et al. Bone mass and strength in older men with type 2 diabetes: the Osteoporotic Fractures in Men Study. J Bone Miner Res 2010;25(2):285–91.
65. Starup-Linde J, Eriksen SA, Lykkeboe S, et al. Biochemical markers of bone turnover in diabetes patients–a meta-analysis, and a methodological study on the effects of glucose on bone markers. Osteoporos Int 2014;25(6):1697–708.
66. Keegan TH, Schwartz AV, Bauer DC, et al. Effect of alendronate on bone mineral density and biochemical markers of bone turnover in type 2 diabetic women: the fracture intervention trial. Diabetes Care 2004;27(7):1547–53.
67. Hunt JV, Smith CC, Wolff SP. Autoxidative glycosylation and possible involvement of peroxides and free radicals in LDL modification by glucose. Diabetes 1990;39(11):1420–4.
68. Hamada Y, Fujii H, Fukagawa M. Role of oxidative stress in diabetic bone disorder. Bone 2009;45(Suppl 1):S35–8.
69. McCabe L, Zhang J, Raehtz S. Understanding the skeletal pathology of type 1 and 2 diabetes mellitus. Crit Rev Eukaryot Gene Expr 2011;21(2):187–206.
70. McCabe LR. Understanding the pathology and mechanisms of type I diabetic bone loss. J Cell Biochem 2007;102(6):1343–57.
71. Hock JM, Krishnan V, Onyia JE, et al. Osteoblast apoptosis and bone turnover. J bone mineral Res 2001;16(6):975–84.
72. Mastrandrea LD, Wactawski-Wende J, Donahue RP, et al. Young women with type 1 diabetes have lower bone mineral density that persists over time. Diabetes Care 2008;31(9):1729–35.
73. Yamagishi S. Role of advanced glycation end products (AGEs) in osteoporosis in diabetes. Curr Drug Targets 2011;12(14):2096–102.
74. Ramasamy R, Yan SF, Schmidt AM. The diverse ligand repertoire of the receptor for advanced glycation endproducts and pathways to the complications of diabetes. Vasc Pharmacol 2012;57(5–6):160–7.
75. Tang SY, Vashishth D. The relative contributions of non-enzymatic glycation and cortical porosity on the fracture toughness of aging bone. J Biomech 2011;44(2):330–6.
76. Tang SY, Vashishth D. Non-enzymatic glycation alters microdamage formation in human cancellous bone. Bone 2010;46(1):148–54.

77. Vashishth D. The role of the collagen matrix in skeletal fragility. Curr Osteoporos Rep 2007;5(2):62–6.
78. Saito M, Marumo K. Collagen cross-links as a determinant of bone quality: a possible explanation for bone fragility in aging, osteoporosis, and diabetes mellitus. Osteoporos Int 2010;21(2):195–214.
79. Baynes JW. Role of oxidative stress in development of complications in diabetes. Diabetes 1991;40(4):405–12.
80. Sroga GE, Wu PC, Vashishth D. Insulin-like growth factor 1, glycation and bone fragility: implications for fracture resistance of bone. PLoS One 2015;10(1): e0117046.
81. Poundarik AA, Wu PC, Evis Z, et al. A direct role of collagen glycation in bone fracture. J Mech Behav Biomed Mater 2015;52:120–30.
82. Weinberg E, Maymon T, Moses O, et al. Streptozotocin-induced diabetes in rats diminishes the size of the osteoprogenitor pool in bone marrow. Diabetes Res Clin Pract 2014;103(1):35–41.
83. Hamada Y, Kitazawa S, Kitazawa R, et al. Histomorphometric analysis of diabetic osteopenia in streptozotocin-induced diabetic mice: a possible role of oxidative stress. Bone 2007;40(5):1408–14.
84. van der Kallen CJ, van Greevenbroek MM, Stehouwer CD, et al. Endoplasmic reticulum stress-induced apoptosis in the development of diabetes: is there a role for adipose tissue and liver? Apoptosis 2009;14(12):1424–34.
85. Kemink SA, Hermus AR, Swinkels LM, et al. Osteopenia in insulin-dependent diabetes mellitus; prevalence and aspects of pathophysiology. J Endocrinol Invest 2000;23(5):295–303.
86. Bouillon R, Bex M, Van Herck E, et al. Influence of age, sex, and insulin on osteoblast function: osteoblast dysfunction in diabetes mellitus. J Clin Endocrinol Metab 1995;80(4):1194–202.
87. Masse PG, Pacifique MB, Tranchant CC, et al. Bone metabolic abnormalities associated with well-controlled type 1 diabetes (IDDM) in young adult women: a disease complication often ignored or neglected. J Am Coll Nutr 2010; 29(4):419–29.
88. Lumachi F, Camozzi V, Tombolan V, et al. Bone mineral density, osteocalcin, and bone-specific alkaline phosphatase in patients with insulin-dependent diabetes mellitus. Ann N Y Acad Sci 2009;1173(Suppl 1):E64–7.
89. Fulzele K, Riddle RC, DiGirolamo DJ, et al. Insulin receptor signaling in osteoblasts regulates postnatal bone acquisition and body composition. Cell 2010; 142(2):309–19.
90. Liu DM, Guo XZ, Tong HJ, et al. Association between osteocalcin and glucose metabolism: a meta-analysis. Osteoporos Int 2015;26(12):2823–33.
91. Kunutsor SK, Apekey TA, Laukkanen JA. Association of serum total osteocalcin with type 2 diabetes and intermediate metabolic phenotypes: systematic review and meta-analysis of observational evidence. Eur J Epidemiol 2015;30(8):599–614.
92. Kanazawa I, Yamaguchi T, Yamauchi M, et al. Serum undercarboxylated osteocalcin was inversely associated with plasma glucose level and fat mass in type 2 diabetes mellitus. Osteoporos Int 2011;22(1):187–94.
93. Kanazawa I, Yamaguchi T, Yamamoto M, et al. Serum osteocalcin level is associated with glucose metabolism and atherosclerosis parameters in type 2 diabetes mellitus. J Clin Endocrinol Metab 2009;94(1):45–9.
94. Neumann T, Hofbauer LC, Rauner M, et al. Clinical and endocrine correlates of circulating sclerostin levels in patients with type 1 diabetes mellitus. Clin Endocrinol 2014;80(5):649–55.

95. van Bezooijen RL, Svensson JP, Eefting D, et al. Wnt but not BMP signaling is involved in the inhibitory action of sclerostin on BMP-stimulated bone formation. J bone mineral Res 2007;22(1):19–28.
96. Boutzios G, Kaltsas G. Immune system effects on the endocrine system. In: De Groot LJ, Beck-Peccoz P, Chrousos G, et al, editors. Endotext. South Dartmouth (MA): MDText.com, Inc.; 2000. Available at: https://www-ncbi-nlm-nih-gov.uml.idm.oclc.org/books/NBK279139/.
97. Halade GV, El Jamali A, Williams PJ, et al. Obesity-mediated inflammatory microenvironment stimulates osteoclastogenesis and bone loss in mice. Exp Gerontol 2011;46(1):43–52.
98. Borst SE. The role of TNF-alpha in insulin resistance. Endocrine 2004;23(2–3):177–82.
99. Katsuki A, Sumida Y, Murashima S, et al. Serum levels of tumor necrosis factor-alpha are increased in obese patients with noninsulin-dependent diabetes mellitus. J Clin Endocrinol Metab 1998;83(3):859–62.
100. Kanis JA, McCloskey EV, Johansson H, et al. A reference standard for the description of osteoporosis. Bone 2008;42(3):467–75.
101. Johnell O, Kanis JA, Oden A, et al. Predictive value of BMD for hip and other fractures. J bone mineral Res 2005;20(7):1185–94.
102. Marshall D, Johnell O, Wedel H. Meta-analysis of how well measures of bone mineral density predict occurrence of osteoporotic fractures. BMJ 1996;312(7041):1254–9.
103. Leslie WD, Hough S. Chapter 3: Fracture risk assessment in diabetes. In: Lecka-Czernik B, Fowlkes JL, editors. Diabetic bone disease. (Switzerland): Springer International; 2016. p. 45–69.
104. Broy SB, Cauley JA, Lewiecki ME, et al. Fracture risk prediction by Non-BMD DXA measures: the 2015 ISCD official positions Part 1: hip geometry. J Clin Densitom 2015;18(3):287–308.
105. McCloskey EV, Oden A, Harvey NC, et al. Adjusting fracture probability by trabecular bone score. Calcified Tissue Int 2015;96(6):500–9.
106. McCloskey EV, Oden A, Harvey NC, et al. A meta-analysis of trabecular bone score in fracture risk prediction and its relationship to FRAX. J bone mineral Res 2016;31(5):940–8.
107. Rosen HN, Vokes TJ, Malabanan AO, et al. The official positions of the International Society for Clinical Densitometry: vertebral fracture assessment. J Clin Densitom 2013;16(4):482–8.
108. Crans GG, Genant HK, Krege JH. Prognostic utility of a semiquantitative spinal deformity index. Bone 2005;37(2):175–9.
109. Clynes MA, Edwards MH, Buehring B, et al. Definitions of Sarcopenia: Associations with Previous Falls and Fracture in a Population Sample. Calcified Tissue Int 2015;97(5):445–52.
110. Binkley N, Cooper C. Sarcopenia, the Next Frontier in Fracture Prevention: Introduction From the Guest Editors. J Clin Densitom 2015;18(4):459–60.
111. Cauley JA. An overview of sarcopenic obesity. J Clin Densitom 2015;18(4):499–505.
112. Al-Ani AN, Cederholm T, Saaf M, et al. Low bone mineral density and fat-free mass in younger patients with a femoral neck fracture. Eur J Clin Invest 2015;45(8):800–6.
113. Albanese CV, Diessel E, Genant HK. Clinical applications of body composition measurements using DXA. J Clin Densitom 2003;6(2):75–85.

114. Meyer HE, Willett WC, Flint AJ, et al. Abdominal obesity and hip fracture: results from the Nurses' Health Study and the Health Professionals Follow-up Study. Osteoporos Int 2016;27(6):2127–36.
115. Yang S, Nguyen ND, Center JR, et al. Association between abdominal obesity and fracture risk: a prospective study. J Clin Endocrinol Metab 2013;98(6): 2478–83.
116. Neumann T, Lodes S, Kastner B, et al. Trabecular bone score in type 1 diabetes-a cross-sectional study. Osteoporos Int 2016;27(1):127–33.
117. Abd El Dayem SM, El-Shehaby AM, Abd El Gafar A, et al. Bone density, body composition, and markers of bone remodeling in type 1 diabetic patients. Scand J Clin Lab Invest 2011;71(5):387–93.
118. Kanis JA, on behalf of the World Health Organization Scientific Group. Assessment of osteoporosis at the primary health-care level. Technical Report. (United Kingdom): WHO Collaborating Centre, University of Sheffield; 2008.
119. Hough FS, Pierroz DD, Cooper C, et al. MECHANISMS IN ENDOCRINOLOGY: Mechanisms and evaluation of bone fragility in type 1 diabetes mellitus. Eur J Endocrinol 2016;174(4):R127–38.
120. Schwartz AV, Vittinghoff E, Bauer DC, et al. Association of BMD and FRAX score with risk of fracture in older adults with type 2 diabetes. JAMA 2011;305(21): 2184–92.
121. Garg R, Chen Z, Beck T, et al. Hip geometry in diabetic women: implications for fracture risk. Metab Clin Exp 2012;61(12):1756–62.
122. Moseley KF, Dobrosielski DA, Stewart KJ, et al. Lean mass predicts hip geometry in men and women with non-insulin-requiring type 2 diabetes mellitus. J Clin Densitom 2011;14(3):332–9.
123. Hamilton CJ, Jamal SA, Beck TJ, et al. Evidence for impaired skeletal load adaptation among Canadian women with type 2 diabetes mellitus: insight into the BMD and bone fragility paradox. Metabolism 2013;62(10):1401–5.
124. Ishii S, Cauley JA, Crandall CJ, et al. Diabetes and femoral neck strength: findings from the Hip Strength Across the Menopausal Transition Study. J Clin Endocrinol Metab 2012;97(1):190–7.
125. Akeroyd JM, Suarez EA, Bartali B, et al. Differences in skeletal and non-skeletal factors in a diverse sample of men with and without type 2 diabetes mellitus. J Diabetes Complications 2014;28(5):679–83.
126. Leslie WD, Aubry-Rozier B, Lamy O, et al, Manitoba Bone Density Program. TBS (trabecular bone score) and diabetes-related fracture risk. J Clin Endocrinol Metab 2013;98(2):602–9.
127. Direk K, Cecelja M, Astle W, et al. The relationship between DXA-based and anthropometric measures of visceral fat and morbidity in women. BMC Cardiovasc Disord 2013;13:25.
128. Porter SA, Massaro JM, Hoffmann U, et al. Abdominal subcutaneous adipose tissue: a protective fat depot? Diabetes care 2009;32(6):1068–75.
129. von Eyben FE, Mouritsen E, Holm J, et al. Intra-abdominal obesity and metabolic risk factors: a study of young adults. Int J Obes Relat Metab Disord 2003;27(8): 941–9.
130. Jensen MD. Role of body fat distribution and the metabolic complications of obesity. J Clin Endocrinol Metab 2008;93(11 Suppl 1):S57–63.
131. Rothney MP, Catapano AL, Xia J, et al. Abdominal visceral fat measurement using dual-energy X-ray: association with cardiometabolic risk factors. Obesity (Silver Spring) 2013;21(9):1798–802.

132. Langsetmo L, Nguyen TV, Nguyen ND, et al. Independent external validation of nomograms for predicting risk of low-trauma fracture and hip fracture. CMAJ 2011;183(2):E107–14.
133. Nguyen ND, Frost SA, Center JR, et al. Development of a nomogram for individualizing hip fracture risk in men and women. Osteoporos Int 2007;18(8): 1109–17.
134. Hippisley-Cox J, Coupland C. Predicting risk of osteoporotic fracture in men and women in England and Wales: prospective derivation and validation of QFractureScores. BMJ 2009;339:b4229.
135. Institute of Medicine. Dietary reference intakes for calcium and vitamin D. Washington, DC: The National Academies Press; 2011.
136. Li K, Kaaks R, Linseisen J, et al. Associations of dietary calcium intake and calcium supplementation with myocardial infarction and stroke risk and overall cardiovascular mortality in the Heidelberg cohort of the European Prospective Investigation into Cancer and Nutrition study (EPIC-Heidelberg). Heart (British Cardiac Society) 2012;98(12):920–5.
137. Bolland MJ, Barber PA, Doughty RN, et al. Vascular events in healthy older women receiving calcium supplementation: randomised controlled trial. BMJ 2008;336(7638):262–6.
138. Bolland MJ, Avenell A, Baron JA, et al. Effect of calcium supplements on risk of myocardial infarction and cardiovascular events: meta-analysis. BMJ 2010;341: c3691.
139. Bolland MJ, Grey A, Avenell A, et al. Calcium supplements with or without vitamin D and risk of cardiovascular events: reanalysis of the Women's Health Initiative limited access dataset and meta-analysis. BMJ 2011;342:d2040.
140. Black DM, Rosen CJ. Clinical Practice. Postmenopausal Osteoporosis. N Engl J Med 2016;374(3):254–62.
141. Gonnelli S, Cepollaro C, Pondrelli C, et al. Bone turnover and the response to alendronate treatment in postmenopausal osteoporosis. Calcified Tissue Int 1999;65(5):359–64.
142. Motyl KJ, McCauley LK, McCabe LR. Amelioration of type I diabetes-induced osteoporosis by parathyroid hormone is associated with improved osteoblast survival. J Cell Physiol 2012;227(4):1326–34.
143. Tsai JN, Uihlein AV, Burnett-Bowie SM, et al. Effects of Two Years of Teriparatide, Denosumab, or Both on Bone Microarchitecture and Strength (DATA-HRpQCT study). J Clin Endocrinol Metab 2016;101(5):2023–30.
144. Iwamoto J, Sato Y, Uzawa M, et al. Three-year experience with alendronate treatment in postmenopausal osteoporotic Japanese women with or without type 2 diabetes. Diabetes Res Clin Pract 2011;93(2):166–73.
145. Johnell O, Kanis JA, Black DM, et al. Associations between baseline risk factors and vertebral fracture risk in the Multiple Outcomes of Raloxifene Evaluation (MORE) Study. J bone mineral Res 2004;19(5):764–72.
146. Saito O, Saito T, Asakura S, et al. Effects of raloxifene on bone metabolism in hemodialysis patients with type 2 diabetes. Int J Endocrinol Metab 2012; 10(2):464–9.
147. Cummings SR, Black DM, Thompson DE, et al. Effect of alendronate on risk of fracture in women with low bone density but without vertebral fractures: results from the Fracture Intervention Trial. JAMA 1998;280(24):2077–82.
148. McClung MR, Boonen S, Torring O, et al. Effect of denosumab treatment on the risk of fractures in subgroups of women with postmenopausal osteoporosis. J bone mineral Res 2012;27(1):211–8.

149. Vestergaard P, Rejnmark L, Mosekilde L. Are antiresorptive drugs effective against fractures in patients with diabetes? Calcified Tissue Int 2011;88(3): 209–14.
150. Kajizono M, Sada H, Sugiura Y, et al. Incidence and risk factors of osteonecrosis of the jaw in advanced cancer patients after treatment with zoledronic acid or denosumab: a retrospective cohort study. Biol Pharm Bull 2015;38(12):1850–5.
151. Khamaisi M, Regev E, Yarom N, et al. Possible association between diabetes and bisphosphonate-related jaw osteonecrosis. J Clin Endocrinol Metab 2007; 92(3):1172–5.
152. Khan AA, Morrison A, Hanley DA, et al. Diagnosis and management of osteonecrosis of the jaw: a systematic review and international consensus. J bone mineral Res 2015;30(1):3–23.
153. Shane E, Burr D, Abrahamsen B, et al. Atypical subtrochanteric and diaphyseal femoral fractures: second report of a task force of the American Society for Bone and Mineral Research. J bone mineral Res 2014;29(1):1–23.
154. Adler RA, El-Hajj Fuleihan G, Bauer DC, et al. Managing Osteoporosis in Patients on Long-Term Bisphosphonate Treatment: Report of a Task Force of the American Society for Bone and Mineral Research. J bone mineral Res 2016; 31(1):16–35.
155. Giusti A, Hamdy NA, Dekkers OM, et al. Atypical fractures and bisphosphonate therapy: a cohort study of patients with femoral fracture with radiographic adjudication of fracture site and features. Bone 2011;48(5):966–71.
156. Lo JC, Huang SY, Lee GA, et al. Clinical correlates of atypical femoral fracture. Bone 2012;51(1):181–4.
157. Schwartz AV, Schafer AL, Grey A, et al. Effects of antiresorptive therapies on glucose metabolism: results from the FIT, HORIZON-PFT, and FREEDOM trials. J bone mineral Res 2013;28(6):1348–54.
158. Vestergaard P. Risk of newly diagnosed type 2 diabetes is reduced in users of alendronate. Calcified Tissue Int 2011;89(4):265–70.
159. Chan DC, Yang RS, Ho CH, et al. The use of alendronate is associated with a decreased incidence of type 2 diabetes mellitus–a population-based cohort study in Taiwan. PLoS One 2015;10(4):e0123279.
160. Toulis KA, Nirantharakumar K, Ryan R, et al. Bisphosphonates and glucose homeostasis: a population-based, retrospective cohort study. J Clin Endocrinol Metab 2015;100(5):1933–40.
161. Yang S, Leslie WD, Morin SN, et al. Antiresorptive Therapy and Newly-Diagnosed Diabetes in Women: A Historical Cohort Study. Diabetes Obes Metab 2016;18(9):875–81.

Primary Hyperparathyroidism

Effects on Bone Health

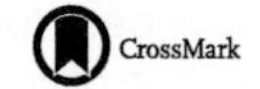

Kyle A. Zanocco, MD, MS[a], Michael W. Yeh, MD[b,*]

KEYWORDS

- Hyperparathyroidism • Parathyroid neoplasms • Parathyroid carcinoma
- Hypercalcemia • Bone density • Osteoporosis

KEY POINTS

- Primary hyperparathyroidism is the most common cause of hypercalcemia in the outpatient setting.
- Many cases of primary hyperparathyroidism are now discovered incidentally with routine blood chemistry screening.
- Hyperparathyroidism results in diminished bone mineral density over time, even in otherwise asymptomatic patients.
- Parathyroidectomy is the only definitive treatment of primary hyperparathyroidism.

INTRODUCTION

Primary hyperparathyroidism (PHPT) is the most common cause of chronic hypercalcemia. With the advent of routine calcium screening, the classical presentation of renal and osseous symptoms has been largely replaced with mild, asymptomatic disease. The optimization of future bone health has therefore emerged as a major treatment consideration for PHPT patients.

EPIDEMIOLOGY

Primary hyperparathyroidism (PHPT) is a common endocrine disorder, affecting 1 in 400 women and 1 in 1200 men in the United States. The annual incidence is 65 per 100,000 women and 25 per 100,000 men. Women are about 3 times more commonly affected by PHPT as men; this sexual dimorphism in epidemiology seems to widen in those older than 50 years. Recently, racial differences in the epidemiology of PHPT

The authors have nothing to disclose.

[a] Section of Endocrine Surgery, UCLA David Geffen School of Medicine, 10833 Le Conte Avenue, 72-182 CHS, Los Angeles, CA 90095, USA; [b] Section of Endocrine Surgery, UCLA David Geffen School of Medicine, 10833 Le Conte Avenue, 72-250 CHS, Los Angeles, CA 90095, USA

* Corresponding author.

E-mail address: myeh@mednet.ucla.edu

Endocrinol Metab Clin N Am 46 (2017) 87–104
http://dx.doi.org/10.1016/j.ecl.2016.09.012 **endo.theclinics.com**

have been found, with the highest rates of disease found in African Americans.[1] Consideration of age, sex, and race yields an approximate prevalence of 1 in 200 women older than 50, and 1 in 100 African-American women older than 50. The prevalence of PHPT has tripled over the last 15 years because of increased rates of biochemical screening and a relatively low rate of cure via surgical treatment (10%–25%).[2]

RISK FACTORS

Major risk factors for the development of primary hyperparathyroidism include exposure to ionizing radiation, prolonged lithium use, and family history.

Individuals with a history of radiation therapy are at increased risk for PHPT. Those who underwent childhood radiation treatment of benign head and neck conditions are at a 3-fold risk of parathyroid neoplasia compared with those in the general population.[3] There is a prolonged latency period lasting 40 to 50 years between radiation for benign disease and the development of parathyroid neoplasia.[4] A shorter latency period of less than 20 years has been observed after higher-dose radiation therapy for malignant diseases.[5] Prior therapeutic breast irradiation is also associated with hyperparathyroidism. The side of breast radiation treatment correlates with the side of subsequent parathyroid adenoma development.[6]

The mood stabilizer lithium alters the setpoint of calcium regulation by antagonizing the calcium-sensing receptor.[7] In the presence of lithium, higher serum calcium concentrations are required to inhibit parathyroid hormone (PTH) secretion. This alteration has been postulated to result in the chronic stimulus of parathyroid tissue, leading to increased parathyroid volume and the possibility of adenomatous transformation.[8]

Approximately 5% of PHPT cases are familial.[9] Several syndromes and their corresponding molecular genetics responsible for neoplastic transformation of parathyroid tissue are described in the following section. In the remaining kindreds with PHPT who lack the features of these well-known syndromes, the term *familial isolated hyperparathyroidism* has been applied.[10] The genetic underpinnings of this distinct clinical entity have yet to be defined.

PATHOPHYSIOLOGY

Pathogenesis of Autonomous Parathyroid Production

PHPT is caused by 3 distinct types of parathyroid lesions. The distribution of pathologic lesions responsible for PHPT is displayed in **Fig. 1**. The most common pathologic

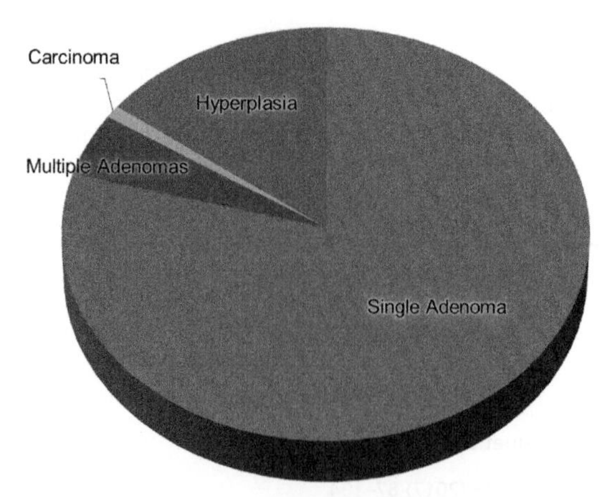

Fig. 1. The distribution of responsible lesions in primary hyperparathyroidism. A single gland adenoma causes 80% of cases. Parathyroid carcinoma occurs in less than 1% of cases.

lesion, occurring in approximately 80% of cases, is a single gland adenoma. This benign tumor consists of an encapsulated proliferation of autonomously functioning chief or oncocytic cells. Double adenomata may be seen in about 5% of cases. Parathyroid hyperplasia, which is responsible for approximately 15% of cases, is commonly described as a benign proliferation of parenchymal cells occurring uniformly in all parathyroid glands; however, heterogeneous nodularity and asymmetric gland size are observed in practice.[11] Parathyroid carcinoma is an exceedingly rare cause of PHPT, occurring in less than 1% of cases.[12]

Molecular Pathogenesis of Hyperparathyroidism

Elucidation of the molecular genetics of familial hyperparathyroidism during the last 3 decades has improved understanding of sporadic parathyroid tumorigenesis. The genes responsible for inherited and sporadic parathyroid disorders leading to primary hyperparathyroidism are described in **Table 1**.

Tumor suppressor genes MEN1 and HRPT2

Inactivating germline mutations of multiple endocrine neoplasia type 1 (MEN1), a tumor suppressor gene that encodes the nuclear protein menin, cause MEN1.[13,14] Patients with this autosomal dominant genetic syndrome have parathyroid, anterior pituitary, pancreatic, and foregut tumors. Most parathyroid tumors in MEN1 patients have a somatic mutation of the remaining wild-type allele.[15] Multiple, recurrent tumors are common throughout an MEN1 patient's lifetime.[16] Somatic mutations in MEN1 are frequent events in sporadic parathyroid adenomas. Up to one-third of sporadic parathyroid adenomas have a mutation in at least 1 MEN1 allele.[17–19]

In contrast to the MEN1 gene, somatic mutations in the parafibromin-encoding HRPT2 tumor-suppressor gene are infrequent events in parathyroid adenomas and frequent in sporadic parathyroid carcinomas.[20] Germline-inactivating mutations of HRPT2, also known as *CDC73*, are common in the autosomal dominant hyperparathyroidism jaw tumor (HPT-JT) syndrome, consisting of parathyroid tumors, ossifying fibromas of the mandible and maxilla, and kidney syndromes.[21]

Oncogenes RET and CCND1/PRAD1

The proto-oncogene RET encodes a widely expressed receptor tyrosine kinase. Germline RET mutations are responsible for MEN types 2A and 2B and familial medullary thyroid cancer.[22] Although a variety of activating RET mutations express a spectrum of phenotypes in these syndromes, the development of parathyroid adenomas seen in MEN2A most commonly arises from mutations at codon 634 on chromosome 10.[23,24] Somatic RET mutations in sporadic parathyroid adenomas are extraordinarily rare.[25]

The cyclin D1 (CCND1) oncogene was discovered by genetic analysis of sporadic parathyroid tumors.[26] This gene is overexpressed in one-third of sporadic adenomas and 90% of parathyroid cancers owing to chromosomal rearrangement within the PTH gene locus.[27]

The calcium-sensing receptor and familial hypocalciuric hypercalcemia

Mutations of the calcium-sensing receptor gene (CASR) cause a spectrum of disruption in calcium homeostasis. At one extreme are homozygous inactivating CASR mutations resulting in neonatal severe hyperparathyroidism (NSHPT).[28] Infants with NSHPT present with extreme hypercalcemia and respiratory failure in the first days of life, and early total parathyroidectomy is often necessary.[29] Pathologic examination of the excised glands demonstrates chief cell hyperplasia.[30]

Table 1
Affected genes in syndromic and sporadic parathyroid tumors

Gene	Protein Encoded	Associated Hyperparathyroid Syndrome	Features of Syndromic Parathyroid Tumors	Defect in Sporadic Parathyroid Tumors
MEN1	Menin	Multiple endocrine neoplasia type 1	Multiple, asymmetric tumors	Inactivation in 25%–35% of benign tumors
HRPT2/CDC73	Parafibromin	Hyperparathyroidism-jaw tumor syndrome	Single tumor common, 15% malignant	Inactivation in 70% of cancers
RET	c-Ret	Multiple endocrine neoplasia type 2A	Single tumor common	Mutation exceedingly rare
CCND1/PRAD1	Cyclin D1	NA	NA	Overexpression results from DNA rearrangement involving PTH gene
CASR	Calcium-sensing receptor	FHH with heterozygous inactivation; NSHPT with homozygous inactivation	FHH: near-normal size and surgical pathology NSHPT: Marked enlargement of multiple glands	Decreased expression common; mutation exceedingly rare

Abbreviation: NA, not applicable.

Data from Sharretts JM, Simonds WF. Clinical and molecular genetics of parathyroid neoplasms. Best Pract Res Clin Endocrinol Metab 2010;24(3):493.

The mildest forms of familial hypocalciuric hypercalcemia (FHH) represent the other extreme. FHH is an autosomal dominant disorder caused by a multitude of different heterozygous inactivating mutations of CASR.[31] The resulting calcium set point alteration causes elevated serum calcium with normal or elevated serum PTH levels. FHH is frequently confused with PHPT; however, parathyroidectomy does not improve hypercalcemia in this largely asymptomatic condition. Furthermore, unlike PHPT, FHH is not associated with loss of bone mineral density (BMD).[32] If FHH patients do become symptomatic from hypercalcemia, the current recommended treatment is calcimimetic therapy.[33]

Somatic mutation of CASR is exceedingly rare in sporadic parathyroid adenomas.[34] However, decreased expression of CASR is common and likely contributes to inappropriate PTH release in these tumors.[35]

Skeletal Pathogenesis in Primary Hyperparathyroidism

Diminished bone mineral density

The PTH excess caused by PHPT leads to diminished BMD over time via upregulated osteoclast activity.[36,37] Continuous serum elevation in PTH increases osteoblast surface expression of receptor activator of nuclear factor κ-B ligand (RANKL), which, in turn, stimulates osteoclastogenesis. PTH also exerts an inhibitory effect on expression of osteoprotegerin, a decoy inhibitor of RANKL, with the net effect of additional osteoclastogenesis.[38] Although the overt abnormalities of bone pain, skeletal deformity, and fragility fracture are becoming unusual in the era of densitometry screening and routine serum chemistry testing, BMD is typically reduced even in PHPT patients with incidentally detected mild biochemical disease.[39]

Bone structure deficits in primary hyperparathyroidism

Densitometric profiles and bone biopsy studies indicate a preferential negative effect of PHPT on cortical bone thickness and relative preservation of trabecular density.[39–41] However, epidemiologic data show increased fracture risk at both trabecular (eg, vertebral) and cortical sites in PHPT.[37,42–45] These discordant data suggest that PHPT decreases structural strength in both cortical and trabecular bone networks. This phenomenon has been investigated by high-resolution peripheral quantitative computed tomography, a research modality that characterizes skeletal microarchitecture in both cortical and trabecular compartments and volumetric bone density.[46] In PHPT patients, high-resolution peripheral quantitative computed tomography shows microarchitectural deterioration and decreased volumetric density of both cortical and trabecular sites.[47] These findings suggest that perceived relative sparing of trabecular BMD is merely an artifact produced by inadvertent inclusion of disordered cortical remnants in the analysis of trabecular density by standard noninvasive volumetric bone density measurement techniques.[47–49]

CLINICAL FEATURES

Presentation of Primary Hyperparathyroidism

The most common overt clinical features of PHPT are renal stone disease and fracture resulting from diminished bone quality.[50] Rarely, severe sequelae of hypercalcemia have been reported.[51] The advent of routine multichannel serum chemistry testing in the 1970s fundamentally altered the disease presentation of PHPT.[52] It is now typical for PHPT to be diagnosed incidentally without any overt clinical signs or symptoms.[53] This entity was officially labeled *asymptomatic PHPT* at a National Institutes of Health Consensus Development Conference in 1990.[54] The term *mild asymptomatic PHPT* refers to asymptomatic patients with a serum calcium that does not exceed

1 mg/dL above the laboratory upper limit of normal, which is typically a threshold of 11.3 to 11.5 mg/dL. Several nonclassical cardiovascular and neurocognitive manifestations are variably attributed to mild PHPT and have been the subject of discussion during 3 subsequent international workshops on asymptomatic PHPT.[50,55,56] Although the association of PHPT and these nonspecific domains has not been officially recognized, it remains an area of active investigation.[50]

Renal Manifestations

Although the incidence of symptomatic nephrolithiasis has decreased from more than 50% of PHPT patients in the era predating routine serum calcium testing to less than 20% today, calcium kidney stones continue to be the most common overt clinical manifestation of the disease.[53,57,58] Subclinical nephrolithiasis and nephrocalcinosis, the mineralization of kidney tissue, are both seen radiographically in an additional 7% of asymptomatic PHPT patients.[59] Renal impairment manifested by a diminished glomerular filtration rate is observed in approximately 20% of PHPT patients.[60] Those who remain untreated may be at increased risk for renal failure; however, prospective data have not shown this phenomenon.[36,60–64]

Skeletal Manifestations

Severity of bone disease is correlated with the duration and severity of PHPT. In even the mildest biochemical cases of PHPT, bone mineral density declines over time.[36] Fragility fracture, defined as fracture resulting from traumatic energy of less than a fall from standing height, is the most common skeletal manifestation of PHPT.[65,66] In the developed world, osteitis fibrosa cystica, also known as *Von Recklinghausen's disease of the bone*, is a vanishingly rare complication of severe longstanding PHPT. Osteitis fibrosa cystica produces characteristic bony swellings known as *brown tumors*, which are hemosiderin-laden osteoclastic cysts.[67] Bone pain, deformity, and fracture are additional hallmarks of the disease.[68] These clinical features continue to appear as presenting signs of PHPT in developing nations without widespread access to serum calcium screening.[69–71]

Hypercalcemic Manifestations

In our experience, clinical features of PTH-mediated hypercalcemia typically become apparent when serum calcium levels exceed 13 mg/dL. The velocity of calcium fluctuation is also an important predictor of symptomatic hypercalcemia. The chronic elevation of calcium typically observed in PHPT produces less dramatic symptoms compared with the rapid calcium increases of malignancy.[72] Early symptoms include fatigue, polydipsia, polyuria, difficulty concentrating, and depression. Gastrointestinal effects of nausea, constipation, and pancreatitis are also observed.[51] In rare cases, severe complications of hypercalcemia ensue, producing acute kidney injury, bradyarrhythmias, shortening of the QT interval, stupor, and coma.[51,73]

Nonclassical Manifestations

Hypertension has been associated with PHPT in several large retrospective series.[74–78] However, prospective studies have not consistently found that definitive surgical treatment of PHPT reduces mean blood pressure in these patients.[79–82] Although increased cardiovascular morbidity and mortality have been reported in patients with severe biochemical disease, these outcomes are not strongly associated with the mild presentation of PHPT that is now common.[83–88]

Several nonspecific neurocognitive symptoms have been implicated in mild PHPT. Although there is considerable overlap with many other common medical and psychiatric disorders, weakness, depression, intellectual weariness, memory loss, decreased concentration, anxiety, irritability, and sleep disturbance have all been reported.[89–92]

DIFFERENTIAL DIAGNOSIS

The diagnosis of PHPT should be entertained in any patient with hypercalcemia. PHPT is the most likely cause of hypercalcemia in the outpatient setting.[1,93–95] **Box 1** lists other causes of hypercalcemia in their order of frequency. In hypercalcemia caused by PHPT, serum PTH levels are either high or inappropriately normal. PTH levels within the normal 95% reference range are inappropriate in the setting of hypercalcemia and indicate nonsuppressible parathyroid activity. FHH has a similar serum biochemical profile as PHPT and should be suspected in patients with long-standing hypercalcemia or a family history of hypercalcemia. Although patients with PHPT typically have elevated or normal urinary calcium levels, a 24-hour urinary calcium of less than 100 mg and a calcium/creatinine clearance ratio of less than 0.01 raises the strong possibility of FHH.[96]

The clinician is occasionally presented with diagnostic uncertainty regarding the primary or secondary nature of parathyroid hormone excess. Chronic kidney disease, medications, malabsorption syndromes, and vitamin D deficiency are common secondary causes of elevated PTH.[66] Correctable secondary causes should be addressed if the diagnosis of PHPT is unclear. For example, normocalcemic patients with concurrent hyperparathyroidism and vitamin D deficiency will occasionally become hypercalcemic with vitamin D supplementation, unmasking traditional hypercalcemic primary hyperparathyroidism.[97] However, if the parathyroid hormone excess is secondary to vitamin D deficiency, parathyroid hormone levels should normalize with correction of the vitamin D level.

An additional important diagnostic consideration in a patient with biochemically confirmed PHPT is the rare possibility of parathyroid carcinoma. As opposed to the mild presentation of PHPT usually associated with benign parathyroid pathology, parathyroid carcinoma typically produces high calcium and parathyroid levels.[66,98–100]

Box 1
The differential diagnosis of hypercalcemia

PHPT

Malignancy

Hypervitaminosis D

Thiazide diuretics

Hyperthyroidism

Hypothyroidism

Milk-alkali syndrome

FHH

Adrenal insufficiency

Renal disease

Granulomatous disease: sarcoidosis, tuberculosis, fungal granulomas

Immobilization

A palpable neck mass is present in many of these cases.[98,100] When these signs are present, a more extensive imaging workup including computed tomography (CT) and positron emission tomography is indicated to detect metastatic disease and guide therapy.[101]

TREATMENT

Confirmation of Biochemical Diagnosis

Incidental hypercalcemia should prompt a repeat serum calcium draw. In addition to calcium, serum PTH, creatinine, and 25-hydroxyvitamin D levels should be obtained when PHPT is suspected.[66] It is rarely necessary to correct total serum calcium levels for abnormal serum albumin levels; however, the following equation is used in these cases:

$$\text{Corrected calcium (mg/dL)} = (0.8[4.0\text{-albumin (g/dL)}]) + \text{total calcium (mg/dL)}$$

A 24-hour urine collection is also recommended to aid in the differential diagnosis of FHH (see above) and to prompt a urinary biochemical stone profile if marked hypercalciuria (>400 mg every 24 h) is present.[50,66]

Treatment of Hypercalcemia

In the rare instances in which patients with biochemically severe PHPT have symptomatic hypercalcemia, inpatient hospitalization and immediate therapeutic intervention are required.[73] Volume contraction resulting from calcium-induced natriuresis should be corrected with intravenous saline boluses.[102] After normalization of volume status, loop diuretics can be used to enhance sodium and calcium excretion. Cinacalcet, a calcimimetic frequently used to lower serum PTH levels in secondary hyperparathyroidism, is approved by the US Food and Drug Administration for the treatment of hypercalcemia in patients with parathyroid carcinoma and PHPT who are unable to undergo parathyroidectomy. The intravenous bisphosphonates ibandronate, pamidronate, and zoledronic acid are used to inhibit further bone resorption.

Localization Studies

Although many localization studies area available to assist in the operative planning of parathyroidectomy, localization studies should never be used to determine the diagnosis of PHPT or influence the decision to refer a patient for surgical consultation.[66] Preoperative ultrasonography should be performed on all PHPT patients to both localize parathyroid disease and diagnose thyroid neoplasia that could require surgical attention. Technetium 99m sestamibi scintigraphy has been used to identify pathologic parathyroid enlargement for the last 3 decades. The reported sensitivity of this test is highly variable but approaches 80% when performed at high-volume centers.[103] Sestamibi scanning is particularly valuable for ruling out ectopic adenomas located in the mediastinum. Parathyroid protocol CT scanning has emerged in the last 10 years as the most sensitive imaging modality and is most useful in the identification of multigland disease and planning of reoperative parathyroid surgery with otherwise negative imaging.[104]

Surgical Management of Primary Hyperparathyroidism

Surgical parathyroidectomy remains the only definitive treatment of PHPT.[66,105] Parathyroidectomy is usually performed under general anesthesia, although groups have reported using local anesthesia plus sedation (monitored anesthetic care) with good results.[106,107] A 2.5-cm transverse cervical incision is typically used, through which either a limited (less than 4 gland) exploration or 4-gland exploration may be conducted (see Controversies in later discussion). Intraoperative PTH monitoring may be used to assess the completeness of parathyroid resection.[66] In experienced hands, the rate of complications such as postoperative hematoma, recurrent laryngeal nerve injury, and hypoparathyroidism is less than 1%.[108]

The success rate of initial parathyroid surgery, as defined by sustained eucalcemia for at least 6 months postoperatively, varies widely from 70% to 98% and is largely a function of surgeon experience.[109] Although the exact volume-outcome function has not been defined, a useful rule of thumb is that a surgeon should perform at least 1 parathyroidectomy per month to achieve good outcomes and at least 1 parathyroidectomy per week to achieve superior outcomes.[110] Parathyroid surgery can usually be completed in less than 1 hour, and an increasing proportion of these cases is being performed on an outpatient bases.[111] Recovery is rapid, with most patients returning to normal activities on the day after surgery. Reoperative parathyroid surgery, for those patients with persistent or recurrent disease, is highly challenging and should only be performed in expert centers.

PROGNOSIS

The prognosis of PHPT rests largely on how it is managed. Contemporary data on the natural history of untreated PHPT are scant. Biochemical disease progression seems to occur in some of patients[112]; however, many if not most patients will subsequently have osteoporosis and increased fracture risk over time if untreated.[36,37] PHPT is associated with a markedly increased risk of nephrolithiasis, approximately 5 times that of the general population.[113] Limited data suggest that mild PHPT does not cause renal function to decline.[114] Several retrospective studies found an association between PHPT and excess mortality, which may be attributable to cardiovascular disease.[115–117]

Patients with PHPT who undergo successful surgical treatment experience improvements in BMD, which translate into substantially decreased risks of hip fracture and any fracture.[37] The risk of nephrolithiasis decreases steeply after parathyroidectomy, but does not reach baseline until approximately 10 years after surgery.[118] Surgical treatment of PHPT arrests renal function deterioration in patients with renal disease.[119] Patients who undergo parathyroidectomy also experience durable improvements in quality of life, as measured by validated tools designed to characterize the vague, nonclassic symptoms of hyperparathyroidism.[120]

Medical therapies have limited efficacy in treating PHPT. Cinacalcet, a calcimimetic agent, normalizes serum calcium levels but has no beneficial effect on BMD.[121] Bisphosphonates improve BMD in patients with PHPT[122] but do not reduce fracture risk. Indeed, bisphosphonate treatment seems to be associated with increased fracture risk in patients with PHPT compared with observation, although this finding requires further study.[37]

CURRENT CONTROVERSIES

Limited Exploration Versus 4-Gland Exploration

Before the 1980s, bilateral (4-gland) exploration was performed for all patients with PHPT. Advances in parathyroid imaging, most notably sestamibi scanning and ultrasound scan, enabled limited (less than 4-gland) exploration to be performed in patients suspected of having an underlying single adenoma.[123] Limited exploration gained popularity through the 1990s as intraoperative PTH monitoring became increasingly available as a rapid and practical indicator of when surgery could be concluded without examining all of the parathyroid glands.[124] Short-term eucalcemia rates for limited exploration and 4-gland exploration were found to be equivalent and consistently greater than 95% in expert centers.[125,126]

The trend toward limited exploration seemed to reverse somewhat after 2010, because of several large-scale studies showing increased rates of long-term disease recurrence in patients undergoing limited exploration, presumably attributable to the presence of additional hypersecreting glands not discovered during limited exploration.[127–129] An increased rate of eucalcemic PTH elevations has been found in patients treated with limited exploration,[130] but the clinical significance of this finding remains unclear. Currently, both limited exploration and bilateral exploration are considered acceptable surgical approaches to patients with PHPT.[66]

Surgery for Asymptomatic Patients

Currently, surgery is recommended for all symptomatic patients with PHPT and select asymptomatic patients who meet one or more consensus criteria.[50] The current consensus criteria include:

- Serum calcium 1.0 mg/dL greater than upper limit of normal
- BMD by dual-energy X-ray absorptiometry with T-score less than 2.5 at lumbar spine, total hip, femoral neck, or distal one-third radius
- Vertebral fracture by radiograph, CT, MRI, or vertebral fracture assessment
- Creatinine clearance less than 60 mL/min
- 24-hour urine calcium greater than 400 mg/dL and increased stone risk by biochemical stone risk analysis
- Presence of nephrolithiasis or nephrocalcinosis by radiograph, ultrasound scan, or CT
- Age less than 50 years

In community practice, PHPT is undertreated: approximately half of patients with PHPT meet consensus criteria for surgery at the time of diagnosis, and about half of those actually undergo surgery.[2] Lack of adherence to the consensus guidelines may be driven by low physician awareness of the guidelines.[131] Several of the individual consensus criteria are supported by low-quality evidence from outdated studies[114] or reports with single-digit sample sizes.[132] In a recent large-scale study examining fracture risk in PHPT, subgroup analysis was performed to compare treatment effects in patients who met consensus guidelines for surgery and those who did not. Parathyroidectomy was associated with reduced fracture risk in both groups of patients.[37] Because fracture risk is likely the dominant clinical concern in the management of PHPT, experts may wish to re-assess eligibility for parathyroid surgery in light of these new data.

FUTURE CONSIDERATIONS

Priority topics for future investigation include the natural history of mild asymptomatic PHPT and the effectiveness of novel pharmacologic therapies. As discussed in the previous section, parathyroidectomy seems to be associated with reduced fracture risk in asymptomatic PHPT patients deemed eligible for observation by current guidelines.[37] The comparative effectiveness of observation versus surgery for mild asymptomatic PHPT needs to be studied prospectively with an emphasis on fracture-related outcomes and quality of life.

The RANK ligand inhibitor denosumab was approved in the United States in 2010 for the treatment of high-risk osteoporosis in postmenopausal women and patients undergoing endocrine therapy for breast and prostate malignancies.[133] Although the mechanism of action of this monoclonal antibody makes it an attractive potential treatment of parathyroid-mediated loss of bone density, protocol-based study in PHPT patients is necessary.

SUMMARY

The presentation of PHPT has changed from nephrolithiasis and severe osseous complications to mild, minimally symptomatic disease. The incidence is likely to continue increasing with the routine biochemical screening of our aging population. When presented with asymptomatic PHPT, the diagnosing clinician should recognize that their patient's future bone health hangs in the balance. Parathyroidectomy is the only definitive treatment of primary hyperparathyroidism. In the hands of an experienced parathyroid surgeon, this procedure is now frequently performed on an outpatient basis with excellent long-term results.

REFERENCES

1. Yeh MW, Ituarte PH, Zhou HC, et al. Incidence and prevalence of primary hyperparathyroidism in a racially mixed population. J Clin Endocrinol Metab 2013;98(3):1122–9.
2. Yeh MW, Wiseman JE, Ituarte PH, et al. Surgery for primary hyperparathyroidism: are the consensus guidelines being followed? Ann Surg 2012;255(6):1179–83.
3. Cohen J, Gierlowski TC, Schneider AB. A prospective study of hyperparathyroidism in individuals exposed to radiation in childhood. JAMA 1990;264(5):581–4.
4. Stephen AE, Chen KT, Milas M, et al. The coming of age of radiation-induced hyperparathyroidism: evolving patterns of thyroid and parathyroid disease after head and neck irradiation. Surgery 2004;136(6):1143–53.
5. McMullen T, Bodie G, Gill A, et al. Hyperparathyroidism after irradiation for childhood malignancy. Int J Radiat Oncol Biol Phys 2009;73(4):1164–8.
6. Woll ML, Mazeh H, Anderson BM, et al. Breast radiation correlates with side of parathyroid adenoma. World J Surg 2012;36(3):607–11.
7. Shen F-H, Sherrard DJ. Lithium-induced hyperparathyroidism: an alteration of the set-point. Ann Intern Med 1982;96(1):63–5.
8. Mallette LE, Khouri K, Zengotita H, et al. Lithium Treatment Increases Intact and Midregion Parathyroid Hormone and Parathyroid Volume. J Clin Endocrinol Metab 1989;68(3):654–60.
9. Sharretts JM, Simonds WF. Clinical and molecular genetics of parathyroid neoplasms. Best Pract Res Clin Endocrinol Metab 2010;24(3):491–502.
10. Simonds WF, James-Newton LA, Agarwal SK, et al. Familial isolated hyperparathyroidism: clinical and genetic characteristics of 36 kindreds. Medicine 2002;81(1):1–26.
11. Akerstrom G, Rudberg C, Grimelius L, et al. Histologic parathyroid abnormalities in an autopsy series. Hum Pathol 1986;17(5):520–7.
12. Cope O. The study of hyperparathyroidism at the Massachusetts General Hospital. N Engl J Med 1966;274(21):1174–82.
13. Guru SC, Goldsmith PK, Burns AL, et al. Menin, the product of the MEN1 gene, is a nuclear protein. Proc Natl Acad Sci U S A 1998;95(4):1630–4.
14. Heppner C, Kester MB, Agarwal SK, et al. Somatic mutation of the MEN1 gene in parathyroid tumours. Nat Genet 1997;16(4):375–8.

15. Lemos MC, Thakker RV. Multiple endocrine neoplasia type 1 (MEN1): analysis of 1336 mutations reported in the first decade following identification of the gene. Hum Mutat 2008;29(1):22–32.
16. Pieterman CR, van Hulsteijn LT, den Heijer M, et al. Primary hyperparathyroidism in MEN1 patients: a cohort study with longterm follow-up on preferred surgical procedure and the relation with genotype. Ann Surg 2012;255(6):1171–8.
17. Miedlich S, Krohn K, Lamesch P, et al. Frequency of somatic MEN1 gene mutations in monoclonal parathyroid tumours of patients with primary hyperparathyroidism. Eur J Endocrinol 2000;143(1):47–54.
18. Scarpelli D, D'Aloiso L, Arturi F, et al. Novel somatic MEN1 gene alterations in sporadic primary hyperparathyroidism and correlation with clinical characteristics. J Endocrinol Invest 2004;27(11):1015–21.
19. Uchino S, Noguchi S, Sato M, et al. Screening of the Men1 gene and discovery of germ-line and somatic mutations in apparently sporadic parathyroid tumors. Cancer Res 2000;60(19):5553–7.
20. Shattuck TM, Välimäki S, Obara T, et al. Somatic and germ-line mutations of the HRPT2 gene in sporadic parathyroid carcinoma. N Engl J Med 2003;349(18): 1722–9.
21. Carpten J, Robbins C, Villablanca A, et al. HRPT2, encoding parafibromin, is mutated in hyperparathyroidism–jaw tumor syndrome. Nat Genet 2002;32(4): 676–80.
22. Arighi E, Borrello MG, Sariola H. RET tyrosine kinase signaling in development and cancer. Cytokine Growth Factor Rev 2005;16(4):441–67.
23. Wells SA Jr, Asa SL, Dralle H, et al. Revised American Thyroid Association guidelines for the management of medullary thyroid carcinoma: the American Thyroid Association Guidelines Task Force on medullary thyroid carcinoma. Thyroid 2015;25(6):567–610.
24. Eng C, Clayton D, Schuffenecker I, et al. The relationship between specific RET proto-oncogene mutations and disease phenotype in multiple endocrine neoplasia type 2: International RET Mutation Consortium analysis. JAMA 1996;276(19):1575–9.
25. Komminoth P, Roth J, Muletta-Feurer S, et al. RET proto-oncogene point mutations in sporadic neuroendocrine tumors. J Clin Endocrinol Metab 1996;81(6): 2041–6.
26. Rosenberg C, Kim H, Shows T, et al. Rearrangement and overexpression of D11S287E, a candidate oncogene on chromosome 11q13 in benign parathyroid tumors. Oncogene 1991;6(3):449–53.
27. Vasef MA, Brynes RK, Sturm M, et al. Expression of cyclin D1 in parathyroid carcinomas, adenomas, and hyperplasias: a paraffin immunohistochemical study. Mod Pathol 1999;12(4):412–6.
28. Pollak MR, Brown EM, Chou Y-HW, et al. Mutations in the human Ca 2+-sensing receptor gene cause familial hypocalciuric hypercalcemia and neonatal severe hyperparathyroidism. Cell 1993;75(7):1297–303.
29. Pearce S, Steinmann B. Casting new light on the clinical spectrum of neonatal severe hyperparathyroidism. Clin Endocrinol 1999;50(6):691–3.
30. Al-Shanafey S, Al-Hosaini R, Al-Ashwal A, et al. Surgical management of severe neonatal hyperparathyroidism: one center's experience. J Pediatr Surg 2010; 45(4):714–7.
31. Pidasheva S, D'Souza-Li L, Canaff L, et al. CASRdb: calcium-sensing receptor locus-specific database for mutations causing familial (benign) hypocalciuric

hypercalcemia, neonatal severe hyperparathyroidism, and autosomal dominant hypocalcemia. Hum Mutat 2004;24(2):107–11.
32. Christensen SE, Nissen PH, Vestergaard P, et al. Skeletal consequences of familial hypocalciuric hypercalcaemia vs. primary hyperparathyroidism. Clin Endocrinol 2009;71(6):798–807.
33. Mayr B, Schnabel D, Dorr HG, et al. Genetics in endocrinology: gain and loss of function mutations of the calcium-sensing receptor and associated proteins: current treatment concepts. Eur J Endocrinol 2016;174(5):R189–208.
34. Cetani F, Pinchera A, Pardi E, et al. No evidence for mutations in the calcium-sensing receptor gene in sporadic parathyroid adenomas. J Bone Miner Res 1999;14(6):878–82.
35. Farnebo F, Enberg U, Grimelius L, et al. Tumor-Specific Decreased Expression of Calcium Sensing Receptor Messenger Ribonucleic Acid in Sporadic Primary Hyperparathyroidism 1. J Clin Endocrinol Metab 1997;82(10):3481–6.
36. Rubin MR, Bilezikian JP, McMahon DJ, et al. The natural history of primary hyperparathyroidism with or without parathyroid surgery after 15 years. J Clin Endocrinol Metab 2008;93(9):3462–70.
37. Yeh MW, Zhou H, Adams AL, et al. The Relationship of Parathyroidectomy and Bisphosphonates With Fracture Risk in Primary Hyperparathyroidism: An Observational Study. Ann Intern Med 2016;164(11):715–23.
38. Ma YL, Cain RL, Halladay DL, et al. Catabolic effects of continuous human PTH (1–38) in vivo is associated with sustained stimulation of RANKL and inhibition of osteoprotegerin and gene-associated bone formation. Endocrinology 2001; 142(9):4047–54.
39. Silverberg SJ, Shane E, de la Cruz L, et al. Skeletal disease in primary hyperparathyroidism. J Bone Miner Res 1989;4(3):283–91.
40. Parisien M, Silverberg SJ, Shane E, et al. The histomorphometry of bone in primary hyperparathyroidism: preservation of cancellous bone structure. J Clin Endocrinol Metab 1990;70(4):930–8.
41. Dempster DW, Muller R, Zhou H, et al. Preserved three-dimensional cancellous bone structure in mild primary hyperparathyroidism. Bone 2007;41(1):19–24.
42. Khosla S, Melton LJ 3rd, Wermers RA, et al. Primary hyperparathyroidism and the risk of fracture: a population-based study. J Bone Miner Res 1999;14(10): 1700–7.
43. Vestergaard P, Mollerup CL, Frokjaer VG, et al. Cohort study of risk of fracture before and after surgery for primary hyperparathyroidism. BMJ 2000; 321(7261):598–602.
44. Vignali E, Viccica G, Diacinti D, et al. Morphometric vertebral fractures in postmenopausal women with primary hyperparathyroidism. J Clin Endocrinol Metab 2009;94(7):2306–12.
45. Yu N, Donnan PT, Flynn RW, et al. Increased mortality and morbidity in mild primary hyperparathyroid patients. The Parathyroid Epidemiology and Audit Research Study (PEARS). Clin Endocrinol (Oxf) 2010;73(1):30–4.
46. Boutroy S, Bouxsein ML, Munoz F, et al. In vivo assessment of trabecular bone microarchitecture by high-resolution peripheral quantitative computed tomography. J Clin Endocrinol Metab 2005;90(12):6508–15.
47. Vu TD, Wang XF, Wang Q, et al. New insights into the effects of primary hyperparathyroidism on the cortical and trabecular compartments of bone. Bone 2013;55(1):57–63.
48. Hansen S, Beck Jensen JE, Rasmussen L, et al. Effects on bone geometry, density, and microarchitecture in the distal radius but not the tibia in women with

primary hyperparathyroidism: A case-control study using HR-pQCT. J Bone Miner Res 2010;25(9):1941–7.
49. Stein EM, Silva BC, Boutroy S, et al. Primary hyperparathyroidism is associated with abnormal cortical and trabecular microstructure and reduced bone stiffness in postmenopausal women. J Bone Miner Res 2013;28(5):1029–40.
50. Bilezikian JP, Brandi ML, Eastell R, et al. Guidelines for the management of asymptomatic primary hyperparathyroidism: summary statement from the Fourth International Workshop. J Clin Endocrinol Metab 2014;99(10):3561–9.
51. Ahmad S, Kuraganti G, Steenkamp D. Hypercalcemic crisis: a clinical review. Am J Med 2015;128(3):239–45.
52. Heath H 3rd, Hodgson SF, Kennedy MA. Primary hyperparathyroidism. Incidence, morbidity, and potential economic impact in a community. N Engl J Med 1980;302(4):189–93.
53. Silverberg SJ, Clarke BL, Peacock M, et al. Current issues in the presentation of asymptomatic primary hyperparathyroidism: proceedings of the Fourth International Workshop. J Clin Endocrinol Metab 2014;99(10):3580–94.
54. NIH conference. Diagnosis and management of asymptomatic primary hyperparathyroidism: consensus development conference statement. Ann Intern Med 1991;114(7):593–7.
55. Bilezikian JP, Potts JT Jr, Fuleihan Gel H, et al. Summary statement from a workshop on asymptomatic primary hyperparathyroidism: a perspective for the 21st century. J Clin Endocrinol Metab 2002;87(12):5353–61.
56. Bilezikian JP, Khan AA, Potts JT Jr. Third International Workshop on the Management of Asymptomatic Primary H. Guidelines for the management of asymptomatic primary hyperparathyroidism: summary statement from the third international workshop. J Clin Endocrinol Metab 2009;94(2):335–9.
57. Silverberg SJ, Shane E, Jacobs TP, et al. Nephrolithiasis and bone involvement in primary hyperparathyroidism. Am J Med 1990;89(3):327–34.
58. Pak CY, Nicar MJ, Peterson R, et al. A lack of unique pathophysiologic background for nephrolithiasis of primary hyperparathyroidism. J Clin Endocrinol Metab 1981;53(3):536–42.
59. Suh JM, Cronan JJ, Monchik JM. Primary hyperparathyroidism: is there an increased prevalence of renal stone disease? AJR Am J Roentgenol 2008;191(3):908–11.
60. Tassone F, Gianotti L, Emmolo I, et al. Glomerular filtration rate and parathyroid hormone secretion in primary hyperparathyroidism. J Clin Endocrinol Metab 2009;94(11):4458–61.
61. Yu N, Donnan PT, Leese GP. A record linkage study of outcomes in patients with mild primary hyperparathyroidism: the Parathyroid Epidemiology and Audit Research Study (PEARS). Clin Endocrinol 2011;75(2):169–76.
62. Ambrogini E, Cetani F, Cianferotti L, et al. Surgery or surveillance for mild asymptomatic primary hyperparathyroidism: a prospective, randomized clinical trial. J Clin Endocrinol Metab 2007;92(8):3114–21.
63. Lundstam K, Heck A, Mollerup C, et al. Effects of parathyroidectomy versus observation on the development of vertebral fractures in mild primary hyperparathyroidism. J Clin Endocrinol Metab 2015;100(4):1359–67.
64. Rao DS, Phillips ER, Divine GW, et al. Randomized controlled clinical trial of surgery versus no surgery in patients with mild asymptomatic primary hyperparathyroidism. J Clin Endocrinol Metab 2004;89(11):5415–22.

65. Sanders K, Pasco J, Ugoni A, et al. The exclusion of high trauma fractures may underestimate the prevalence of bone fragility fractures in the community: the Geelong Osteoporosis Study. J Bone Miner Res 1998;13(8):1337–42.
66. Wilhelm SM, Wang TS, Ruan DT, et al. The American association of endocrine surgeons guidelines for definitive management of primary hyperparathyroidism. JAMA surgery 2016;151(10):959–68.
67. Mohan M, Neelakandan RS, Siddharth D, et al. An unusual case of brown tumor of hyperparathyroidism associated with ectopic parathyroid adenoma. Eur J Dent 2013;7(4):500.
68. Morton JJ. The generalized type of osteitis fibrosa cystica: von recklinghausen's disease. Arch Surg 1922;4(3):534–66.
69. Mishra S, Agarwal G, Kar D, et al. Unique clinical characteristics of primary hyperparathyroidism in India. Br J Surg 2001;88(5):708–14.
70. Zhao L, Liu J-M, He X-Y, et al. The changing clinical patterns of primary hyperparathyroidism in Chinese patients: data from 2000 to 2010 in a single clinical center. J Clin Endocrinol Metab 2013;98(2):721–8.
71. Bandeira F, Griz L, Caldas G, et al. From mild to severe primary hyperparathyroidism: the Brazilian experience. Arq Bras Endocrinol Metabol 2006;50(4): 657–63.
72. Stewart AF. Hypercalcemia associated with cancer. N Engl J Med 2005;352(4): 373–9.
73. Khosla S. Hypercalcemia and hypocalcemia. In: Kasper DFA, Hauser S, Longo D, et al, editors. Harrison's principles of internal medicine. 19th edition. New York: McGraw-Hill; 2015. p. 313–5.
74. Vaidya A, Curhan GC, Paik JM, et al. Hypertension, antihypertensive medications, and risk of incident primary hyperparathyroidism. J Clin Endocrinol Metab 2015;100(6):2396–404.
75. Zhao G, Ford ES, Li C, et al. Independent associations of serum concentrations of 25-hydroxyvitamin D and parathyroid hormone with blood pressure among US adults. J Hypertens 2010;28(9):1821–8.
76. Van Ballegooijen AJ, Kestenbaum B, Sachs MC, et al. Association of 25-hydroxyvitamin D and parathyroid hormone with incident hypertension: MESA (Multi-Ethnic Study of Atherosclerosis). J Am Coll Cardiol 2014;63(12):1214–22.
77. Yagi S, Aihara K, Kondo T, et al. High serum parathyroid hormone and calcium are risk factors for hypertension in Japanese patients. Endocr J 2014;61(7): 727–33.
78. Nainby-Luxmoore J, Langford H, Nelson N, et al. A case-comparison study of hypertension and hyperparathyroidism. J Clin Endocrinol Metab 1982;55(2): 303–6.
79. Feldstein CA, Akopian M, Pietrobelli D, et al. Long-term effects of parathyroidectomy on hypertension prevalence and circadian blood pressure profile in primary hyperparathyroidism. Clin Exp Hypertens 2010;32(3):154–8.
80. Heyliger A, Tangpricha V, Weber C, et al. Parathyroidectomy decreases systolic and diastolic blood pressure in hypertensive patients with primary hyperparathyroidism. Surgery 2009;146(6):1042–7.
81. Nilsson I-L, Åberg J, Rastad J, et al. Maintained normalization of cardiovascular dysfunction 5 years after parathyroidectomy in primary hyperparathyroidism. Surgery 2005;137(6):632–8.
82. Piovesan A, Molineri N, Casasso F, et al. Left ventricular hypertrophy in primary hyperparathyroidism. Effects of successful parathyroidectomy. Clin Endocrinol 1999;50(3):321–8.

83. Soreide JA, van Heerden JA, Grant CS, et al. Survival after surgical treatment for primary hyperparathyroidism. Surgery 1997;122(6):1117–23.
84. Wermers RA, Khosla S, Atkinson EJ, et al. Survival after the diagnosis of hyperparathyroidism: a population-based study. Am J Med 1998;104(2):115–22.
85. Hedback G, Tisell LE, Bengtsson BA, et al. Premature death in patients operated on for primary hyperparathyroidism. World J Surg 1990;14(6):829–35 [discussion: 836].
86. Ogard CG, Engholm G, Almdal TP, et al. Increased mortality in patients hospitalized with primary hyperparathyroidism during the period 1977-1993 in Denmark. World J Surg 2004;28(1):108–11.
87. Palmer M, Adami HO, Bergstrom R, et al. Mortality after surgery for primary hyperparathyroidism: a follow-up of 441 patients operated on from 1956 to 1979. Surgery 1987;102(1):1–7.
88. Vestergaard P, Mollerup CL, Frokjaer VG, et al. Cardiovascular events before and after surgery for primary hyperparathyroidism. World J Surg 2003;27(2): 216–22.
89. Eigelberger MS, Cheah WK, Ituarte PH, et al. The NIH criteria for parathyroidectomy in asymptomatic primary hyperparathyroidism: are they too limited? Ann Surg 2004;239(4):528–35.
90. Roman SA, Sosa JA, Mayes L, et al. Parathyroidectomy improves neurocognitive deficits in patients with primary hyperparathyroidism. Surgery 2005; 138(6):1121–8 [discussion: 1128–9].
91. Kahal H, Aye M, Rigby AS, et al. The effect of parathyroidectomy on neuropsychological symptoms and biochemical parameters in patients with asymptomatic primary hyperparathyroidism. Clin Endocrinol (Oxf) 2012;76(2):196–200.
92. Zanocco K, Butt Z, Kaltman D, et al. Improvement in patient-reported physical and mental health after parathyroidectomy for primary hyperparathyroidism. Surgery 2015;158(3):837–45.
93. Lafferty FW. Differential diagnosis of hypercalcemia. J Bone Miner Res 1991; 6(S2):S51–9.
94. Boonstra CE, Jackson CE. Hyperparathyroidism detected by routine serum calcium analysis: prevalence in a clinic population. Ann Intern Med 1965;63(3): 468–74.
95. Christensson T, Hellström K, Wengle B, et al. Prevalence of hypercalcaemia in a health screening in Stockholm. Acta Med Scand 1976;200(1–6):131–7.
96. Christensen SE, Nissen PH, Vestergaard P, et al. Discriminative power of three indices of renal calcium excretion for the distinction between familial hypocalciuric hypercalcaemia and primary hyperparathyroidism: a follow-up study on methods. Clin Endocrinol 2008;69(5):713–20.
97. Cusano NE, Silverberg SJ, Bilezikian JP. Normocalcemic primary hyperparathyroidism. J Clin Densitom 2013;16(1):33–9.
98. Erovic BM, Goldstein DP, Kim D, et al. Parathyroid cancer: outcome analysis of 16 patients treated at the princess Margaret hospital. Head Neck 2013;35(1):35–9.
99. Harari A, Waring A, Fernandez-Ranvier G, et al. Parathyroid carcinoma: a 43-year outcome and survival analysis. J Clin Endocrinol Metab 2011;96(12): 3679–86.
100. Schaapveld M, Jorna FH, Aben KK, et al. Incidence and prognosis of parathyroid gland carcinoma: a population-based study in The Netherlands estimating the preoperative diagnosis. Am J Surg 2011;202(5):590–7.
101. Wei CH, Harari A. Parathyroid carcinoma: update and guidelines for management. Curr Treat Options Oncol 2012;13(1):11–23.

102. Adami S, Parfitt A. Calcium-induced natriuresis: physiologic and clinical implications. Calcif Tissue Int 2000;66(6):425–9.
103. Cheung K, Wang TS, Farrokhyar F, et al. A meta-analysis of preoperative localization techniques for patients with primary hyperparathyroidism. Ann Surg Oncol 2012;19(2):577–83.
104. Cham S, Sepahdari AR, Hall KE, et al. Dynamic Parathyroid Computed tomography (4DCT) facilitates reoperative parathyroidectomy and enables cure of missed hyperplasia. Ann Surg Oncol 2015;22(11):3537–42.
105. Udelsman R, Akerstrom G, Biagini C, et al. The surgical management of asymptomatic primary hyperparathyroidism: proceedings of the fourth international workshop. J Clin Endocrinol Metab 2014;99(10):3595–606.
106. Carling T, Donovan P, Rinder C, et al. Minimally invasive parathyroidectomy using cervical block: reasons for conversion to general anesthesia. Arch Surg 2006;141(4):401–4 [discussion: 404].
107. Udelsman R, Donovan PI. Open minimally invasive parathyroid surgery. World J Surg 2004;28(12):1224–6.
108. Carty SE. Prevention and management of complications in parathyroid surgery. Otolaryngol Clin North Am 2004;37(4):897–907.xi.
109. Yeh MW, Wiseman JE, Chu SD, et al. Population-level predictors of persistent hyperparathyroidism. Surgery 2011;150(6):1113–9.
110. Stavrakis AI, Ituarte PH, Ko CY, et al. Surgeon volume as a predictor of outcomes in inpatient and outpatient endocrine surgery. Surgery 2007;142(6): 887–99 [discussion: 887–99].
111. Abdulla AG, Ituarte PH, Harari A, et al. Trends in the frequency and quality of parathyroid surgery: analysis of 17,082 cases over 10 years. Ann Surg 2015; 261(4):746–50.
112. Yu N, Leese GP, Smith D, et al. The natural history of treated and untreated primary hyperparathyroidism: the parathyroid epidemiology and audit research study. QJM 2011;104(6):513–21.
113. Rejnmark L, Vestergaard P, Mosekilde L. Nephrolithiasis and renal calcifications in primary hyperparathyroidism. J Clin Endocrinol Metab 2011;96(8): 2377–85.
114. Hendrickson CD, Castro Pereira DJ, Comi RJ. Renal impairment as a surgical indication in primary hyperparathyroidism: do the data support this recommendation? J Clin Endocrinol Metab 2014;99(8):2646–50.
115. Yu N, Leese GP, Donnan PT. What predicts adverse outcomes in untreated primary hyperparathyroidism? The parathyroid epidemiology and audit research study (PEARS). Clin Endocrinol (Oxf) 2013;79(1):27–34.
116. Macfarlane DP, Yu N, Donnan PT, et al. Should 'mild primary hyperparathyroidism' be reclassified as 'insidious': is it time to reconsider? Clin Endocrinol (Oxf) 2011;75(6):730–7.
117. Nilsson IL, Wadsten C, Brandt L, et al. Mortality in sporadic primary hyperparathyroidism: nationwide cohort study of multiple parathyroid gland disease. Surgery 2004;136(5):981–7.
118. Mollerup CL, Vestergaard P, Frokjaer VG, et al. Risk of renal stone events in primary hyperparathyroidism before and after parathyroid surgery: controlled retrospective follow up study. BMJ 2002;325(7368):807.
119. Tassone F, Guarnieri A, Castellano E, et al. Parathyroidectomy halts the deterioration of renal function in primary hyperparathyroidism. J Clin Endocrinol Metab 2015;100(8):3069–73.

120. Pasieka JL, Parsons L, Jones J. The long-term benefit of parathyroidectomy in primary hyperparathyroidism: a 10-year prospective surgical outcome study. Surgery 2009;146(6):1006–13.
121. Peacock M, Bolognese MA, Borofsky M, et al. Cinacalcet treatment of primary hyperparathyroidism: biochemical and bone densitometric outcomes in a five-year study. J Clin Endocrinol Metab 2009;94(12):4860–7.
122. Sankaran S, Gamble G, Bolland M, et al. Skeletal effects of interventions in mild primary hyperparathyroidism: a meta-analysis. J Clin Endocrinol Metab 2010; 95(4):1653–62.
123. Palazzo FF, Sadler GP. Minimally invasive parathyroidectomy. BMJ 2004; 328(7444):849–50.
124. Irvin GL 3rd. American Association of Endocrine Surgeons. Presidential address: chasin' hormones. Surgery 1999;126(6):993–7.
125. Bergenfelz A, Lindblom P, Tibblin S, et al. Unilateral versus bilateral neck exploration for primary hyperparathyroidism: a prospective randomized controlled trial. Ann Surg 2002;236(5):543–51.
126. McGill J, Sturgeon C, Kaplan SP, et al. How does the operative strategy for primary hyperparathyroidism impact the findings and cure rate? A comparison of 800 parathyroidectomies. J Am Coll Surg 2008;207(2):246–9.
127. Schneider DF, Mazeh H, Sippel RS, et al. Is minimally invasive parathyroidectomy associated with greater recurrence compared to bilateral exploration? Analysis of more than 1,000 cases. Surgery 2012;152(6):1008–15.
128. Norman J, Lopez J, Politz D. Abandoning unilateral parathyroidectomy: why we reversed our position after 15,000 parathyroid operations. J Am Coll Surg 2012; 214(3):260–9.
129. Siperstein A, Berber E, Barbosa GF, et al. Predicting the success of limited exploration for primary hyperparathyroidism using ultrasound, sestamibi, and intraoperative parathyroid hormone: analysis of 1158 cases. Ann Surg 2008; 248(3):420–8.
130. Pasieka JL. What should we tell our patients? Lifetime guarantee or is it 5- to 10-year warranty on a parathyroidectomy for primary hyperparathyroidism? World J Surg 2015;39(8):1928–9.
131. Mahadevia PJ, Sosa JA, Levine MA, et al. Clinical management of primary hyperparathyroidism and thresholds for surgical referral: a national study examining concordance between practice patterns and consensus panel recommendations. Endocr Pract 2003;9(6):494–503.
132. Silverberg SJ, Brown I, Bilezikian JP. Age as a criterion for surgery in primary hyperparathyroidism. Am J Med 2002;113(8):681–4.
133. McClung MR, Lewiecki EM, Cohen SB, et al. Denosumab in postmenopausal women with low bone mineral density. N Engl J Med 2006;354(8):821–31.

The Effects of Bariatric Surgery on Bone Metabolism

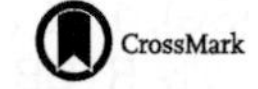

Naina Sinha Gregory, MD

KEYWORDS

- Obesity • Bariatric surgery • Adipokines • Gut hormones • Bone turnover markers • DXA

KEY POINTS

- Bariatric surgery seems to have detrimental effects on skeletal health through multiple mechanisms.
- The degree of bone loss seems to be related to the degree of malabsorption created with the varying procedures.
- Malabsorption of calcium and vitamin D in addition to a decrease in mechanical loading contributes to bone loss and changes in bone markers.
- The weight loss following surgery affects levels of adipokines, which have been found to have direct effects on bone metabolism.
- The anatomic changes following these surgeries affect gastrointestinal hormone secretion, which affects bone metabolism.

INTRODUCTION

Most recent estimates reveal that more than one-third (34.9%) of the US adult population is obese (body mass index [BMI], >30 kg/m^2). The subset of adults with extreme obesity (BMI>40 kg/m^2) continues to increase, with most recent estimates of 6.3%.[1] Obesity is associated with increased rates of several comorbidities, including type 2 diabetes, hypertension, dyslipidemia, coronary heart disease, sleep apnea, and stroke. In addition, there is an associated increase in rates of breast, endometrial, prostate, and colon cancers.[2] Bariatric surgery is an effective treatment of obesity and its associated conditions, leading to improvement or complete remission of diabetes, hypertension, dyslipidemia, and sleep apnea.[3] The numbers of these procedures continues to increase, with 179,000 performed in the United States in 2013. Of these, 34.2% were Roux-en-Y gastric bypass (RYGB), 42.1% sleeve gastrectomy

---

Disclosures: The author has nothing to disclose.
Division of Endocrinology, Department of Medicine, New York Presbyterian Hospital, Weill Cornell Medical College, 211 East 80th Street, New York, NY 10075, USA
E-mail address: sinhana@med.cornell.edu

Endocrinol Metab Clin N Am 46 (2017) 105–116
http://dx.doi.org/10.1016/j.ecl.2016.09.011
endo.theclinics.com
0889-8529/17/

(SG), 14% adjustable gastric banding (AGB), and 1% the duodenal switch.[4] Historically RYGB procedures accounted for most of the procedures performed over the past decade but the number of SG procedures has been steadily increasing.

Obesity has long been considered protective against bone disease, with higher BMI levels associated with increased bone density. However, vitamin D deficiency and increased parathyroid hormone levels are prevalent in obese individuals. The prevalence of vitamin D deficiency in obese individuals varies from 20% to 85%.[5] Possible explanations include lack of sufficient sun exposure and sequestration of vitamin D in adipose tissue.[6] In contrast with the improvement in many obesity-related conditions seen following bariatric surgery, vitamin D deficiency and secondary hyperparathyroidism do not improve and can even be further accelerated, especially with certain surgical procedures that have a significant malabsorptive component.[7]

Early bariatric procedures were more malabsorptive than the ones currently being performed and were associated with significant rates of vitamin and mineral deficiencies. The jejunoileal bypass and biliopancreatic diversion involved more extensive intestinal bypass[8] (**Fig. 1**). These early procedures were associated with significant skeletal loss attributable in large part to osteomalacia.[9]

The current surgeries being performed are less malabsorptive. In addition, more attention to skeletal health is being performed preoperatively. Vitamin D status is

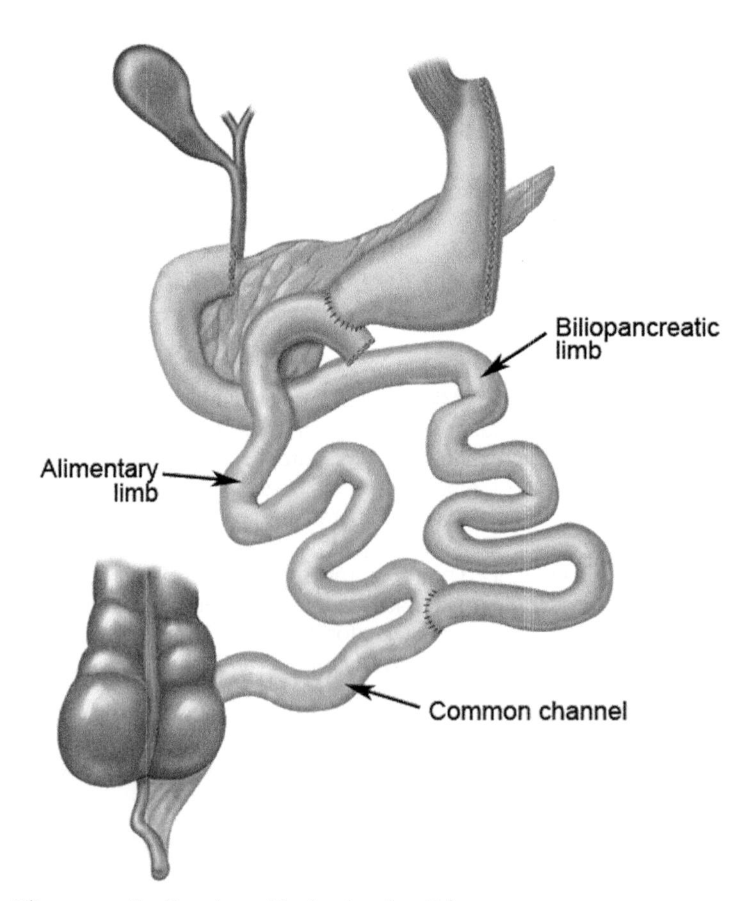

Fig. 1. Biliopancreatic diversion with duodenal switch.

now frequently being assessed and deficiencies corrected before surgery. Calcium supplementation is routinely given postoperatively. All of these factors must be taken into account when evaluating the impact of these procedures on bone health.

MECHANICAL UNLOADING

Mechanical loading of bone is associated with a decrease in sclerostin levels.[10] Sclerostin is known to have a negative impact on bone formation through the Wnt/B catenin pathway. Sclerostin antagonizes this pathway, which is involved in osteoblast function.[11] Mechanical loading of bone decreases sclerostin gene expression in osteocytes. Weight loss is associated with mechanical unloading and is expected to lead to increased sclerostin levels and associated bone loss. Studies evaluating sclerostin levels following diet-induced weight loss have shown an increase in sclerostin levels. These increases were prevented with resistance training.[12] There has been 1 study measuring sclerostin levels following RYGB and SG. Rapid and sustained increases in sclerostin level that were associated with significant loss in bone mineral density (BMD) were reported.[13] Sclerostin antibodies are currently being evaluated as a treatment of osteoporosis and may be an effective treatment of weight loss–associated bone loss.

CHANGES IN GASTROINTESTINAL HORMONE LEVELS

The RYGB procedure involves a significant alteration in anatomy in which a gastric pouch is connected to the proximal jejunum (Roux limb). The section of the intestine that is bypassed is referred to as the biliopancreatic limb and contains the biliary and pancreatic secretions. With this change in anatomy, the secretions of many gut hormones are affected.

Ghrelin is a gut hormone secreted by the gastric mucosa. Levels increase before meals and are suppressed following meals.[14] Ghrelin is known to be a stimulator of growth hormone (GH). GH is known to promote bone formation.[15] Ghrelin may positively affect bone metabolism through this GH axis but also seems to promote bone formation directly. Many in vitro studies have confirmed an effect of enhanced proliferation on osteoblasts.[16] Bariatric surgeries that remove the gastric fundus when creating a gastric pouch have been shown to decrease ghrelin levels.[17] Although most studies have shown a decrease in ghrelin following RYGB, there have been a few studies in which ghrelin levels have not changed or have been increased.[18] These inconsistent results have been explained by variations in the surgical creation of the gastric pouches and possible interference with vagal nerve function.[19] Decreased ghrelin levels are expected to have a negative impact on bone metabolism following surgery.

Glucose-dependent insulinotropic polypeptide (GIP) is a gut hormone secreted by the K cells in the proximal small intestine. Obesity is associated with increased levels of this hormone.[20] GIP has been shown in vitro to have antiapoptotic effects on osteoblasts in addition to an inhibitory effect on osteoclast resorption, both of which have a positive impact on bone metabolism.[21] Surgeries involving bypass of the proximal small bowel are expected to decrease GIP levels, which would negatively affect bone metabolism. Studies to date have generally shown decreased GIP levels but the impact on bone metabolism has not been clearly examined.[22]

Glucagonlike peptide-1 (GLP-1) is a gut hormone secreted by the L cells of the distal ileum and colon. It is known to have a potent effect on insulin secretion.[23] It also seems to have an impact on bone metabolism. Initial studies examining GLP-1 showed increased bone resorption through a calcitonin-dependent pathway.[24]

Further studies have revealed a positive impact on osteoblasts through a GPI/IPG (inositol phosphoglycan)-coupled receptor.[25] GLP-1 levels are increased following RYGB and this increase may positively affect bone metabolism, but further studies are needed for clarification.[26]

Peptide YY (PYY) is another gut hormone secreted by the L cells of the distal ileum and colon. It is known to reduce appetite and is found at lower levels in obesity.[27] Increased levels of PYY have been found in anorexia and are associated with low levels of bone turnover markers. PYY has been found to be negatively correlated with the bone formation marker PINP (Procollagen Type 1 N-Terminal Propertied).[28] These studies suggest a negative correlation between PYY and bone formation but animal models have revealed conflicting results.[29] RYGB has been associated with an increase in PYY levels. This increase in PYY levels has been associated with increases in CTX (C-terminal telopeptide) levels following RYGB.[30] Further studies are needed to evaluate the impact of this increase in PYY on bone metabolism.

Amylin is a hormone cosecreted with insulin from the beta cells of the pancreas. It is found at higher levels in obesity.[31] Amylin has been shown to enhance osteoblast proliferation and to inhibit osteoclast function, leading to a positive impact on bone metabolism.[32] Initial studies have described decreased amylin levels following RYGB but additional studies are needed to confirm these findings.[33] A decrease in amylin levels is expected to have a negative impact on bone metabolism.

Insulin is a hormone secreted by the beta cells of the pancreas. Studies have shown both positive and negative effects of insulin on bone metabolism. Insulin is known to promote osteoblast proliferation through the MAPK (mitogen-activated protein kinase) and PI3K (Phosphatidylinositol-3 kinase) pathway. Its anabolic effect also occurs through the insulinlike growth factor-1 pathway.[34] It also has an inhibitory effect on resorption through the insulin receptors on osteoclasts.[35] In contrast with these positive effects, insulin decreases osteoprotegerin level, which favors bone resorption.[36] Insulin levels have been positively associated with BMD. Many studies have shown decreased insulin levels following RYGB.[26] The expected impact would be negative on bone metabolism but further investigation is needed.

CHANGES IN FAT-DERIVED HORMONES

The number of roles of fat cells and their many functions continues to grow. Fat cells secrete many hormones called adipokines. Recently is has been discovered that there is much communication between fat and bone. Adipokines, including adiponectin and leptin, have been examined in the post–bariatric surgery population.

Levels of adiponectin have been found to be lower in obesity. It is involved in insulin sensitivity and fatty acid metabolism. It also has a role in bone metabolism and is secreted at low levels from bone-forming cells.[37] To date the exact role of adiponectin on bone remains unclear. Most studies have shown an inverse relationship between BMD and adiponectin,[38] which may be one of the factors explaining the protective effect of fat on bone. This relationship has not been confirmed in in vivo studies, in which adiponectin has been shown to inhibit osteoclast growth and increase osteoblast proliferation.[39] An increase in adiponectin has been seen post-RYGB but its impact on bone remains to be described. One study found a correlation between the increase in adiponectin and the decrease in BMD following RYGB surgery but additional studies have not confirmed this finding.[40]

Leptin is another hormone that is secreted by fat cells. Levels of leptin are proportional to fat stores. It has a role in energy expenditure and appetite regulation. There is an underlying leptin resistance in obese individuals so that there is inadequate suppression of appetite despite high levels of leptin.[41] Leptin receptors have been found on osteoblasts and osteoclasts and have an overall anabolic effect. It promotes osteoblast differentiation and matrix mineralization. It also inhibits osteoclast differentiation leading to an inhibition of bone resorption.[42] Leptin levels following surgery are decreased, with one study reporting the reduction in leptin to be positively correlated with the increase in bone resorption markers.[26] There is some evidence that there may be a negative impact on bone through a central effect of leptin through a sympathetic pathway, but further investigation is needed.[43]

EFFECT OF SURGERY ON BONE MARKERS, BONE DENSITY, AND FRACTURE RISK

Roux-en-Y Gastric Bypass

RYGB is a combination restrictive and malabsorptive procedure. It has been the most commonly performed bariatric procedure in the past decade. The first part involves formation of a gastric pouch roughly 20 to 30 cm^3 in volume, which comprises the restrictive component. This pouch is anastomosed further downstream to the proximal jejunum. This bypass of most of the stomach and duodenum accounts for the malabsorptive component (**Fig. 2**). The excess weight loss averages 65% to 70% with this procedure.[4]

Early reports of the effect of this procedure on skeletal health included hypocalcemia, osteitis fibrosa cystica, and osteomalacia.[44] Many studies found a marked

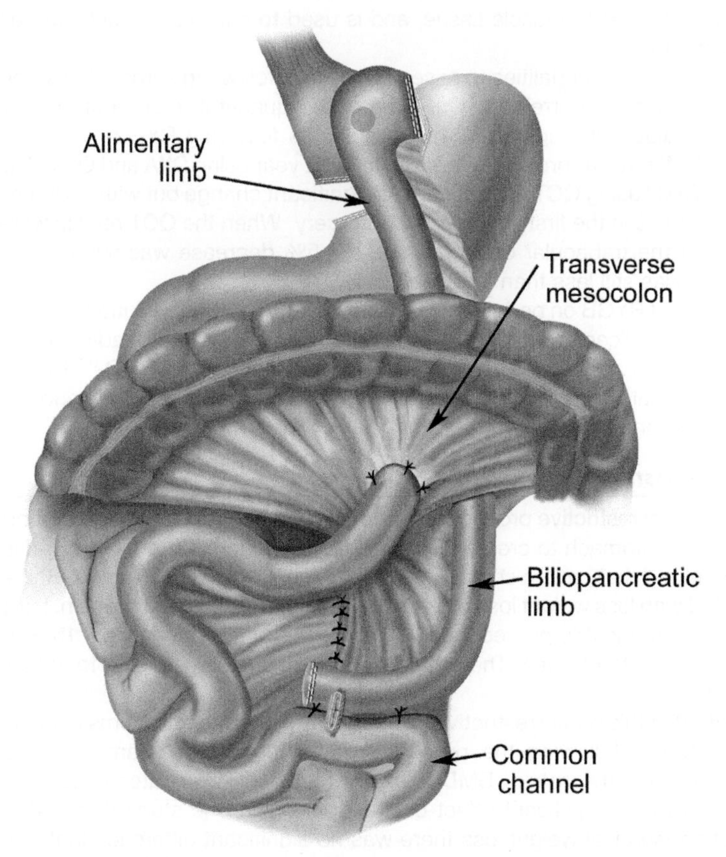

Fig. 2. Roux-en-Y gastric bypass.

increase in bone resorption markers as early as 3 months following surgery. This increase in resorption was found to persist 2 years following surgery.[45] An increase in markers of bone formation has also been seen but the increase in resorption markers has been greater. This finding suggests that the overall net effect favors bone loss following surgery.

When bone density using dual energy x-ray absorptiometry (DXA) methodology was used, RYGB was associated with significant decreases in both spine and hip, with more pronounced decreases found at the hip. On average the rate of bone loss following surgery approaches 10% per year at the hip and 5% at the spine. The effect on wrist DXA has been variable.[46]

When examining these studies, the limitations of DXA in the setting of obesity and weight loss must be taken into consideration. Most DXA scanners have a weight limit of 160 kg (350 lb), although newer models can go up to 200 kg (450 lb). Changes in soft tissue also affect accuracy of measurement. The accuracy of DXA measurements varies as body composition changes. The impact on the accuracy cannot be predicted and varies based on the different manufacturers of the DXA and the technology used (eg, fan beam vs pencil beam).[47] Fan-beam scanners are particularly prone to projection artifact, in which a change in the distance from source to the bone can alter measurements. This artifact can be a significant limitation given the amount of weight loss following these bariatric procedures. Another significant limitation of using DXA in this population is the 2-component ratio. This ratio refers to the DXA calculations that involve ratios of fat to muscle tissue, and is used to calculate muscle, fat, and bone measurements.[48]

When alternative modalities to assess bone loss following surgery have been used, the results have not correlated. One study used quantitative computed tomography (QCT) to evaluate the spine and hip in subjects following RYGB. The decrease in the spine BMD was approximately 3% in the first year using DXA and QCT. The results of the hip BMD using QCT did not show a significant change but with DXA there was a decrease of 8% in the first year following surgery. When the QCT results were further analyzed at the trabecular compartment, a 4.5% decrease was seen, although the magnitude was still less than that seen with DXA.[49]

The effect of RYGB on peripheral bone density using high-resolution peripheral QCT has shown significant decreases in volumetric BMD at both the radius and the tibia. Further analysis revealed a decrease in cortical volumetric BMD.[50] Resorption at the endocortical layer was also described. Increased cortical porosity and decreased tibial bone strength has also been found.

Adjustable Gastric Banding

AGB is a purely restrictive procedure in which a silicone band is placed around the top portion of the stomach to create a smaller gastric pouch (**Fig. 3**). The band limits the amount of food that can be consumed at one time. Compared with RYGB, the AGB is associated with less weight loss overall and a higher rate of weight regain. It is the third most common bariatric procedure performed, accounting for roughly 15% of all surgeries in the United States. The excess weight loss averages 40% to 45% with this procedure.[4]

The effect of this purely restrictive procedure on the skeleton seems to be less detrimental. Studies following the procedure have found less dramatic increases in markers of bone resorption. BMD changes revealed lower rates of loss in the hip (3%–5%) with no significant effect on the spine.[51] In one study that had a control group of nonsurgical weight loss there was no significant difference in the decrease in BMD when the 2 groups were compared.[52]

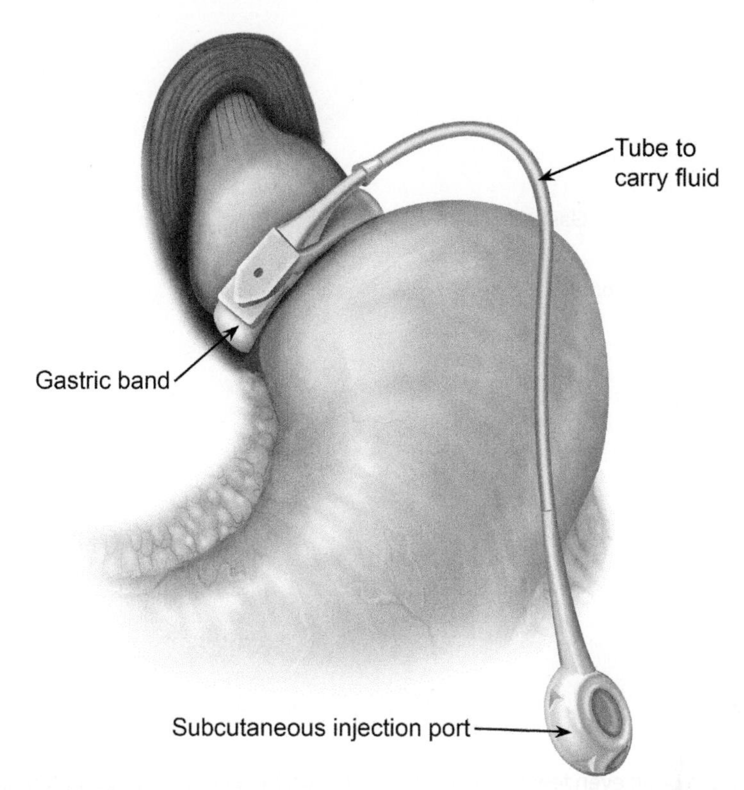

Fig. 3. Jones band.

There are fewer studies examining the effect of this procedure on whole-body BMD and the results have not been consistent. Most have found significant bone loss in the 2 years following surgery but some have found no loss and others have found an increase in BMD.[53] The lack of a control group to help distinguish the effect of weight loss versus the effect of the restrictive procedure is a major limitation in the studies and prevents a strong conclusion from being drawn.

Sleeve Gastrectomy

SG is another purely restrictive procedure and involves the creation of a tubular gastric pouch. Approximately 75% of the stomach is removed (**Fig. 4**). It results is almost the same amount of weight loss as the RYGB with a lower complication rate and less postoperative nutritional deficiency. It is also associated with similar reductions in obesity-related comorbidities, including type 2 diabetes, hypertension, hyperlipidemia, and sleep apnea.[54] As a result of this, the SG is now the second most common bariatric surgery worldwide and the number of surgeries being performed continues to increase every year. The excess weight loss averages 50% to 60% with this procedure.[4]

There have been few studies examining the effect of SG on bone metabolism, in part because of its recent increase in popularity. The few studies that have been done have shown decreases in DXA that are more pronounced in the hip that at the spine (7% vs 3%).[55] One study found increases in spine BMD. Closer examination of this population showed a marked increase in vitamin D deficiency preoperatively versus postoperatively.

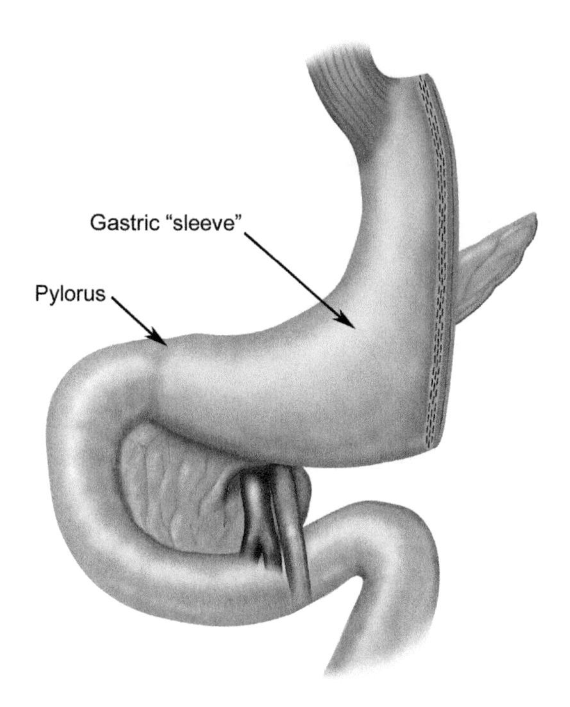

Fig. 4. SG.

There have been even fewer studies examining on the effect on bone metabolism of SG versus RYGB. The studies that have been done have shown a slightly lower degree of bone loss with the SG, but statistical significance was not reached.[56] Further studies are needed to characterize the effect of SG on skeletal health.

LIMITATIONS OF THE CURRENT STUDIES

Although there have been several studies evaluating the effect of the various bariatric procedures on bone metabolism and skeletal health, many questions remain. The studies have had numerous limitations that render their conclusions difficult to interpret. Most of the studies have followed small numbers of subjects, with the average being 30 subjects per study. Most of the studies did not have a control group. In addition, most of the studies did not have a bone density measurement before surgery. The modality used to measure BMD was primarily DXA, which is fraught with compounding factors in interpretation, as previously described. Very few used QCT methodology, which is the modality less affected by changes in body composition.

FRACTURE RISK FOLLOWING BARIATRIC SURGERY

It is important to determine whether the bone loss following these bariatric procedures is associated with an increased fracture risk. Obese patients are known to have higher BMD, therefore it is unclear whether the bone loss following surgery has any clinical significance. There have been few studies of fracture risk. The first did not find an increase in fracture risk in the first 2 years compared with weight-matched controls. Most of these subjects had the AGB, which is known to have the least negative impact on bone metabolism.[57] Another study did find an increased fracture risk with most of the cohort undergoing RYGB but there were no weight-based controls, making interpretation of fracture risk difficult.[58] A recent 12-year cohort study showed a 1.2-fold increased risk in the surgical group versus the control group. The more malabsorptive surgeries had a significantly higher fracture risk within 2 years following surgery.[59]

CLINICAL CONSIDERATIONS

The overall impact of these procedures on bone metabolism seems to be negative, although the studies to date have had limitations and further clinical studies are needed, especially to establish whether decreases in BMD are associated with increased fracture risk.

In the interim, attention should be paid to skeletal health in this at-risk population. Supplementation with calcium and vitamin D is currently recommended, with guidelines suggesting 1500 mg of calcium citrate in divided doses and a starting dose of 3000 international units (IU) of vitamin D.[60] Some patients may need higher doses of supplementation (50,000–100,000 IU/d) to avoid secondary hyperparathyroidism. The reasons for the varying amount of supplementation are unclear but do point to the importance of regular monitoring in these patients.

Patients with obesity and those who have undergone bariatric surgery are known to be at higher risk of falls.[61] They also have been found to fracture at higher BMD and lower FRAX (Fracture Risk Assessment Tool) scores, which points to the possible need for different thresholds for treatment in this population.[62] Special treatment considerations are needed in the bariatric population. No studies to date have examined osteoporosis treatments in postbariatric patients. It is unclear whether the bone loss seen following these procedures would respond to the current available treatments. Oral bisphosphonates, with their known low absorption rate, may not be the ideal therapy, especially when the possibility of gastric or esophageal erosions in the setting of gastrointestinal surgery is a concern. Current and future treatment options should be evaluated in this population.

SUMMARY

The number of bariatric surgeries being performed continues to increase every year. It is important that the impact of these procedures on skeletal health and fracture risk is closely examined. The mechanisms of bone loss following these surgeries are multifactorial and include decreased calcium and vitamin D absorption associated with secondary hyperparathyroidism, decreased mechanical loading, and changes in the levels of adipokines and gastrointestinal hormones. The duration of the increased markers of bone resorption following surgery and its long-term impact on fracture risk is not known. Further prospective studies are needed to clearly elucidate the roles of the various hormone and bone markers in determining the effects of these surgeries.

REFERENCES

1. Ogden C, Carroll M, Kit B, et al. Prevalence of childhood and adult obesity in the United States, 2011-2012. JAMA 2014;311(8):806–14.
2. Guh D, Zhang W, Bansback N, et al. The incidence of co-morbidities related to obesity and overweight: a systematic review and meta-analysis. BMC Public Health 2009;9:88.
3. Buchwald H, Avidor Y, Braunwald E, et al. Bariatric surgery: a systematic review and meta-analysis. JAMA 2004;292:1724–37.

4. Estimate of bariatric surgery numbers 2011-2014. American Society for Metabolic and Bariatric surgery. Available at: https://asmbs.org. Accessed May 28, 2016.
5. Wortsman J, Matsuoka L, Holick M. Decreased bioavailability of vitamin D in obesity. Am J Clin Nutr 2000;72(3):690–3.
6. Bell N, Epstein S, Greene A, et al. Evidence for alteration of the vitamin D-endocrine system in obese subjects. J Clin Invest 1985;76:370–3.
7. Ybarra J, Sanchez-Hernandez J, Gich I, et al. Unchanged hypovitaminosis D and secondary hyperparathyroidism in morbid obesity after bariatric surgery. Obes Surg 2005;15:330–5.
8. Tsiftsis D, Mylonas P, Mead N, et al. Bone mass decreased in morbidly obese women after long limb biliopancreatic diversion and marked weight loss without secondary hyperparathyroidism: a physiologic adaptation to weight loss? Obes Surg 2009;19(11):1497–502.
9. Parfitt A, Podenphant J, Villanueva A, et al. Metabolic bone disease with and without osteomalacia after intestinal bypass surgery: a bone histomorphometric study. Bone 1985;6(4):211–20.
10. Robling A, Bellido T, Turner C. Mechanical stimulation in vivo reduces osteocyte expression of sclerostin. J Musculoskelet Neuronal Interact 2006;6:354.
11. Bonewald L, Johnson M. Osteocytes, mechanosensing and Wnt signaling. Bone 2008;42:606–15.
12. Armamento-Villareal R, Sadler C, Napoli N, et al. Weight loss in obese older adults increases serum sclerostin and impairs hip geometry but both are prevented by exercise training. J Bone Miner Res 2012;27:1215–21.
13. Muschitz C, Kocijan R, Marterer C, et al. Sclerostin levels and changes in bone metabolism after bariatric surgery. J Clin Endocrinol Metab 2015;100(3):891–901.
14. Date Y, Kojima M, Hosada H, et al. Ghrelin, a novel growth hormone-releasing acylated peptide, is synthesized in a distinct endocrine cell type in the gastrointestinal tract. Endocrinology 2000;141:4255–61.
15. Ohlsson C, Bengtsson B, Isaksson O, et al. Growth hormone and bone. Endocr Rev 1998;19:55–79.
16. Fukushima N, Hanada R, Teranishi H, et al. Ghrelin directly regulates bone formation. J Bone Miner Res 2005;20:790–8.
17. Cummings D, Weigle D, Frayo R, et al. Plasma ghrelin levels after diet-induced weight loss or gastric bypass surgery. N Engl J Med 2002;346:1623–30.
18. Pournaras D, le Roux C. Ghrelin and metabolic surgery. Int J Pept 2010;2010.
19. le Roux C, Neary N, Halsey T, et al. Ghrelin does not stimulate food intake in patients with surgical procedures involving vagotomy. J Clin Endocrinol Metab 2005;90:4521–4.
20. Vilsbøll T, Krarup T, Sonne J, et al. Incretin secretion in relation to meal size and body weight in healthy subjects and people with type 1 and type 2 diabetes mellitus. J Clin Endocrinol Metab 2003;88:2706–13.
21. Tsukiyama K, Yamada Y, Yamada C, et al. Gastric inhibitory polypeptide as an endogenous factor promoting new bone formation after food ingestion. Mol Endocrinol 2006;20:1644–51.
22. Rao R, Kini S. GIP and bariatric surgery. Obes Surg 2011;21:244–52.
23. Meloni A, DeYoung M, Lowe C, et al. GLP-1 receptor activated insulin secretion from the pancreatic beta-cells: mechanism and glucose dependence. Diabetes Obes Metab 2013;15(1):15–27.
24. Yamada C, Yamada Y, Tsukiyama K, et al. The murine glucagon-like peptide-1 receptor is essential for control of bone resorption. Endocrinology 2008;149:574–9.

25. Nuche-Berenguer B, Portal-Nunez S, Moreno P, et al. Presence of a functional receptor for GLP-1 in osteoblastic cells, independent of the cAMP-linked GLP-1 receptor. J Cell Physiol 2010;225:585–92.
26. Dirksen C, Jørgensen N, Bojsen-Moller K, et al. Mechanisms of improved glycaemic control after Roux-en-Y gastric bypass. Diabetologia 2012;55:1890–901.
27. le Roux C, Batterham R, Aylwin S, et al. Attenuated peptide YY release in obese subjects is associated with reduced satiety. Endocrinology 2006;147:3–8.
28. Russell M, Stark J, Nayak S, et al. Peptide YY in adolescent athletes with amenorrhea, eumenorrheic athletes and non-athletic controls. Bone 2009;45:104–9.
29. Wortley K, Garcia K, Okamoto H, et al. Peptide YY regulates bone turnover in rodents. Gastroenterology 2007;133:1534–43.
30. Yu E, Wewalka M, Ding S, et al. Effects of gastric bypass banding on bone remodeling in obese patients with type 2 diabetes. J Clin Endocrinol Metab 2016;101(2):714–22.
31. Roth J. Amylin and the regulation of appetite and adiposity: recent advances in receptor signaling, neurobiology and pharmacology. Curr Opin Endocrinol Diabetes Obes 2013;20(1):8–13.
32. Villa I, Rubinacci A, Ravasi F, et al. Effects of amylin on human osteoblast-like cells. Peptides 1997;18:537–40.
33. Bose M, Teixeira J, Olivan B, et al. Weight loss and incretin responsiveness improve glucose control independently after gastric bypass surgery. J Diabetes 2010;2:47–55.
34. Yang J, Zhang X, Wang W, et al. Insulin stimulates osteoblast proliferation and differentiation through ERK and P13K in MG-63 cells. Cell Biochem Funct 2010;28:334–41.
35. Thomas D, Udagawa N, Hards D, et al. Insulin receptor expression in primary and cultured osteoclast-like cells. Bone 1998;23:181–6.
36. Ferron M, Wei J, Yoshizawa T, et al. Insulin signaling in osteoblasts integrates bone remodeling and energy metabolism. Cell 2010;142:296–308.
37. Berner H, Lyngstadaas S, Spahr A, et al. Adiponectin and its receptors are expressed in bone-forming cells. Bone 2004;35:842–9.
38. Biver E, Salliot C, Combescure C, et al. Influence of adipokines and ghrelin on bone mineral density and fracture risk: a systematic review and meta-analysis. J Clin Endocrinol Metab 2011;96:2703–13.
39. Oshima K, Nampei A, Matsuda M, et al. Adiponectin increases bone mass by suppressing osteoclast and activating osteoblast. Biochem Biophys Res Commun 2005;331:520–6.
40. Carrasco F, Ruz M, Rojas P, et al. Changes in bone mineral density, body composition and adiponectin levels in morbidly obese patients after bariatric surgery. Obes Surg 2009;19:41–6.
41. Considine R, Sinha M, Heiman M, et al. Serum immunoreactive-leptin concentrations in normal-weight and obese humans. N Engl J Med 1996;334:292–5.
42. Karsenty G. Convergence between bone and energy homeostasis: leptin regulation of bone mass. Cell Metab 2006;4:341–8.
43. Takeda S, Elefteriou F, Levasseur R, et al. Leptin regulates bone formation via the sympathetic nervous system. Cell 2002;111:305–17.
44. Crowley L, Seay J, Mullin G. Late effects of gastric bypass for obesity. Am J Gastroenterol 1984;79(11):850–60.
45. Coates P, Fernstrom J, Fernstrom M, et al. Gastric bypass surgery for morbid obesity leads to an increase in bone turnover and a decrease in bone mass. J Clin Endocrinol Metab 2004;89(3):1061–5.

46. Fleischer J, Stein E, Bessler M, et al. The decline in hip bone density after gastric bypass surgery is associated with extent of weight loss. J Clin Endocrinol Metab 2008;93(10):3735–40.
47. Blake G, Parker J, Buxton F, et al. Dual X-ray absorptiometry: a comparison between fan beam and pencil beam scans. Br J Radiol 1993;66(790):902–6.
48. Knapp K, Welsman J, Hopkins S, et al. Obesity increases precision errors in dual-energy X-ray absorptiometry measurements. J Clin Densitom 2012;15(3):315–9.
49. Yu E, Bouxsein M, Roy A, et al. Bone loss after bariatric surgery: discordant results between DXA and QCT bone density. J Bone Miner Res 2014;29(3):542–50.
50. Stein E, Carrelli A, Young P, et al. Bariatric surgery results in cortical bone loss. J Clin Endocrinol Metab 2013;98(2):541–9.
51. Giusti V, Gasteyger C, Suter M, et al. Gastric banding induces negative bone remodelling in the absence of secondary hyperparathyroidism: potential role of serum C telopeptides for follow-up. Int J Obes (London) 2005;29(12):1429–35.
52. Dixon J, Strauss B, Laurie C, et al. Changes in body composition with weight loss: obese subjects randomized to surgical and medical programs. Obesity (Silver Spring) 2007;15(5):1187–98.
53. Guney E, Kisakol G, Ozgen G, et al. Effect of weight loss on bone metabolism: comparison of vertical banded gastroplasty and medical intervention. Obes Surg 2003;13(3):383–8.
54. Li J, Lai D, Ni B, et al. Comparison of laparoscopic Roux-en-Y gastric bypass with laparoscopic sleeve gastrectomy for morbid obesity or type 2 diabetes mellitus: a meta-analysis of randomized controlled trials. Can J Surg 2013;56(6):E158–64.
55. Ruiz-Tovar J, Oller I, Priego P, et al. Short- and mid-term changes in bone mineral density after laparoscopic sleeve gastrectomy. Obes Surg 2013;23:861–6.
56. Vilarrasa N, Gordejuela A, Gomez-Vaquero C, et al. Effect of bariatric surgery on bone mineral density: comparison of gastric bypass and sleeve gastrectomy. Obes Surg 2013;23(12):2086–91.
57. Lalmohamed A, De Vries F, Bazelier M, et al. Risk of fracture after bariatric surgery in the United Kingdom: population-based, retrospective cohort study. BMJ 2012;345:e5085.
58. Nakamura K, Haglind E, Clowes J, et al. Fracture risk following bariatric surgery: a population-based study. Osteoporos Int 2014;25(1):151–8.
59. Lu C, Chang Y, Chang H, et al. Fracture risk after bariatric surgery: a 12-year nationwide cohort study. Medicine 2015;94(48):e2087.
60. Mechanick J, Youdim A, Jones D, et al. Clinical practice guidelines for the perioperative nutritional, metabolic, and nonsurgical support of the bariatric surgery patient. Endocr Pract 2013;19(2):337–72.
61. Berarducci A, Haines K, Murr M. Incidence of bone loss, falls, and fractures after Roux-en-Y gastric bypass for morbid obesity. Appl Nurs Res 2009;22(1):35–41.
62. Premaor M, Parker R, Cummings S, et al. Predictive value of FRAX for fracture in obese older women. J Bone Miner Res 2013;28(1):188–95.

Premenopausal Osteoporosis

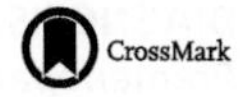

Adi Cohen, MD, MHS

KEYWORDS

- Premenopausal women • Secondary causes of osteoporosis
- Osteoporosis treatment

KEY POINTS

- Premenopausal fractures are rare and may be an important indicator of underlying poor bone quality and future fracture risk.
- Measurement of bone mineral density (BMD) by dual-energy x-ray absorptiometry (DXA) should not be used as the sole guide for diagnosis or treatment of osteoporosis in premenopausal women.
- Timing of peak BMD accrual and expected changes associated with pregnancy and lactation should be considered when interpreting BMD results obtained in premenopausal women.
- Evaluation of low trauma fractures or low BMD should include a thorough evaluation for potential secondary causes.
- Where possible, treatment of the underlying cause should be the focus of management. Premenopausal women with an ongoing cause of bone loss and those who have had, or continue to have, low trauma fractures may require pharmacological intervention.

INTRODUCTION

Osteoporosis is less common in premenopausal women than in postmenopausal women. Both fractures and low BMD, however, do occur in the premenopausal years, and young women with these conditions require specialized clinical considerations. This article reviews the definition, epidemiology, and potential causes of osteoporosis in premenopausal women and also addresses recommendations for evaluation as well as potential treatment strategies. Readers are also referred to previously published reviews on this topic.[1–7]

Dr A. Cohen receives research support from Eli Lilly and Company and Amgen.
Division of Endocrinology, Department of Medicine, Columbia University Medical Center, Columbia University, College of Physicians & Surgeons, PH8-864, 630 West 168th Street, New York, NY 10032, USA
E-mail address: ac1044@columbia.edu

Endocrinol Metab Clin N Am 46 (2017) 117–133
http://dx.doi.org/10.1016/j.ecl.2016.09.007
endo.theclinics.com
0889-8529/17/

DIAGNOSIS OF OSTEOPOROSIS IN PREMENOPAUSAL WOMEN

Premenopausal Fractures

The diagnosis of osteoporosis in a premenopausal woman is most secure when there is a history of low trauma fracture. A fracture is considered low trauma if it is sustained in the setting of trauma equivalent to a fall from a standing height or less. Stress fractures occur in the context of continued skeletal stress and in the absence of a specific traumatic event. Clinical judgment is required to determine whether normal stress on fragile bone or excessive stress on normal bone has led to the pathology. As in all cases of unusual fracture, the diagnosis of osteoporosis should be considered only after osteomalacia (undermineralization due to causes such as severe vitamin D deficiency or hypophosphatemia) and other causes of pathologic fracture (eg, malignancy, avascular necrosis, fibrous dysplasia, and other bone lesion) have been ruled out.

Fractures are substantially less common in premenopausal women than in postmenopausal women.[8–12] Premenopausal fractures may be an important indicator, however, of underlying poor bone quality and future fracture risk. Data from the Study of Osteoporotic Fractures demonstrate that women with a history of premenopausal fracture are 35% more likely to fracture during the postmenopausal years compared with women without a history of premenopausal fracture.[9] In a cross-sectional study of 1284 postmenopausal women in New Zealand, a history of fracture between ages 20 and 50 was associated with a 74% increased risk of fracture after age 50 years.[12] In both studies, these relationships persisted after controlling for several potential confounding variables. Other studies have reported similar findings.[13,14]

Low trauma fractures in premenopausal women are usually related to known risk factors for bone fragility, called secondary causes of osteoporosis (discussed later). Low trauma fracture(s) in a premenopausal woman should lead to an evaluation that includes BMD testing and a thorough evaluation for potential secondary causes.

Interpretation of Bone Mineral Density Measurements in Premenopausal Women

In postmenopausal women, BMD assessment by DXA is a cornerstone of fracture risk prediction models used for therapeutic decision making because of the wealth of longitudinal observational and interventional studies correlating DXA findings with fracture incidence in this population.

In premenopausal women, cross-sectional studies have reported lower BMD by DXA in those with fractures. Premenopausal women with Colles fractures have been found to have significantly lower BMD at the nonfractured radius,[15] lumbar spine, and femoral neck[16] than controls without fractures. Female military recruits and athletes with stress fractures were also found to have lower BMD than controls.[17–19] There are few longitudinal prospective studies, however, relating BMD by DXA to fracture risk in premenopausal women. Because of this, and because fracture rates are much lower in premenopausal than postmenopausal women,[9,11,12] the predictive relationship between BMD and short-term fracture incidence is unclear in premenopausal women. Similarly, the World Health Organization Fracture Risk Assessment Tool provides fracture probability only for those aged 40 and above and is intended to be applied to postmenopausal women. For these reasons, measurement of BMD by DXA should not be used as the sole guide for diagnosis or treatment of osteoporosis in premenopausal women.

Screening BMD by DXA is not recommended in premenopausal women.[20] BMD measurement is recommended in young women with a history of low trauma fracture and in those with known causes of bone loss (discussed later).

Two organizations have provided guidelines regarding DXA interpretation in premenopausal women.

The International Society for Clinical Densitometry (ISCD) recommends use of BMD Z scores (comparison to age-matched norms) rather than T scores (comparison to premenopausal norms) at the lumbar spine, hip, and forearm.[20] A Z score less than or equal to −2.0 should be interpreted as "below the expected range for age" and a Z score greater than −2.0 as "within the expected range for age."[20] The diagnostic categories of "osteopenia" and "osteoporosis" based solely on BMD T score should not be applied in premenopausal women; however, T scores may be used in the perimenopausal period. The ISCD[20] and others[1,3,21,22] have recommended that young, otherwise healthy, women should not be diagnosed with osteoporosis solely on the basis of low areal BMD (aBMD) by DXA, unless there is a history of fragility fracture or a secondary cause of osteoporosis (discussed later).

The International Osteoporosis Foundation (IOF) recommends use of Z score less than −2 to define low bone mass in children, adolescents, those under 20 years, and some over 20 years in the context of delayed puberty. In contrast to ISCD, the IOF recommends use of T scores in those aged 20 to 50 years and suggests use of T score less than −2.5 to define osteoporosis, particularly in those with known secondary causes or in the context of low trauma fractures that provide evidence of bone fragility.[7]

Idiopathic low bone mineral density

Women with low BMD without a history of adult low trauma fracture and without a known cause can be said to have idiopathic low bone density.[23] Based on current recommendations, such women should not be diagnosed with "osteoporosis."

3-D bone imaging and transiliac bone biopsy studies performed by the authors' group, however, have shown that healthy, normally menstruating, premenopausal women with unexplained low BMD and no fractures (idiopathic low BMD) have microarchitectural disruption and decreased estimated bone strength that is similar to a comparable cohort of premenopausal women with idiopathic low trauma fractures, even after correcting for bone size.[23–25] This finding is also supported by data from a group of premenopausal women with constitutional thinness (very low body mass index, normal menses, and no known systemic disease), who were found to have low BMD, smaller bone size, and decreased estimated breaking strength in comparison to normal women.[26] These studies are limited by their small sample size as well as the possibility of referral/ascertainment bias. Although these results may not be generalizable to all premenopausal women with low aBMD by DXA, they suggest that very low BMD may represent a presymptomatic phase of osteoporosis in premenopausal women.

Even though the currently available data suggest that those young women with idiopathic low bone density and no fracture history are likely to have abnormal bone microarchitecture that is consistent with osteoporosis, this does not mean that such a finding should be used to make therapeutic decisions in premenopausal women as in postmenopausal women. This is because (1) currently available data do not allow using BMD by DXA to predict fracture risk in premenopausal women, (2) fracture risk depends greatly on age, and (3) few studies have addressed risks and benefits of osteoporosis medications in premenopausal women. Risks and benefits of osteoporosis medications are likely to differ in premenopausal women compared with postmenopausal women.

Special Considerations Required for Interpretation of Bone Mineral Density Results in Premenopausal Women

Dynamics of peak bone mineral density accrual

BMD in premenopausal women depends primarily on achievement of peak bone mass. Attainment of peak bone mass varies according to gender,[27,28] ethnicity,[29] body size, menarchal age,[30,31] and region of bone. In healthy girls, the peak period of bone mass accrual occurs between ages 11 and 14,[32] and the rate of bone mass accrual slows dramatically by approximately 2 years after menarche.[27] Although at least 90% of peak bone mass is acquired by the late teen years,[32–34] studies have documented small additional gains between the ages of 20 and 29.[35] Moreover, population-based, cross-sectional studies suggest that the timing of peak bone mass accrual may be site specific,[27] with women reaching peak bone mass at the proximal femur in their 20s and at the spine and forearm around age 30.[36] When interpreting BMD measurements in premenopausal women, the possibility that peak bone mass has not yet been achieved must always be considered.

Low BMD in a premenopausal woman may result from the attainment of a peak bone mass that is below average due to genetic predisposition, illnesses, or medications that have a negative impact on bone density accrual. The factors responsible for the attainment of low peak bone mass may, or may not, remain active or measurable at the time of the evaluation. Low BMD in a premenopausal woman that is related to genetic factors that determine peak bone mass or to a previously active secondary cause may not be associated with ongoing bone loss but could be associated with abnormal bone quality (idiopathic low bone mineral density, discussed previously).

Physiologic changes associated with pregnancy and lactation

Changes in bone mass in association with both pregnancy and lactation have been reported in several studies. At the lumbar spine, longitudinal studies document losses of 3% to 5% during a pregnancy and 3% to 10% over a 6-month period of lactation,[37] with recovery of bone mass demonstrated over 6 to 12 months, thereafter, even in the setting of continued lactation.[38,39] At the hip, bone loss of 2% to 4% has been documented over 6 months of lactation.[37] The amount of bone loss during lactation is directly associated with longer durations of lactation and postpartum amenorrhea.[38–41] Both human and rodent studies suggest that patterns of recovery of bone mass after weaning are site specific, with full recovery at the spine but only partial recovery at the femur.[40,42,43] To date, however, longitudinal studies of BMD recovery in humans extend 12 months to 20 months postpartum. Longer duration of follow-up may be required to document the true degree of recovery.

A majority of epidemiologic studies in humans suggest that the net effect of the loss and regain of bone mass during and after lactation does not affect postmenopausal bone mass or long-term fracture risk.[44–46] Other studies show, however, that multiparity and longer periods of lactation are associated with decreased bone mineralization.[47–52] Additionally, studies performed in Turkey, China, and Mexico suggest that there may be an impact of lactation history on postmenopausal BMD in some populations.[48,53,54] Differences in population age, stature, parity, socioeconomic conditions, study duration and design, analysis techniques, and covariates included must be taken into account when interpreting these differing results.

Because of these physiologic bone mass changes associated with reproduction, interpretation of BMD results in premenopausal women must take into account the timing of any recent pregnancy or lactation. Based on available data, BMD at the lumbar spine is likely to have returned to that individual's premenopausal baseline by 12 months' postweaning.[40]

Pregnancy and lactation–associated osteoporosis In some women, premenopausal osteoporosis may first present with low trauma fracture(s), usually at trabecular sites, such as the vertebrae, occurring in the last trimester of pregnancy or during lactation.[41,55–57] Given the physiologic bone mass changes described previously, pregnancy and lactation may represent particularly vulnerable times for the premenopausal woman's skeleton, particularly if low BMD is present before pregnancy.

Premenopausal fractures, however, including those associated with pregnancy and lactation, remain rare, suggesting that additional factors contribute to bone fragility in women who present with fractures during this time. Women with low trauma fractures sustained during pregnancy and/or lactation require the same thorough evaluation for secondary causes as do young women with fractures that are not associated with reproductive events. The authors have included women with pregnancy and lactation–associated osteoporosis, in whom no cause is found after extensive evaluation, in cohorts defined to have idiopathic osteoporosis (IOP).[23,58]

SECONDARY CAUSES OF OSTEOPOROSIS IN PREMENOPAUSAL WOMEN

Most premenopausal women with low trauma fractures or low BMD have an underlying disorder or medication exposure that has interfered with bone mass accrual during adolescence and/or has caused excessive bone loss after reaching peak bone mass. In a population study from Olmsted County, Minnesota, 90% of men and women ages 20 to 44 with osteoporotic fractures and low BMD were found to have a secondary cause.[59] In contrast, several case series of young women with osteoporosis from tertiary centers report that only 50% to 60% have secondary causes,[60–62] likely reflecting referral bias.

Potential secondary causes are listed in **Box 1** and fall into several broad categories: estrogen deficiency, inflammatory diseases, collagen disorders, gastrointestinal diseases, and glucocorticoids and other medication exposures. Many diseases of childhood and young adulthood (eg, gastrointestinal diseases and inflammatory diseases) lead to osteoporosis through multifactorial mechanisms involving the combined effects of malnutrition, systemic inflammation, estrogen deficiency/delayed puberty, and medication effects.

The main goal of the evaluation of a premenopausal woman with low trauma fractures or low BMD is to identify any secondary cause and to institute specific treatment of that cause if it is indicated. Correction or treatment of several of these conditions, including anorexia nervosa,[63] estrogen deficiency, hypercalciuria,[64] celiac disease,[65–67] Crohn disease,[68] endogenous and iatrogenic hypercortisolism, and hyperparathyroidism,[69] has been associated with measureable BMD improvement in some populations, although some have not been specifically studied in premenopausal women.

Evaluation of Premenopausal Women with Low Trauma Fracture and/or Low Bone Mineral Density

Many secondary causes can be identified by a detailed history and physical examination.

Medical history should include information on

- Adult and childhood fractures
- Adult and childhood illnesses and medication exposures
- Menstrual history
- Timing of recent pregnancy or lactation
- Dieting and exercise behavior

Box 1
Secondary causes of osteoporosis in premenopausal women

- Any childhood disease that has affected puberty and/or skeletal development
- Premenopausal amenorrhea (eg, pituitary diseases, medications, or exercise-induced amenorrhea)
- Anorexia nervosa
- Cushing syndrome
- Hyperthyroidism
- Primary hyperparathyroidism
- Vitamin D, calcium, and/or other nutrient deficiency
- Gastrointestinal malabsorption (celiac disease, inflammatory bowel disease, cystic fibrosis, or postoperative states)
- Rheumatoid arthritis, SLE, and other inflammatory conditions
- Connective tissue diseases, for example
  - Osteogenesis imperfecta
  - Marfan syndrome
  - Ehlers-Danlos syndrome
- Diabetes mellitus (types 1 and 2)
- Renal disease
- Liver disease
- Hypercalciuria
- Alcoholism
- Other rare diseases, including mastocytosis, Gaucher disease, hemochromatosis, and hypophosphatasia

Medications (some have not been studied in premenopausal populations)

- Glucocorticoids
- Immunosuppressants (eg, cyclosporine)
- Antiepileptic drugs (in particular cytochrome P450 inducers, such as phenytoin and carbamazepine)
- Cancer chemotherapy
- GnRH agonists (when used to suppress ovulation)
- Depot medroxyprogesterone acetate (Depo-Provera)
- Heparin
- Other medications with probable relationships to osteoporosis: proton pump inhibitors, selective serotonin reuptake inhibitors, and low-molecular-weight heparin

- Gastrointestinal symptoms
- Nephrolithiasis
- Family history of osteoporosis and/or nephrolithiasis

Physical examination should seek signs of

- Nutritional deficiency or eating disorder
- Cushing syndrome
- Thyroid hormone excess

- Connective tissue disorders (eg, osteogenesis imperfecta, Ehlers-Danlos syndrome, and Marfan syndrome)
- Inflammatory conditions (eg, rheumatoid arthritis and systemic lupus erythematosus [SLE])

Laboratory evaluation may target hormonal, calcium metabolism, or gastrointestinal disorders. Recommendations for an initial laboratory evaluation and a more extensive evaluation are given in **Box 2**.

The laboratory evaluation should aim to identify conditions, such as

- Vitamin D and/or calcium deficiency (and laboratory evidence that may distinguish osteomalacia from osteoporosis)
- Hyperthyroidism
- Hyperparathyroidism
- Cushing syndrome
- Early menopause
- Renal or liver disease
- Celiac disease and other forms of malabsorption
- Idiopathic hypercalciuria

Box 2
Laboratory evaluation

Initial laboratory evaluation

- Complete blood cell count
- Electrolytes and renal function
- Serum calcium and phosphate
- Serum albumin, transaminases, and total alkaline phosphatase
- Serum thyroid-stimulating hormone
- Serum 25-hydroxyvitamin D
- PTH
- 24-Hour urine for calcium and creatinine

Additional laboratory evaluation

- Estradiol, luteinizing hormone, follicle-stimulating hormone, and prolactin
- Screening for Cushing syndrome: 24-hour urine for free cortisol (or dexamethasone suppression test)
- Celiac screen (serologies)
- Serum/urine protein electrophoresis
- Erythrocyte sedimentation rate or C-reactive protein
- Vitamin A/retinol level
- Specific testing for other rare conditions (eg, mastocytosis, Gaucher disease, hypophosphatasia, and hemochromatosis)
- If genetic diseases, such as Gaucher disease, hypophosphatasia or osteogenesis imperfecta are considered, genetic testing may be pursued
- Bone turnover markers
- Transiliac crest bone biopsy

Utility of markers of bone turnover and bone biopsy
Bone turnover markers may be measured with the goal of distinguishing those likely to have stable BMD from those with an ongoing process of bone loss, who may have a higher short-term risk of fracture. Those with elevated bone turnover markers may also be more likely to have a diagnosable secondary cause. Bone turnover markers also increase after a fracture, however, and, when bone turnover markers are assessed in women during very early adulthood, they may be elevated as a result of the active bone accrual occurring in that individual and may not reflect a process of bone loss.

Transiliac crest bone biopsy after double tetracycline labeling may be useful in certain clinical scenarios when it is necessary to examine bone remodeling, rule out osteomalacia, differentiate between different types of renal osteodystrophy, or complete an examination for rare secondary causes.

Idiopathic osteoporosis In some cases of low trauma fracture in premenopausal women, no known secondary cause can be found after extensive evaluation. These women are said to have IOP. Based on current guidelines, the term IOP applies only to those with a history of low trauma fractures and not to those with low BMD and no history of fractures. That said, multiple prior studies describing and examining mechanisms of IOP in women and men have included both those with fractures and those with low BMD alone.

Several recent publications have described the bone structural and remodeling characteristics of this group. In studies using central quantitative CT, peripheral high-resolution CT, and micro-CT of transiliac bone biopsy samples, the authors' group has demonstrated markedly thinner cortices; fewer, thinner, more widely separated, and heterogeneously distributed trabeculae; and lower estimated stiffness in IOP women compared with normal controls. Studies of biochemical and bone remodeling characteristics suggest that the pathogenesis of IOP is heterogeneous, with some women exhibiting evidence of low bone turnover whereas others have evidence of high bone turnover. Pathogenesis is likely to be diverse; causes, including excess urinary calcium excretion and insulin-like growth factor 1 (IGF-1) axis abnormalities, have been implicated.[23,70]

TREATMENT CONSIDERATION FOR PREMENOPAUSAL WOMEN WITH LOW TRAUMA FRACTURES AND/OR LOW BONE MINERAL DENSITY

For all patients, it is appropriate to recommend adequate weight-bearing exercise,[71] nutrition, calcium and vitamin D, and lifestyle modifications, such as smoking cessation and avoidance of excess alcohol. Current guidelines from the Institute of Medicine[72] recommend 1000 mg of calcium and 600 IU of vitamin D for premenopausal women. These recommendations could be tailored to the individual based on evaluation of calcium metabolism. Exercise recommendations must also be tailored to the individual patient, because excessive exercise in premenopausal women may lead to weight loss and/or hypothalamic amenorrhea, exacerbating low bone density.

Medications

Combination oral contraceptives
Use of oral contraceptives to replace estrogen in those who are estrogen deficient may have beneficial effects on bone mass,[73–75] although oral reproductive hormone replacement has been shown to be insufficient for the treatment of osteoporosis in anorexia nervosa, a more complex condition.[63,74,76]

In contrast, a majority of studies of oral contraceptives in healthy premenopausal women without preexisting estrogen deficiency show no effect of oral contraceptives on bone mass.[74,77,78] Some studies have also documented an adverse effect of low dose (<30 μg ethinyl estradiol) oral contraceptives on bone mass in very young women/adolescents.[79–81] Based on available data, the effects of oral contraceptives on fracture risk are unclear.[77]

Selective estrogen receptor modulators

Selective estrogen receptor modulators, such as raloxifene and tamoxifen, should not be used to treat bone loss in menstruating women because they block estrogen action on bone and lead to further bone loss.[82,83]

Bisphosphonates

Bisphosphonates have been shown to improve BMD or prevent bone loss in young adults with several conditions, including pregnancy and lactation–associated fractures, breast cancer therapy, glucocorticoid therapy, anorexia nervosa, cystic fibrosis, and thallessemia[55,84–92]; in some cases, premenopausal women were studied specifically.[55,84–88,91,92] Two oral bisphosphonates, alendronate and risedronate, have been approved by the US Food and Drug Administration (FDA) for use in premenopausal women receiving glucocorticoids. Even though trials show favorable short-term BMD outcomes, however, fracture data are rarely available and long-term risks in premenopausal women are unknown.

Bisphosphonates carry a category C rating for safety in pregnancy from the FDA because they accumulate in the skeleton, cross the placenta, and accumulate in the fetal skeleton in a rat model and have been reported to cause toxic effects in pregnant rats.[93] Although a majority of published case reports have documented no adverse maternal and fetal outcomes,[55,94–96] effective contraception should be encouraged during bisphosphonate use, and there is also the potential for adverse effects after stopping bisphosphonates, because they remain in the skeleton for years.

The choice of bisphosphonates in younger women must also take into account increasing concerns about the potential risks of long-term use of these agents.[97,98] In young women, plans for duration of bisphosphonate use must be discussed as part of the process of initiation of this therapy, and the goal should be for the shortest possible duration of bisphosphonate use.

Denosumab

Denosumab is currently approved for the treatment of osteoporosis in postmenopausal women and men at high risk for fracture. Although denosumab may have some advantages in premenopausal populations because of its shorter half-life relative to bisphosphonates and lack of skeletal accumulation, the efficacy and safety of this medication have not been defined in premenopausal women. Denosumab, as marketed for osteoporosis, has been assigned a designation of pregnancy category X; animal studies indicate that denosumab may cause fetal harm.

Teriparatide (parathyroid hormone[1–34])

Teriparatide, or parathyroid hormone (PTH)(1–34), has been used successfully in clinical trials to prevent bone loss or increase BMD in premenopausal women on gonadotropin-releasing hormone (GnRH) agonists for the treatment of endometriosis,[99] in premenopausal women taking glucocorticoids,[100,101] in premenopausal women with IOP,[102,103] and in those with anorexia nervosa.[104] Additionally, a case series documented benefit in pregnancy-associated osteoporosis.[105] All of the studies described previously were limited in terms of sample size and were not large enough to examine fracture risk reduction. In premenopausal women, FDA approval for use of teriparatide is currently encompassed under the FDA approval for the treatment of those with osteoporosis associated with sustained systemic glucocorticoid therapy at high risk for fracture.

Because the long-term effects of teriparatide in young women are not known, use of this medication should be reserved for those at highest risk for fracture or those who are experiencing recurrent fractures. In young women less than 25 years of age, documentation of fused epiphyses is recommended prior to consideration of teriparatide treatment.

Few data are available to guide treatment options for premenopausal women after teriparatide cessation. One study documented BMD gain in premenopausal women who resumed menses after cessation of both long-acting GnRH analog and PTH(1–34).[106] In a study of 13 premenopausal women with IOP and normal gonadal function, followed for 2.0 years ± 0.6 years after teriparatide cessation, BMD declined 4.2% ± 3.9% at the spine and remained stable at the hip.[107] This finding suggests that women with IOP require antiresorptive treatment to prevent bone loss after teriparatide.

Specific Clinical Situations

Idiopathic Low Bone Mineral Density

In premenopausal women with isolated low BMD, no fractures, and no known secondary cause after thorough evaluation, pharmacologic therapy is rarely justified. Although these women may have bone microarchitectural abnormalities underlying their low BMD,[23,24] they are expected to have stable BMD[108] and a low short-term risk of fracture. BMD should be measured at 1-year to 2-year intervals to identify women with declining BMD. Evidence of declining BMD in a premenopausal woman should lead to continued evaluation for secondary causes and, in rare cases, consideration of therapeutic options.

Premenopausal women with idiopathic osteoporosis defined based on fracture history

In premenopausal women with a history of low trauma fracture and no known cause found after extensive evaluation, the use of medications to decrease fracture risk could be considered on a case-by-case basis. Fracture location and frequency as well as BMD trajectory should help guide treatment decisions.

Few data are available to delineate the specific risks or benefits of medications for osteoporosis in women with IOP.

In a study of 9 women with pregnancy and lactation–associated vertebral fractures, bisphosphonate treatment over a median of 24 months was associated with substantial BMD gains.[55] Because bone density is expected to increase postpartum and after weaning in normal women, however, and there was no untreated control group, it is not clear to what extent bisphosphonate use provided an incremental benefit for these patients.

In an observational study of 21 premenopausal women with IOP, teriparatide, 20 μg daily over 24 months, led to BMD increases of 10.8% at the lumbar spine and 6.2% at the total hip.[109] Among this unique cohort, however, a small subset with very low baseline bone turnover had little or no increase in BMD on this medication.[102,109]

Premenopausal women with fractures or low bone mineral density related to known secondary causes

In premenopausal women with low BMD or low trauma fractures and a known secondary cause of osteoporosis, the first goal of management should be to address the underlying cause. Bone density benefits have been shown in the context of intervention for several such secondary causes in premenopausal women:

- Estrogen replacement for those with estrogen deficiency[73–75]
- Discontinuation of medications, for example, depot medroxyprogesterone acetate (Depo-Provera)[110,111]

- Gluten-free diet for celiac disease[65–67]
- Nutritional rehabilitation and weight gain for anorexia nervosa[63]
- Parathyroidectomy for primary hyperparathyroidism[69]

Although thiazides are used for idiopathic hypercalciuria and seem to have beneficial effects on BMD in men,[64] few data are available in young women.

Continuing or severe effects of the secondary cause may lead to a necessity for pharmacologic therapy. Options for treatment are discussed previously.

Glucocorticoid-induced osteoporosis: specific considerations in premenopausal women

Combination estrogen/progestin contraceptives can be considered (if not contraindicated) in premenopausal women with amenorrhea who are or will be treated with glucocorticoids. Alendronate, risedronate, and teriparatide have been approved by the FDA for use in women (including premenopausal women) receiving glucocorticoids. Few premenopausal women, however, participated in the relevant large registration trials for bisphosphonates and teriparatide in glucocorticoid-induced osteoporosis and none of the premenopausal women in those trials fractured.[100,112–114]

Guidelines from the American College of Rheumatology suggest that bisphosphonates or teriparatide could be considered for premenopausal women of childbearing potential with a history of fragility fracture, if there is glucocorticoid exposure of at least 7.5 mg of prednisone or equivalent per day for greater than or equal to 3 months.[115]

A study comparing teriparatide and alendronate for glucocorticoid-induced osteoporosis included some premenopausal women. Overall, teriparatide was associated with significantly greater increases in lumbar spine and total hip BMD and resulted in significantly fewer incident vertebral fractures than alendronate.[101] The BMD responses were similar in premenopausal women as in men and postmenopausal women, but no fractures occurred in either premenopausal group.[100]

SUMMARY

Most premenopausal women with low trauma fracture(s) or low BMD have a secondary cause of osteoporosis or bone loss. Women who present with unexplained fractures or low BMD should have a thorough clinical and laboratory evaluation to search for known causes of fractures and/or bone loss. Where possible, treatment of the underlying cause should be the focus of management. Premenopausal women with an ongoing cause of bone loss and those who have had, or continue to have, low trauma fractures may require pharmacologic intervention. Clinical trials provide evidence of benefits of bisphosphonates and teriparatide for BMD in several types of premenopausal osteoporosis, but studies are small and do not provide evidence regarding fracture risk reduction.

REFERENCES

1. Gourlay ML, Brown SA. Clinical considerations in premenopausal osteoporosis. Arch Intern Med 2004;164:603–14.
2. Khan AA, Syed Z. Bone densitometry in premenopausal women: synthesis and review. J Clin Densitom 2004;7:85–92.
3. Leib ES. Treatment of low bone mass in premenopausal women: when may it be appropriate? Curr Osteoporos Rep 2005;3:13–8.
4. Abraham A, Cohen A, Shane E. Premenopausal bone health: osteoporosis in premenopausal women. Clin Obstet Gynecol 2013;56:722–9.

5. Cohen A, Shane E. Evaluation and management of the premenopausal woman with low BMD. Curr Osteoporos Rep 2013;11:276–85.
6. Cohen A. Premenopausal osteoporosis. In: Marcus R, Cauley J, Dempster D, et al, editors. Osteoporosis. 4th edition. Philadelphia: Elsevier; 2013. p. 1101–12.
7. Ferrari S, Bianchi ML, Eisman JA, et al. Osteoporosis in young adults: pathophysiology, diagnosis, and management. Osteoporos Int 2012;23(12):2735–48.
8. Hui SL, Slemenda CW, Johnston CC Jr. Age and bone mass as predictors of fracture in a prospective study. J Clin Invest 1988;81:1804–9.
9. Hosmer WD, Genant HK, Browner WS. Fractures before menopause: a red flag for physicians. Osteoporos Int 2002;13:337–41.
10. Melton LJ 3rd, Amadio PC, Crowson CS, et al. Long-term trends in the incidence of distal forearm fractures. Osteoporos Int 1998;8:341–8.
11. Thompson PW, Taylor J, Dawson A. The annual incidence and seasonal variation of fractures of the distal radius in men and women over 25 years in Dorset, UK. Injury 2004;35:462–6.
12. Wu F, Mason B, Horne A, et al. Fractures between the ages of 20 and 50 years increase women's risk of subsequent fractures. Arch Intern Med 2002;162:33–6.
13. Honkanen R, Tuppurainen M, Kroger H, et al. Associations of early premenopausal fractures with subsequent fractures vary by sites and mechanisms of fractures. Calcif Tissue Int 1997;60:327–31.
14. Rothberg AD, Matshidze PK. Perimenopausal wrist fracture–an opportunity for prevention and management of osteoporosis. S Afr Med J 2000;90:1121–4.
15. Wigderowitz CA, Cunningham T, Rowley DI, et al. Peripheral bone mineral density in patients with distal radial fractures. J Bone Joint Surg Br 2003;85:423–5.
16. Hung LK, Wu HT, Leung PC, et al. Low BMD is a risk factor for low-energy Colles' fractures in women before and after menopause. Clin Orthop Relat Res 2005;(435):219–25.
17. Lappe J, Davies K, Recker R, et al. Quantitative ultrasound: use in screening for susceptibility to stress fractures in female army recruits. J Bone Miner Res 2005; 20:571–8.
18. Lauder TD, Dixit S, Pezzin LE, et al. The relation between stress fractures and bone mineral density: evidence from active-duty Army women. Arch Phys Med Rehabil 2000;81:73–9.
19. Myburgh KH, Hutchins J, Fataar AB, et al. Low bone density is an etiologic factor for stress fractures in athletes. Ann Intern Med 1990;113:754–9.
20. Lewiecki EM, Gordon CM, Baim S, et al. International society for clinical densitometry 2007 adult and pediatric official positions. Bone 2008;43:1115–21.
21. Licata AA. "Does she or doesn't she...have osteoporosis?" The use and abuse of bone densitometry. Endocr Pract 2000;6:336–7.
22. Lindsay R. Bone mass measurement for premenopausal women. Osteoporos Int 1994;4(Suppl 1):39–41.
23. Cohen A, Dempster D, Recker R, et al. Abnormal bone microarchitecture and evidence of osteoblast dysfunction in premenopausal women with idiopathic osteoporosis. J Clin Endocrinol Metab 2011;96:3095.
24. Cohen A, Liu XS, Stein EM, et al. Bone microarchitecture and stiffness in premenopausal women with idiopathic osteoporosis. J Clin Endocrinol Metab 2009;94:4351–60.
25. Cohen A, Lang TF, McMahon DJ, et al. Central QCT reveals lower volumetric BMD and stiffness in premenopausal women with idiopathic osteoporosis, regardless of fracture history. J Clin Endocrinol Metab 2012;97(11):4244–52.

26. Galusca B, Zouch M, Germain N, et al. Constitutional thinness: unusual human phenotype of low bone quality. J Clin Endocrinol Metab 2008;93:110–7.
27. Bonjour JP, Theintz G, Buchs B, et al. Critical years and stages of puberty for spinal and femoral bone mass accumulation during adolescence. J Clin Endocrinol Metab 1991;73:555–63.
28. Nguyen TV, Maynard LM, Towne B, et al. Sex differences in bone mass acquisition during growth: the Fels Longitudinal Study. J Clin Densitom 2001;4: 147–57.
29. Walker MD, Babbar R, Opotowsky AR, et al. A referent bone mineral density database for Chinese American women. Osteoporos Int 2006;17:878–87.
30. Chevalley T, Rizzoli R, Hans D, et al. Interaction between calcium intake and menarcheal age on bone mass gain: an eight-year follow-up study from prepuberty to postmenarche. J Clin Endocrinol Metab 2005;90:44–51.
31. Rosenthal DI, Mayo-Smith W, Hayes CW, et al. Age and bone mass in premenopausal women. J Bone Miner Res 1989;4:533–8.
32. Theintz G, Buchs B, Rizzoli R, et al. Longitudinal monitoring of bone mass accumulation in healthy adolescents: evidence for a marked reduction after 16 years of age at the levels of lumbar spine and femoral neck in female subjects. J Clin Endocrinol Metab 1992;75:1060–5.
33. Bachrach LK, Hastie T, Wang MC, et al. Bone mineral acquisition in healthy Asian, Hispanic, black, and Caucasian youth: a longitudinal study. J Clin Endocrinol Metab 1999;84:4702–12.
34. Bailey DA, McKay HA, Mirwald RL, et al. A six-year longitudinal study of the relationship of physical activity to bone mineral accrual in growing children: the university of Saskatchewan bone mineral accrual study. J Bone Miner Res 1999;14: 1672–9.
35. Recker RR, Davies KM, Hinders SM, et al. Bone gain in young adult women. JAMA 1992;268:2403–8.
36. Lofman O, Larsson L, Toss G. Bone mineral density in diagnosis of osteoporosis: reference population, definition of peak bone mass, and measured site determine prevalence. J Clin Densitom 2000;3:177–86.
37. Karlsson MK, Ahlborg HG, Karlsson C. Maternity and bone mineral density. Acta Orthop 2005;76:2–13.
38. Karlsson C, Obrant KJ, Karlsson M. Pregnancy and lactation confer reversible bone loss in humans. Osteoporos Int 2001;12:828–34.
39. Sowers M, Corton G, Shapiro B, et al. Changes in bone density with lactation. JAMA 1993;269:3130–5.
40. Kolthoff N, Eiken P, Kristensen B, et al. Bone mineral changes during pregnancy and lactation: a longitudinal cohort study. Clin Sci (Lond) 1998;94:405–12.
41. Kovacs CS. Maternal mineral and bone metabolism during pregnancy, lactation, and post-weaning recovery. Physiol Rev 2016;96:449–547.
42. Liu XS, Ardeshirpour L, VanHouten JN, et al. Site-specific changes in bone microarchitecture, mineralization, and stiffness during lactation and after weaning in mice. J Bone Miner Res 2012;27:865–75.
43. Vajda EG, Bowman BM, Miller SC. Cancellous and cortical bone mechanical properties and tissue dynamics during pregnancy, lactation, and postlactation in the rat. Biol Reprod 2001;65:689–95.
44. Alderman BW, Weiss NS, Daling JR, et al. Reproductive history and postmenopausal risk of hip and forearm fracture. Am J Epidemiol 1986;124:262–7.

45. Cummings SR, Nevitt MC, Browner WS, et al. Risk factors for hip fracture in white women. Study of Osteoporotic Fractures Research Group. N Engl J Med 1995;332:767–73.
46. Michaelsson K, Baron JA, Farahmand BY, et al. Influence of parity and lactation on hip fracture risk. Am J Epidemiol 2001;153:1166–72.
47. Chowdhury S, Sarkar NR, Roy SK. Impact of lactational performance on bone mineral density in marginally-nourished Bangladeshi women. J Health Popul Nutr 2002;20:26–30.
48. Dursun N, Akin S, Dursun E, et al. Influence of duration of total breast-feeding on bone mineral density in a Turkish population: does the priority of risk factors differ from society to society? Osteoporos Int 2006;17:651–5.
49. Hopkinson JM, Butte NF, Ellis K, et al. Lactation delays postpartum bone mineral accretion and temporarily alters its regional distribution in women. J Nutr 2000; 130:777–83.
50. Laskey MA, Prentice A. Bone mineral changes during and after lactation. Obstet Gynecol 1999;94:608–15.
51. Lissner L, Bengtsson C, Hansson T. Bone mineral content in relation to lactation history in pre- and postmenopausal women. Calcif Tissue Int 1991;48:319–25.
52. More C, Bettembuk P, Bhattoa HP, et al. The effects of pregnancy and lactation on bone mineral density. Osteoporos Int 2001;12:732–7.
53. Khoo CC, Woo J, Leung PC, et al. Determinants of bone mineral density in older postmenopausal Chinese women. Climacteric 2011;14:378–83.
54. Rojano-Mejia D, Aguilar-Madrid G, Lopez-Medina G, et al. Risk factors and impact on bone mineral density in postmenopausal Mexican mestizo women. Menopause 2011;18:302–6.
55. O'Sullivan SM, Grey AB, Singh R, et al. Bisphosphonates in pregnancy and lactation-associated osteoporosis. Osteoporos Int 2006;17:1008–12.
56. Blanch J, Pacifici R, Chines A. Pregnancy-associated osteoporosis: report of two cases with long-term bone density follow-up. Br J Rheumatol 1994;33: 269–72.
57. Kovacs CS, Ralston SH. Presentation and management of osteoporosis presenting in association with pregnancy or lactation. Osteoporos Int 2015;26:2223–41.
58. Cohen A, Recker RR, Lappe J, et al. Premenopausal women with idiopathic low-trauma fractures and/or low bone mineral density. Osteoporos Int 2011;23(1): 171–82.
59. Khosla S, Lufkin EG, Hodgson SF, et al. Epidemiology and clinical features of osteoporosis in young individuals. Bone 1994;15:551–5.
60. Moreira Kulak CA, Schussheim DH, McMahon DJ, et al. Osteoporosis and low bone mass in premenopausal and perimenopausal women. Endocr Pract 2000;6:296–304.
61. Peris P, Guanabens N, Martinez de Osaba MJ, et al. Clinical characteristics and etiologic factors of premenopausal osteoporosis in a group of Spanish women. Semin Arthritis Rheum 2002;32:64–70.
62. Cohen A, Fleischer J, Freeby MJ, et al. Clinical characteristics and medication use among premenopausal women with osteoporosis and low BMD: the experience of an osteoporosis referral center. J Womens Health (Larchmt) 2009;18: 79–84.
63. Miller KK, Lee EE, Lawson EA, et al. Determinants of skeletal loss and recovery in anorexia nervosa. J Clin Endocrinol Metab 2006;91:2931–7.

64. Adams JS, Song CF, Kantorovich V. Rapid recovery of bone mass in hypercalciuric, osteoporotic men treated with hydrochlorothiazide. Ann Intern Med 1999; 130:658–60.
65. Ciacci C, Maurelli L, Klain M, et al. Effects of dietary treatment on bone mineral density in adults with celiac disease: factors predicting response. Am J Gastroenterol 1997;92:992–6.
66. Mautalen C, Gonzalez D, Mazure R, et al. Effect of treatment on bone mass, mineral metabolism, and body composition in untreated celiac disease patients. Am J Gastroenterol 1997;92:313–8.
67. McFarlane XA, Bhalla AK, Robertson DA. Effect of a gluten free diet on osteopenia in adults with newly diagnosed coeliac disease. Gut 1996;39:180–4.
68. Mauro M, Radovic V, Armstrong D. Improvement of lumbar bone mass after infliximab therapy in Crohn's disease patients. Can J Gastroenterol 2007;21: 637–42.
69. Lumachi F, Camozzi V, Ermani M, et al. Bone mineral density improvement after successful parathyroidectomy in pre- and postmenopausal women with primary hyperparathyroidism: a prospective study. Ann N Y Acad Sci 2007;1117:357–61.
70. Peris P, Ruiz-Esquide V, Monegal A, et al. Idiopathic osteoporosis in premenopausal women. Clinical characteristics and bone remodelling abnormalities. Clin Exp Rheumatol 2008;26:986–91.
71. Wallace BA, Cumming RG. Systematic review of randomized trials of the effect of exercise on bone mass in pre- and postmenopausal women. Calcif Tissue Int 2000;67:10–8.
72. Ross AC, Manson JE, Abrams SA, et al. The 2011 report on dietary reference intakes for calcium and vitamin D from the Institute of Medicine: what clinicians need to know. J Clin Endocrinol Metab 2011;96:53–8.
73. Cundy T, Ames R, Horne A, et al. A randomized controlled trial of estrogen replacement therapy in long-term users of depot medroxyprogesterone acetate. J Clin Endocrinol Metab 2003;88:78–81.
74. Liu SL, Lebrun CM. Effect of oral contraceptives and hormone replacement therapy on bone mineral density in premenopausal and perimenopausal women: a systematic review. Br J Sports Med 2006;40:11–24.
75. Sagsveen M, Farmer JE, Prentice A, et al. Gonadotrophin-releasing hormone analogues for endometriosis: bone mineral density. Cochrane Database Syst Rev 2003;(4):CD001297.
76. Sim LA, McGovern L, Elamin MB, et al. Effect on bone health of estrogen preparations in premenopausal women with anorexia nervosa: a systematic review and meta-analyses. Int J Eat Disord 2010;43:218–25.
77. Lopez LM, Grimes DA, Schulz KF, et al. Steroidal contraceptives: effect on bone fractures in women. Cochrane Database Syst Rev 2011;(6):CD006033.
78. Wei S, Winzenberg T, Laslett LL, et al. Oral contraceptive use and bone. Curr Osteoporos Rep 2011;9:6–11.
79. Cromer BA. Bone mineral density in adolescent and young adult women on injectable or oral contraception. Curr Opin Obstet Gynecol 2003;15:353–7.
80. Polatti F, Perotti F, Filippa N, et al. Bone mass and long-term monophasic oral contraceptive treatment in young women. Contraception 1995;51:221–4.
81. Scholes D, Ichikawa L, LaCroix AZ, et al. Oral contraceptive use and bone density in adolescent and young adult women. Contraception 2010;81:35–40.
82. Powles TJ, Hickish T, Kanis JA, et al. Effect of tamoxifen on bone mineral density measured by dual-energy x-ray absorptiometry in healthy premenopausal and postmenopausal women. J Clin Oncol 1996;14:78–84.

83. Vehmanen L, Elomaa I, Blomqvist C, et al. Tamoxifen treatment after adjuvant chemotherapy has opposite effects on bone mineral density in premenopausal patients depending on menstrual status. J Clin Oncol 2006;24:675–80.
84. Fuleihan Gel H, Salamoun M, Mourad YA, et al. Pamidronate in the prevention of chemotherapy-induced bone loss in premenopausal women with breast cancer: a randomized controlled trial. J Clin Endocrinol Metab 2005;90:3209–14.
85. Golden NH, Iglesias EA, Jacobson MS, et al. Alendronate for the treatment of osteopenia in anorexia nervosa: a randomized, double-blind, placebo-controlled trial. J Clin Endocrinol Metab 2005;90:3179–85.
86. Miller KK, Grieco KA, Mulder J, et al. Effects of risedronate on bone density in anorexia nervosa. J Clin Endocrinol Metab 2004;89:3903–6.
87. Nakayamada S, Okada Y, Saito K, et al. Etidronate prevents high dose glucocorticoid induced bone loss in premenopausal individuals with systemic autoimmune diseases. J Rheumatol 2004;31:163–6.
88. Nzeusseu Toukap A, Depresseux G, Devogelaer JP, et al. Oral pamidronate prevents high-dose glucocorticoid-induced lumbar spine bone loss in premenopausal connective tissue disease (mainly lupus) patients. Lupus 2005;14:517–20.
89. Conwell LS, Chang AB. Bisphosphonates for osteoporosis in people with cystic fibrosis. Cochrane Database Syst Rev 2012;(4):CD002010.
90. Skordis N, Ioannou YS, Kyriakou A, et al. Effect of bisphosphonate treatment on bone mineral density in patients with thalassaemia major. Pediatr Endocrinol Rev 2008;6(Suppl 1):144–8.
91. Okada Y, Nawata M, Nakayamada S, et al. Alendronate protects premenopausal women from bone loss and fracture associated with high-dose glucocorticoid therapy. J Rheumatol 2008;35:2249–54.
92. Yeap SS, Fauzi AR, Kong NC, et al. A comparison of calcium, calcitriol, and alendronate in corticosteroid-treated premenopausal patients with systemic lupus erythematosus. J Rheumatol 2008;35:2344–7.
93. Minsker DH, Manson JM, Peter CP. Effects of the bisphosphonate, alendronate, on parturition in the rat. Toxicol Appl Pharmacol 1993;121:217–23.
94. Levy S, Fayez I, Taguchi N, et al. Pregnancy outcome following in utero exposure to bisphosphonates. Bone 2009;44:428–30.
95. Ornoy A, Wajnberg R, Diav-Citrin O. The outcome of pregnancy following pre-pregnancy or early pregnancy alendronate treatment. Reprod Toxicol 2006; 22:578–9.
96. Munns CF, Rauch F, Ward L, et al. Maternal and fetal outcome after long-term pamidronate treatment before conception: a report of two cases. J Bone Miner Res 2004;19:1742–5.
97. Khosla S, Burr D, Cauley J, et al. Bisphosphonate-associated osteonecrosis of the jaw: report of a task force of the American Society for Bone and Mineral Research. J Bone Miner Res 2007;22:1479–91.
98. Shane E, Burr D, Ebeling PR, et al. Atypical subtrochanteric and diaphyseal femoral fractures: report of a task force of the American Society for Bone and Mineral Research. J Bone Miner Res 2010;25:2267–94.
99. Finkelstein JS, Klibanski A, Arnold AL, et al. Prevention of estrogen deficiency-related bone loss with human parathyroid hormone-(1-34): a randomized controlled trial. JAMA 1998;280:1067–73.
100. Langdahl BL, Marin F, Shane E, et al. Teriparatide versus alendronate for treating glucocorticoid-induced osteoporosis: an analysis by gender and menopausal status. Osteoporos Int 2009;20:2095–104.

101. Saag KG, Shane E, Boonen S, et al. Teriparatide or alendronate in glucocorticoid-induced osteoporosis. N Engl J Med 2007;357:2028–39.
102. Cohen A, Stein EM, Recker RR, et al. Teriparatide for idiopathic osteoporosis in premenopausal women: a pilot study. J Clin Endocrinol Metab 2013;98:1971–81.
103. Nishiyama KK, Cohen A, Young P, et al. Teriparatide increases strength of the peripheral skeleton in premenopausal women with idiopathic osteoporosis: a pilot HR-pQCT study. J Clin Endocrinol Metab 2014;99:2418–25.
104. Fazeli PK, Wang IS, Miller KK, et al. Teriparatide increases bone formation and bone mineral density in adult women with anorexia nervosa. J Clin Endocrinol Metab 2014;99:1322–9.
105. Choe EY, Song JE, Park KH, et al. Effect of teriparatide on pregnancy and lactation-associated osteoporosis with multiple vertebral fractures. J Bone Miner Metab 2012;30:596–601.
106. Finkelstein JS, Arnold AL. Increases in bone mineral density after discontinuation of daily human parathyroid hormone and gonadotropin-releasing hormone analog administration in women with endometriosis. J Clin Endocrinol Metab 1999;84:1214–9.
107. Cohen A, Kamanda-Kosseh M, Recker RR, et al. Bone density after teriparatide discontinuation in premenopausal idiopathic osteoporosis. J Clin Endocrinol Metab 2015;100:4208–14.
108. Peris P, Monegal A, Martinez MA, et al. Bone mineral density evolution in young premenopausal women with idiopathic osteoporosis. Clin Rheumatol 2007;26:958–61.
109. Cohen A, Young P, Stein EM, et al. Absence of the anabolic window characterizes premenopausal women with idiopathic osteoporosis who do not respond to teriparatide. In: American Society for Bone and Mineral Research Annual Meeting. Oral Presentation 1102. Minneapolis, MN, October 14, 2012.
110. Kaunitz AM, Miller PD, Rice VM, et al. Bone mineral density in women aged 25-35 years receiving depot medroxyprogesterone acetate: recovery following discontinuation. Contraception 2006;74:90–9.
111. Scholes D, LaCroix AZ, Ichikawa LE, et al. Change in bone mineral density among adolescent women using and discontinuing depot medroxyprogesterone acetate contraception. Arch Pediatr Adolesc Med 2005;159:139–44.
112. Adachi JD, Bensen WG, Brown J, et al. Intermittent etidronate therapy to prevent corticosteroid-induced osteoporosis. N Engl J Med 1997;337:382–7.
113. Saag KG, Emkey R, Schnitzer TJ, et al. Alendronate for the prevention and treatment of glucocorticoid-induced osteoporosis. Glucocorticoid-Induced Osteoporosis Intervention Study Group. N Engl J Med 1998;339:292–9.
114. Wallach S, Cohen S, Reid DM, et al. Effects of risedronate treatment on bone density and vertebral fracture in patients on corticosteroid therapy. Calcif Tissue Int 2000;67:277–85.
115. Grossman JM, Gordon R, Ranganath VK, et al. American College of Rheumatology 2010 recommendations for the prevention and treatment of glucocorticoid-induced osteoporosis. Arthritis Care Res (Hoboken) 2010;62:1515–26.

Assessing Vitamin D Status in African Americans and the Influence of Vitamin D on Skeletal Health Parameters

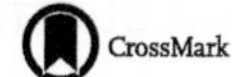

Albert Shieh, MD, MSCR[a,b,*], John F. Aloia, MD[c]

KEYWORDS

- Vitamin D • African American • 25-Hydroxyvitamin D • Calcium absorption
- Parathyroid hormone • Bone mineral density

KEY POINTS

- Despite having lower total 25-hydroxyvitamin D (25OHD) levels compared with white Americans (WAs), African Americans (AAs) have higher bone mineral density and lower fracture risk.
- It was previously proposed that this may be explained by the possibility that AAs may have lower total, but comparable free, 25OHD levels compared with WAs; these earlier findings may have resulted from vitamin D binding protein isoform-dependent variations in assay performance.
- AAs have higher intestinal calcium absorption efficiency and lower urinary calcium excretion compared with WAs.
- AAs may have skeletal resistance to secondary hyperparathyroidism. The threshold 25OHD level below which PTH secretion increases substantially is generally lower in AAs than in WAs.
- AAs have higher BMD and lower fracture risk. Epidemiologic studies suggest an inverse relation between vitamin D status and BMD in WAs, but not in AAs.

The authors have nothing to disclose.

[a] Division of Geriatrics, Department of Medicine, David Geffen School of Medicine, University of California, Los Angeles, 10945 LeConte Avenue, Suite 2339, Los Angeles, CA 90095-1687, USA; [b] Division of Endocrinology, Diabetes, and Hypertension, Department of Medicine, David Geffen School of Medicine, University of California, Los Angeles, 10945 LeConte Avenue, Suite 2339, Los Angeles, CA 90095-1687, USA; [c] Department of Medicine, Bone Mineral Research and Treatment Center, Dean Winthrop University Hospital Clinical Campus, Stony Brook University School of Medicine, 222 Station Plaza North, Suite 510, Mineola, NY 11501, USA
* Corresponding author. 10945 LeConte Avenue, Suite 2339, Los Angeles, CA 90095-1687.
E-mail address: ashieh@mednet.ucla.edu

Endocrinol Metab Clin N Am 46 (2017) 135–152
http://dx.doi.org/10.1016/j.ecl.2016.09.006 endo.theclinics.com
0889-8529/17/

INTRODUCTION

The classical endocrine function of vitamin D is to facilitate intestinal calcium absorption, prevent secondary hyperparathyroidism, and maintain skeletal strength. Vitamin D status is assessed clinically by measuring serum 25-hydroxyvitamin D (25OHD) concentrations.[1,2] In epidemiologic studies, lower 25OHD levels are associated with increased parathyroid hormone (PTH) secretion, decreased bone mineral density (BMD), and increased fracture risk.[3–10] Randomized clinical trials have confirmed that adequate vitamin D intake in combination with calcium prevents fragility fractures in those most at risk for nutritional deficiency.[11]

In the United States, there is a significant disparity in vitamin D status among individuals of African versus European descent. In particular, African Americans (AAs) consistently have lower 25OHD levels compared with white Americans (WAs) throughout the life cycle.[12] Despite these lower 25OHD levels, AAs tend to have greater BMD and lower fracture risk than their WA counterparts.[13,14] Given the importance of vitamin D in helping to maintain skeletal health, this finding has been described as a paradox.[12]

In recent years, it has been proposed that this paradox may be explained by the possibility that although total 25OHD levels (protein-bound 25OHD + free 25OHD) are lower among AAs, free 25OHD levels are comparable with those in WAs.[15,16] This article begins with a review of classical and nonclassical vitamin D physiology. The theoretic rationale for using total versus free 25OHD as a marker of vitamin D status is discussed, and whether total versus free 25OHD is a better marker of vitamin D status in racially/ethnically diverse populations is reviewed. Finally, the effects of vitamin D status and vitamin D supplementation on markers of vitamin D bioactivity (intestinal calcium absorption, PTH secretion, BMD, fracture risk) are described.

VITAMIN D PHYSIOLOGY

Sources of Vitamin D

Vitamin D is obtained through sunlight exposure and oral intake (food or supplement). With sunlight exposure, solar ultraviolet B (UVB) radiation (wavelength spectrum 280–320 nm) penetrates the skin and converts 7-deydrocholesterol to pre–vitamin D_3. Pre–vitamin D_3 is then converted to vitamin D_3 in a thermosensitive, but nonenzymatic, reaction.[17] The rate of endogenous vitamin D_3 synthesis is determined by intensity of UVB and skin pigmentation. UVB intensity varies depending on season (less in winter) and latitude (less with greater distance from equator).[18] Increased melanin in the skin limits UVB access to 7-deydrocholesterol.[19] Dietary sources of vitamin D are limited (vitamin D_3 from fatty fish and egg yolks; vitamin D_2 from shiitake mushrooms). Supplemental vitamin D can also be obtained as vitamin D_2 (ultraviolet irradiation of ergosterol from yeast) and vitamin D_3 (ultraviolet irradiation of 7-dehydrocholesterol from lanolin).[20] Most clinical guidelines treat vitamin D_2 and vitamin D_3 as therapeutically equivalent based on early reports that both analogues reverse vitamin D-deficient rickets in children.[1,2,21]

Classical Endocrine Vitamin D Physiology

The canonical endocrine function of vitamin D is to facilitate intestinal calcium absorption. Under the classical paradigm, vitamin D (D_2 or D_3) is converted to 25OHD (produced in nanogram per milliliter concentrations) in the liver by the CYP2R1 hydroxylase. 25OHD is then converted to 1,25-dihydroxyvitamin D (1,25$(OH)_2$D) in the kidney by the CYP27B1 hydroxylase (produced in picogram per milliliter concentrations). The latter reaction occurs when filtered 25OHD, bound to the vitamin D binding protein (DBP), is internalized by the renal epithelial cell from the glomerular filtrate by a megalin-mediated mechanism.[22] $1,25(OH)_2D$ subsequently circulates to the intestinal enterocyte and, acting in an endocrine fashion, enhances intestinal calcium absorption. In vitamin D–deficient states, intestinal calcium absorption efficiency is decreased, leading to a small decline in serum calcium concentration, and increased PTH secretion by the parathyroid cell (secondary hyperparathyroidism).[12,23,24] Although $1,25(OH)_2D$ is considered the activated form of vitamin D, the major metabolite of 25OHD is actually 24,25-dihyroxyvitamin D ($24,25(OH)_2D$) (produced in nanogram per milliliter concentrations by the CYP24A1 hydroxylase). The biologic activity of $24,25(OH)_2D$ remains controversial, but is generally viewed as a 25OHD catabolite whose synthesis is strongly associated with 25OHD concentrations and is (in part) regulated by the vitamin D receptor[25] (**Fig. 1**).

Nonclassical Vitamin D Physiology

A potential role for vitamin D–directed bioactivity in tissues beyond those involved in calcium homeostasis derives from two major findings. First, CYP27B1, the hydroxylase that converts 25OHD to $1,25(OH)_2D$, is expressed in many extrarenal tissues throughout the body.[26,27] Second, the vitamin D receptor, which is activated by $1,25(OH)_2D$, to mediate vitamin D–directed gene expression is found in virtually all tissues.[28] Under the nonclassical paradigm, substrate 25OHD, produced by CYP2R1 within the hepatocyte, is internalized by a vitamin D target cell.[29] 25OHD is then converted in an intracrine fashion within the vitamin D target cell to $1,25(OH)_2D$ by locally expressed CYP27B1 hydroxylase.[29,30]

Vitamin D Binding Protein

DBP is synthesized in the liver and binds to all vitamin D metabolites in circulation. The mechanism by which substrate 25OHD enters a vitamin D target cell depends on whether 25OHD is DPB-bound or free (unbound to DBP or other serum proteins, such as albumin); and whether the target cell expresses megalin. Under classical vitamin D physiology, 25OHD is internalized by the renal epithelial cell where it is converted to $1,25(OH)_2D$. Because the renal epithelial cell expresses megalin (a cell surface receptor for DBP), 25OHD entry enters this target cell bound to DBP via a

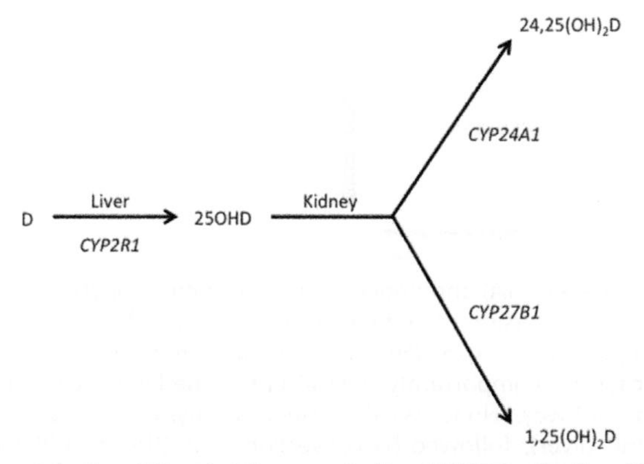

Fig. 1. Vitamin D metabolism. Vitamin D is converted to 25OHD by the liver. 25OHD is then converted to either $1,25(OH)_2D$ or $24,25(OH)_2D$ by the kidney. 1,25(OH)2D synthesis is increased by low serum phosphate, low serum calcium, and high PTH levels. In contrast, $24,25(OH)_2D$ synthesis is increased by high serum phosphate, high serum calcium, and high FGF23.

megalin.[22] Under nonclassical vitamin D physiology, some extrarenal tissues (eg, placenta, mammary gland, parathyroid gland) also express megalin.[31] It is therefore theoretically possible that 25OHD also enters these target cell bound to DBP. This pathway, however, has not been shown to be functionally intact in vivo. In contrast, most extrarenal tissues do not express megalin.[31] In these tissues, the “free-hormone hypothesis” proposes that 25OHD enters vitamin D target cells by simple diffusion in its free form, unbound to DBP or other serum proteins[30] (**Fig. 2**). This concept involving

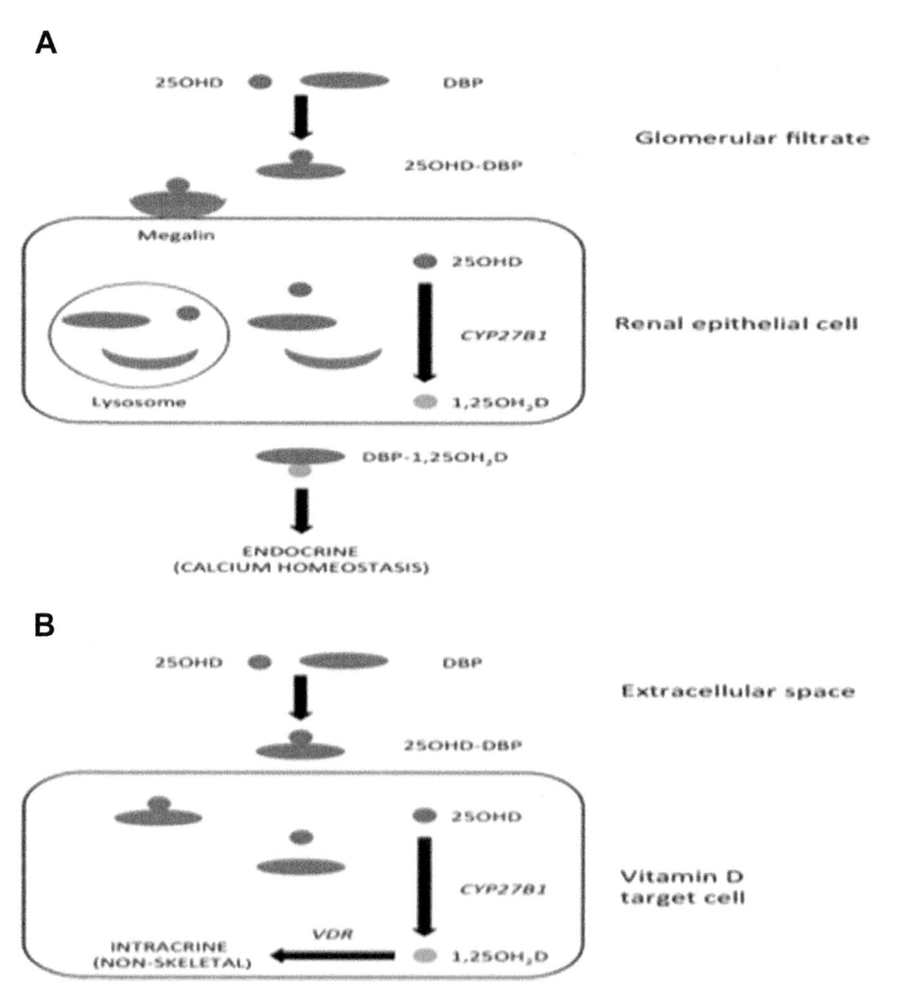

Fig. 2. Schematic of classical (*A*) and nonclassical (*B*) vitamin D physiology. Classical vitamin D physiology involves conversion of vitamin D to 25OHD (liver), followed by conversion of 25OHD to 1,25(OH)$_2$D (kidney). 1,25(OH)$_2$D then acts in an endocrine fashion to facilitate intestinal calcium absorption. Importantly, 25OHD enters the kidney cell bound to DBP via a megalin-mediated pathway. Nonclassical vitamin D physiology involves conversion of vitamin D to 25OHD (liver), followed by conversion of 25OHD to 1,25(OH)2D within the vitamin D target cell. 1,25(OH)$_2$D then mediates vitamin D–directed gene expression within the target cell. Mechanism of 25OHD entry into the target cell is controversial. In cells that express megalin, 25OHD may enter bound to DBP. In cells that do not express megalin, 25OHD may enter via diffusion. VDR, vitamin D receptor.

unbound hormone has been applied clinically to thyroid hormone, cortisol, and sex steroid hormones, where medications or concurrent comorbidities may influence levels of the respective hormone-binding globulin.

ASSESSING VITAMIN D STATUS

25-Hydroxyvitamin D as a Marker of Vitamin D Status

Several vitamin D metabolites exist within the systemic circulation. However, 25OHD is the metabolite that is measured clinically to assess an individual's vitamin D status.[20] 25OHD has a longer half-life (~3 weeks and longer), and is associated in epidemiologic studies with various clinical markers of vitamin D bioactivity (eg, PTH, BMD, fracture risk).[5,6,9,10,32–34] Circulating 25OHD may be bound to serum carrier proteins (mostly DBP or albumin) or free.[35] An individual's vitamin D status is determined by measuring his or her total 25OHD concentration.

AAs have consistently been shown to have lower vitamin D status as assessed by total 25OHD than WAs across the lifespan in regional and national epidemiologic studies using a variety of thresholds for low 25OHD (**Fig. 3**). For example, in National Health and Nutrition Examination Survey (NHANES), 92% of AA children between 1 and 11 years had 25OHD levels less than 20 ng/mL, compared with 59% of WAs.[36] Also in NHANES, 42.4% of AA adolescents and adults between 15 and 49 years had 25OHD levels less than 15 ng/mL, compared with 4.2% of WAs.[37] The cause of lower 25OHD levels in AAs is multifactorial. Increased melanin in the skin limits absorption of UVB radiation and formation of pre–vitamin D_3.[19] AAs also consume less dietary vitamin D.[38]

Interpretation of the clinical vitamin D literature requires recognition that it is difficult to accurately measure 25OHD levels, and variability exists between different assay methodologies. The most common assays used in clinical laboratories are antibody-based or high-performance liquid chromatography–based coupled with UV (ultraviolet) or mass spectrometric detection. Multiple sources of variability between assays have been reported, and include differences in methodology for vitamin D metabolite separation from DBP, cross-reactivity to 25OHD2, cross-reactivity to 3-epi-25OHD3 and other vitamin D metabolites, and matrix interferences.[39] This in turn, leads to underestimation and overestimation of 25OHD values. Many have argued

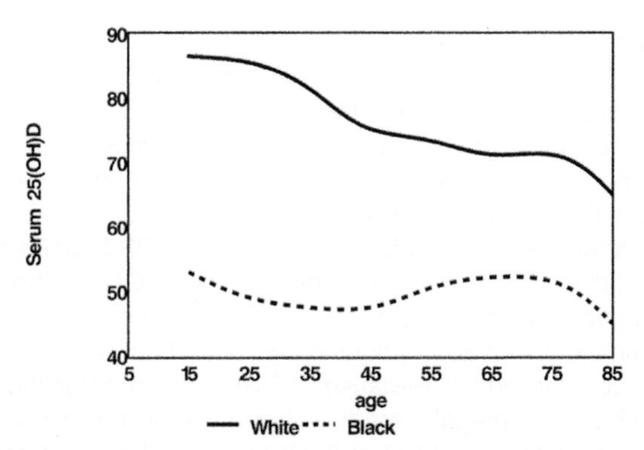

Fig. 3. Serum 25OHD level in African Americans versus white persons by age among participants in the National Health and Nutrition Examination Survey. (*From* Aloia JF. African Americans, 25-hydroxyvitamin D, and osteoporosis: a paradox. Am J Clin Nutr 2008;88(Suppl):546S; with permission.)

that poor 25OHD measurement standardization limits efforts to develop clinical and public health vitamin D guidelines. The Vitamin D Standardization Program, an international collaborative effort founded in 2010, aims to address this problem.[40,41]

Theoretic Arguments for Measuring Total Versus Free/Bioavailable 25-Hydroxyvitamin D as a Marker of Vitamin D Status

The question of whether measuring total versus free 25OHD is superior for assessing an individual's vitamin D status arises from several considerations. First, more than 99.9% of circulating total 25OHD is bound to serum proteins (mostly DBP and albumin).[35] 25OHD binds with greater affinity to DBP ($K_a = 7 \times 10^8$ M^{-1}) than to albumin ($K_a = 6 \times 10^5$ M^{-1}).[35] Free 25OHD refers to 25OHD (<0.1%) that is not bound to a serum carrier protein. Bioavailable 25OHD refers to 25OHD (~10%) that is free or bound to albumin.[30] Second, there are different isoforms of DBP that may vary in total quantity expressed and binding avidity for vitamin D metabolites. Variations in DBP were first described based on different isoelectric focusing migration patterns of a then-unidentified serum protein.[42] Initially referred to as Group-Specific Component (Gc)1F, Gc1S, and Gc2, these proteins are now recognized as isoforms of DBP.[43,44] DBP isoform may be important because Gc alleles have distinct racial distribution patterns.[30,45] For example, individuals of African and Asian descent more frequently express the Gc1F isoform, whereas those of European descent more frequently express the Gc2 isoform.[30] Each isoform results from variations in the DBP amino acid sequence that may alter their binding avidity for vitamin D metabolites. In particular, Gc1F has been reported to have the highest avidity for vitamin D metabolites, and Gc2 has the lowest.[43,44] This, however, has not been consistently shown.[46]

An area of intensive vitamin D research at present time focuses on whether total versus free/bioavailable 25OHD represents a superior marker of vitamin D status in vivo. Before presenting the currently available human clinical data and its implications in AAs specifically, we first explore the theoretic physiologic rationale for measuring one versus the other. In classical vitamin D physiology, $1,25(OH)_2D$ is synthesized when DBP-bound 25OHD is internalized by the renal epithelial cell via a megalin-mediated mechanism and then converted to the active metabolite by CYP27B1.[22] Based on this, one would posit that total 25OHD represents the better marker of vitamin D status of classical vitamin D bioactivity. In nonclassical vitamin D physiology, it has been proposed that $1,25(OH)_2D$ is synthesized in nonmegalin-expressing tissues when free 25OHD is internalized by the target cell via simple diffusion and then converted to the active metabolite by locally expressed CYP27B1.[30] Based on this, one would posit that free 25OHD represents a better marker of vitamin D status of nonclassical vitamin D bioactivity.

This may, however, be an oversimplification. For example, it is unclear whether 25OHD only enters megalin-expressing tissues (eg, renal epithelial cell) bound to DBP, or if some 25OHD enters the target cell in free unbound form. The physiologic plausibility of the latter is suggested by experiments in DBP knockout mice in whom total 25OHD and total $1,25(OH)_2D$ are (as expected) low.[47] Of note, however, provided that there is adequate vitamin D intake through the diet, the skeletal phenotype (and presumably intestinal calcium absorption) in DBP knockout animals is similar to that of their wild-type counterparts.[47] Because 25OHD cannot enter the renal epithelial cell bound to DBP via the megalin-mediated pathway in these animals, it may be that physiologically relevant quantities of 25OHD enters the target cell in its free unbound form. Although this argues for a broader physiologic role for free/bioaviable 25OHD, there remain important reservations regarding the free hormone hypothesis.[48,49]

Determining Free/Bioavailable 25-Hydroxyvitamin D Levels

There are direct and indirect methods for determining free/bioavailable 25OHD levels. The direct method involves direct assay of the free 25OHD metabolite. The indirect method uses mathematical modeling to calculate free/bioavailable 25OHD levels by applying binding coefficients for DBP and albumin to measurements of total 25OHD, DBP, and albumin.[45,50] The accuracy of this approach, therefore, is contingent on reliable estimates of DBP avidity for vitamin D metabolites and reliable measurements of 25OHD, DBP, and albumin. With respect to estimates of DBP avidity, there is concern that use of a single average binding coefficient for DBP leads to inaccurate estimations of free/bioavailable 25OHD because DBP avidity for 25OHD may vary depending on DBP isoform.[51] Indeed, free 25OHD levels estimated using this approach consistently exceed those obtained by direct measurement.[51,52]

With respect to absolute DBP concentration, there is considerable variability depending on type of DBP assay used. The most reliable methods for DBP quantification are liquid chromatography–tandem mass spectrometry and proteomic analysis.[52,53] Other commonly reported methods include monoclonal (R&D Systems, Minneapolis, MN) and polyclonal (Genway, San Diego, CA; Immunodiagnostik, Germany) antibody-based enzyme-linked immunosorbent assay (ELISA).[45,52,53] Earlier studies using the monoclonal ELISA reported that AAs had lower levels of DBP compared with WAs.[45] However, the monoclonal ELISA has been recently shown to underestimate the Gc1F isoform (expressed more commonly in individuals of African descent).[45,52] In contrast, when measured by polyclonal ELISA, liquid chromatography–tandem mass spectrometry, or proteomic analysis, DBP levels are similar between AAs and WAs.[16,52–55] This has led some investigators to argue for reconsideration of conclusions drawn from studies in which free/bioavailable 25OHD was estimated using DBP measurements by monoclonal ELISA, especially if the Gc1F isoform was prevalent among study participants.[52]

Given the challenges associated with mathematical estimates of free/bioavailable 25OHD, there is an increasing preference to use directly measured free 25OHD in basic and clinical studies. Although a dialysis-based assay has previously been reported,[35] it is labor-intensive and time-consuming. More recently, several antibody-based methodologies have become available, but are neither commercially available nor fully validated. One of the more commonly used assays is an ELISA (Future Diagnostics, Netherlands). Free 25OHD levels obtained by direct measurement via this assay strongly correlate with calculated free 25OHD levels estimated when DBP levels are measured by liquid chromatography–tandem mass spectrometry, proteomic analysis, or polyclonal ELISA ($r \geq 0.8$).[52]

Clinical Utility of Determining Free/Bioavailable 25-Hydroxyvitamin D in African Americans

One of the first large-scale clinical studies comparing total and bioavailable 25OHD levels across race/ethnicity involved a community-based cohort of 2085 AA and WA participants.[45] Using previously collected serum, the investigators first determined each study participant's DBP genotype. Among homozygous participants, they estimated bioavailable 25OHD concentration from measurements of total 25OHD, DBP (monoclonal ELISA), and albumin. Total 25OHD and DBP levels were lower in AAs compared with WAs (25OHD, 15.6 $\pm$ 0.2 ng/mL vs 25.8 $\pm$ 0.4 ng/mL; $P<.001$) (DBP, 168 $\pm$ 3 μg/mL vs 335 $\pm$ 5 μg/mL; $P<.001$). Among homozygous patients, however, calculated bioavailable 25OHD levels were similar in AAs and WAs (2.9 $\pm$ 0.1 pg/mL vs 3.1 $\pm$ 0.1 pg/mL; $P = .7$). This led the authors to propose an attractive explanation for the seeming paradox of lower total 25OHD and superior skeletal health parameters among AAs: despite having lower total 25OHD levels, AAs have lower DBP levels, and therefore similar free/bioavailable 25OHD levels compared with WAs.[45] However, DBP was quantified by monoclonal ELISA. Because this ELISA underestimates the Gc1F DBP isoform, and this isoform is prevalent among individuals of African and Asian descent, it is possible that the calculated bioavailable 25OHD in AA participants overestimated the true bioavailable 25OHD.[52,53]

Since this study, several additional studies have compared total and directly measured 25OHD levels across race/ethnicity. Two representative studies are highlighted here.[16,52] In a sample of 164 healthy postmenopausal AA and WA women propensity-matched for age and body mass index, total 25OHD levels were lower in AAs compared with WAs (19.5 $\pm$ 4.7 ng/mL vs 26.9 $\pm$ 6.4 ng/mL; $P<.0001$). In this study, DBP was quantified by monoclonal and polyclonal ELISAs. DBP was lower in AAs compared with WAs when assessed by monoclonal ELISA (151.4 $\pm$ 73.2 μg/mL vs 264.8 $\pm$ 95.5 μg/mL; $P<.0001$), but similar when assessed by polyclonal ELISA (378 $\pm$ 82 μg/mL vs 351 $\pm$ 66 μg/mL; $P = .02$). Interestingly, directly measured free 25OHD was nearly identical in AAs and WAs (5.25 $\pm$ 1.2 pg/mL vs 5.25 $\pm$ 1.3 pg/mL; $P = .9$).[16] These findings are intriguing for several reasons. Assuming that polyclonal ELISA measurement of DBP is accurate, DBP levels in AAs and WAs are similar. One would therefore assume, that if total 25OHD levels are lower in AA, free 25OHD levels also should be lower. This, however, was not seen. The exact reasons for this discrepancy remain unclear.

More recently, total 25OHD, DBP (monoclonal and polyclonal ELISA), calculated free 25OHD, and directly measured free 25OHD was determined in 1057 community-dwelling men of African and European ancestry residing in the United States, United Kingdom, and Gambia.[52] Again, DBP levels were lower in AA versus WA men when measured by monoclonal ELISA, but similar by polyclonal ELISA. Polyclonal ELISA results correlated closely with those by proteomic analysis. Among AAs, calculated free 25OHD based on polyclonal ELISA measurement of DBP and directly measured free 25OHD levels were lower compared with WAs (all $P<.001$). Total 25OHD was highly correlated with calculated free 25OHD levels (polyclonal DBP ELISA, $r>0.9$), and the latter tracked closely with directly measured free 25OHD levels ($r>0.8$). The authors concluded that total 25OHD remained a useful marker of vitamin D status irrespective of race/ethnicity and DBP genotype.[52]

Although this topic continues to be actively investigated, the totality of the emerging literature seems to suggest that (1) prior reports of higher free/bioavailable 25OHD levels in AAs likely resulted from DBP isoform-dependent variations in assay performance, (2) total and free 25OHD levels track closely with one another, and (3) total 25OHD measurement likely remains a useful marker of vitamin D status even in diverse populations. It remains to be seen, however, whether dynamic changes in markers of vitamin D bioactivity correlate more closely with change in total versus free 25OHD.[55,56] This in turn may be dependent on outcome of interest (ie, classical vs nonclassical vitamin D action).

24,25-Hydroxyvitamin D and the Vitamin D Metabolite Ratio as a Marker of Vitamin D Status

Some investigators recently proposed that $24,25(OH)_2D$ and the ratio of $24,25(OH)_2D$ to 25OHD (vitamin D metabolite ratio [VMR]) can serve as useful markers of vitamin D status.[57–60] One early study to explore this possibility administered 4000 IU/day of vitamin D_3 versus placebo for 6 weeks to healthy young adults, and found that serum $24,25(OH)_2D$ and 25OHD concentrations were highly correlated ($r = 0.91$). This prompted the investigators to wonder whether $24,25(OH)_2D$ could serve as an alternative measure of vitamin D status.[57] A subsequent study reported that the ratio of

$24,25(OH)_2D$ to 25OHD (VMR) was markedly decreased when serum 25OHD levels were less than 10 ng/mL.[59] This was interpreted to mean that VMR may serve as a functional marker of 25OHD substrate availability. More recently, absolute serum 25OHD and $24,25(OH)_2D$ concentrations were found to be lower among AAs versus WAs, but VMR was similar between groups. The correlation between VMR and PTH was also similar between groups. This led the investigators to propose that VMR may be a useful marker of vitamin D status independent of race/ethnicity.[60] Further studies of VMR are required to determine its clinical utility.

MARKER OF CLASSICAL VITAMIN D BIOACTIVITY

Calcium Economy

The classical endocrine function of vitamin D is to mediate calcium homeostasis. The amount of dietary calcium retained by the body is a function of calcium absorbed (intestine) and calcium excreted (urine, feces). Intestinal calcium absorption and calcium excretion have been studied in AAs. With respect to calcium absorption, AAs have either similar or higher intestinal calcium absorption compared with WAs.[61–66] These findings are generally associated with lower calcium intake, 25OHD (one exception), similar or higher PTH, and higher $1,25(OH)_2D$ levels among AAs versus WAs. With respect to calcium excretion, most studies have focused on urine. Lower urinary calcium excretion in AAs has been consistently reported.[61–66]

Taken in totality, the literature seems to suggest that across all segments of the lifespan calcium retention is greater in AAs compared with WAs secondary to comparable with higher intestinal calcium absorption efficiency and lower urinary calcium excretion. This occurs despite lower 25OHD levels in AAs. The finding of higher $1,25(OH)_2D$ levels in AAs is of interest. It is classically understood that increased PTH drives renal synthesis of $1,25(OH)_2D$. However, in several of the previously mentioned studies, PTH levels were similar between AAs and WAs.[61–66] Another race/ethnicity-driven mechanism may therefore be contributing. One possibility is that FGF-23 (an osteocyte-derived factor that suppresses $1,25(OH)_2D$ production) may be lower in AAs than WAs.[67] It is also classically understood that $1,25(OH)_2D$ increases intestinal calcium absorption efficiency. However, even in studies in which intestinal calcium absorption efficiency is similar between AAs and WAs, $1,25(OH)_2D$ is higher in the former. This has led some to propose that AAs may have intestinal resistance to $1,25(OH)_2D$.[64] Indeed, there are variants of the vitamin D receptor that modify the intestinal calcium absorption efficiency.[68] Whether these variants have a specific race/ethnic distribution has not been defined.

From a clinical standpoint, the question that most cross-sectional and vitamin D intervention studies have attempted to address is whether vitamin D status influences intestinal calcium absorption and whether the association is different in AAs versus WAs. Without consideration for race/ethnicity, the totality of the literature suggests that a threshold change in calcium absorption likely exists at 25OHD levels less than 10 ng/mL.[65,69–71] At higher 25OHD levels, multiple prospective dose-response studies have now shown that vitamin D supplementation either effects no or relatively small increases in intestinal calcium absorption.[69,72] With respect to whether the 25OHD/intestinal calcium absorption association is different in AAs versus WAs, randomized control trial data are fairly limited. In 323 AA and WA children, administration of 400 to 4000 IU/day of vitamin D_3 did not increase calcium absorption in either race/ethnicity (baseline 25OHD was 28 ng/mL).[73] In 198 adolescent females, 400 to 2400 IU/day of vitamin D_3 similarly did not improve calcium absorption. Baseline 25OHD level was 11.6 ng/mL in AA participants.[69]

Secondary Hyperparathyroidism

Classically, it is believed that vitamin D deficiency leads to decreased intestinal calcium absorption, transiently decreased serum calcium, and increased PTH secretion (secondary hyperparathyroidism).[12,23,24] Along these lines, an inverse relationship between PTH and 25OHD has been reported.[3–5] 25OHD may also have a direct genomic effect on the parathyroid gland.[74,75] Differences in PTH level between AAs and WAs have also been reported. In middle-aged adults from NHANES, mean PTH level was 42.6 pg/mL in 1792 AAs versus 38.3 pg/mL in 4026 WAs.[10] In older adults from the Health ABC study, mean PTH was 44.2 pg/mL in 1023 AAs versus 35.3 pg/mL in 1615 WAs.[6] In both studies, 25OHD was lower in AAs. In the first study, calcium intake was recorded, and was lower in AAs.[10] Although these and other studies report that AAs have higher PTH levels than WAs, other studies have not.[6,10,65,66,76] Taken in totality, however, the literature suggests that AAs have similar to higher PTH levels compared with WAs, usually in association with lower 25OHD levels. Inconsistencies between studies may be because AA and WA subjects were not propensity-matched for covariates that influence PTH secretion (eg, calcium intake).

From a clinical standpoint, two questions have generated interest. First, why do AAs have stronger skeletal health parameters despite higher PTH levels?[12] Second, what is the threshold 25OHD level below which serum PTH levels begin to increase, and is this threshold different in AAs? With respect to the first question, it has been proposed that AAs have skeletal resistance to PTH.[77–79] This is based on the finding that despite having similar to higher PTH levels than WAs, AAs have lower bone turnover when assessed biochemically and histomorphometrically.[78,79] To test this hypothesis, human (1–34)PTH was administered to 15 AA and 18 WA premenopausal women over 24 hours. Increase in bone resorption markers was significantly higher in WAs than in AAs. Change in bone formation markers was similar between groups.[78]

With respect to the inverse relation between PTH and 25OHD, the threshold 25OHD level below which PTH increases is generally lower in AAs. In two studies conducted at the same center, the threshold 25OHD level that represents the PTH inflection point was between 14 and 16 ng/mL in AA, compared with 24 ng/mL in WAs.[80,81] In the Multicenter Osteoarthritis Study, the threshold 25OHD levels were 20 ng/mL in AAs and 30 ng/mL WAs.[82] In NHANES, the threshold 25OHD was also lower in AAs versus WAs.[9] Although the different studies reported different thresholds, presumably because of variability in assay methodology and calcium intake (another variable that influences PTH secretion), the totality of the literature suggests that AAs tend to have different threshold 25OHD levels for PTH increase. The precise mechanism behind this finding is not well understood, but one could speculate that polymorphisms in the calcium sensing receptor or vitamin D receptor could play a role. Another possibility is that higher PTH levels may have anabolic actions, especially in the setting of skeletal resistance.

SKELETAL PHENOTYPE IN AFRICAN AMERICANS

Fracture Risk

In the Study of Osteoporotic Fractures, a prospective cohort study of 7970 postmenopausal women (65–99 years), AA participants had 30% to 40% lower incidence of nonvertebral fracture at every BMD tertile compared with WAs.[14] Similarly, in the National Osteoporosis Risk Assessment study, a prospective study of 197,848 postmenopausal women, major osteoporotic fracture risk was 48% lower among AAs compared with WAs.[13]

Data on the influence of vitamin D status and fracture in AAs are limited and mostly observational. In AA children, a case-control study reported that a 25OHD level less than 20 ng/mL was associated with a 3.46-fold increased odds of fracture after adjustment of relevant covariates.[83] In the ARIC Study of 12,781 middle-aged WA and AA participants, baseline 25OHD level less than 20 ng/mL was associated with 21% and 35% greater hazard for any and hip fracture requiring hospitalization, respectively, over 20 years of follow-up.[34] Of note, 25OHD was measured only at baseline, and it is unclear whether serum levels remained constant over the study period.

Bone Mineral Density

BMD accounts for 80% of a bone's strength. Data from a longitudinal study of femoral BMD in children (6–16 years) and adults from NHANES confirm that AAs have higher BMD than WAs throughout all segments of the lifespan.[12] BMD loss begins at approximately the same age in AAs and WAs. In the multiethnic Study of Women Across the Nation, cumulative BMD loss from 5 years before to 5 years after the final menstrual period was greater in WA (−9.11%) versus AA (−8.0%) women.[84] In the National Osteoporosis Risk Assessment study, a prospective study of 197,848 postmenopausal women, AA participants had one-half the prevalence of osteoporosis.[13] The higher BMD reported in AAs does not seem to be an artifact of larger bone size.[85] After age 75, however, rate of BMD loss may be more rapid in AAs than WAs.[12]

From a clinical standpoint, two principal questions have been addressed. First, does vitamin D status affect BMD in AAs? Second, does vitamin D supplementation improve BMD or prevent BMD loss in AAs? In NHANES, BMD was negatively associated with 25OHD in WAs, but not AAs.[9] Similar results were reported in 331 AA and 421 AA men with mean 25OHD levels of 25 ng/mL and 37 ng/mL, respectively.[7] A smaller VA study of 112 AA patients found that total hip BMD was positively associated with 25OHD only at levels less than 15 ng/mL.[8] In one prospective vitamin D supplementation trial of postmenopausal women, vitamin D3 at 800 IU/day for 2 years (baseline 25OHD <20 ng/mL) followed by 2000 IU/day for 1 year (mean baseline 25OHD 18.8 ng/mL) did not slow BMD decline.[86] Another similar study in which mean participant baseline 25OHD was 11.6 ng/mL reported similar findings.[87] One potential area of further study may be in the effects of vitamin D on BMD loss in late postmenopausal AA women specifically over 75 years because BMD loss after this age may be faster in AAs.

Bone Microarchitecture

Bone microarchitecture is an important component of bone quality, which in turn is associated with fracture risk. Interracial/ethnic differences in bone microarchitecture as assessed by imaging and histomorphometry have been reported. For example, in 314 early pubertal adolescents, cortical volumetric BMD at the tibial diaphysis was greater in AAs, and tibial strength was 17% higher. Higher bone formation and lower bone resorption marker levels were also noted in AA participants.[88] In premenopausal women, histomorphometric study of iliac biopsies in 55 women did not reveal any difference in bone volume, microstructure, or turnover between AA and WA participants. However, total formation period within each remodeling unit was longer in AAs, possibly allowing greater deposition of bone mineral.[89] In 1067 adults in Multi-Ethnic Study of Atherosclerosis, trabecular volumetric BMD was higher in AAs despite lower 25OHD levels.[90]

The association between vitamin D status and bone microarchitecture is inconsistent. For example, in Multi-Ethnic Study of Atherosclerosis, volumetric trabecular BMD was lower among WAs with 25OHD levels less than 20 ng/mL versus greater than or equal to 30 ng/mL, but not in AAs.[90] Similarly, in the MrOS study, cortical parameters increased with increasing serum 25OHD levels in WAs, but not in Africans. Of note, the 25OHD levels were higher in African (34.7 ng/mL) versus WA (27.6 ng/mL) study participants.[91]

VITAMIN D SUPPLEMENTATION

There remains controversy over the optimal serum 25OHD level necessary for preventing adverse skeletal health outcomes. For skeletal health, the Institute of Medicine recommends maintaining a serum 25OHD level of 20 ng/mL.[1] Based on the evidence presented previously, however, race/ethnicity-specific recommendations may be warranted, but currently do not exist.

Studies have assessed the 25OHD dose response to vitamin D supplementation in AAs. In adolescents, 400 IU/day of vitamin D_3 was sufficient to raise mean 25OHD levels from 13 ng/mL to 24 ng/mL over 16 weeks; 2000 IU/day raised mean 25OHD levels from 13 ng/mL to 34 ng/mL over 16 weeks.[92] In adults, 1640 and 4000 IU/day of vitamin D_3 were estimated to be required to raise serum 25OHD concentrations from less than 20 ng/mL to greater than 20 ng/mL and 30 ng/mL, respectively.[93–95] An amount of 4800 IU/day of vitamin D_3 increased 25OHD levels to 50 ng/mL.[69] 25OHD response to vitamin D supplementation was found to be similar in AAs compared with WAs in children and adults.[69,73] One error common to these studies is that investigators aim to estimate the amount of vitamin D needed to ensure that nearly all within the population achieve the recommended dietary allowance–associated serum 25OHD level. The goal, however, should be to estimate the amount needed such that most of the population achieves the estimated average requirement–associated serum 25OHD level. The former has been critiqued for leading to overestimation of vitamin D intake needs within the population and increasing the possibility of adverse effects because it may result in a proportion of the population's intake to exceed the tolerable upper intake level (**Fig. 4**).[96,97] The Institute of Medicine–recommended serum 25OHD threshold is achieved with 800 IU of vitamin D per day. However, because obesity is prevalent among AAs, higher intake levels may be needed to achieve a specific 25OHD level.[98]

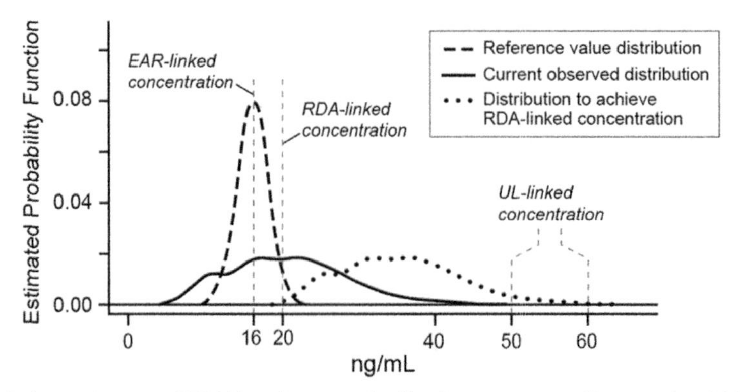

Fig. 4. Estimated serum 25OHD reference distribution corresponding to the EAR-linked 25OHD value (16 ng/mL) compared with observed serum 25OHD distribution in adults 19 to 70 years (NHANES 2005–2006) and observed serum 25OHD distribution shifted such that 97.5% of the sample achieves the RDA-linked 25OHD value (20 ng/mL). Shifting the 25OHD distribution such that 95.7% of the population achieves the RDA-linked 25OHD value causes a portion of the population's intake to exceed the tolerable upper intake level. EAR, estimated average requirement; RDA, recommended dietary allowance; UL, upper limit. (*From* Taylor CL, Carriquiry AL, Bailey RL, et al. Appropriateness of the probability approach with a nutrient status biomarker to assess population inadequacy: a study using vitamin D. Am J Clin Nutr 2013;97:72–8; with permission.)

SUMMARY

This article reviews classical and nonclassical vitamin D physiology, describes whether total versus free 25OHD is a better marker of vitamin D status in AAs, and summarizes the influence of vitamin D status and vitamin D supplementation on markers of vitamin D bioactivity (intestinal calcium absorption, PTH secretion, BMD, fracture) in AAs. Key points are summarized next:

- Classical vitamin D physiology involves conversion of vitamin D to 25OHD (liver), followed by conversion of 25OHD to 1,25$(OH)_2$D (kidney). 1,25$(OH)_2$D then facilitates intestinal calcium absorption. Importantly, 25OHD enters the kidney cell bound to DBP via a megalin-mediated pathway.
- Nonclassical vitamin D physiology involves conversion of vitamin D to 25OHD (liver), followed by conversion of 25OHD to 1,25(OH)2D within the vitamin D target cell. 1,25$(OH)_2$D then mediates vitamin D–directed gene expression within the target cell. Mechanism of 25OHD entry into the target cell is controversial. In cells that express megalin, 25OHD may enter bound to DBP. In cells that do not express megalin, 25OHD may enter via diffusion.
- Free 25OHD is determined by mathematical modeling or direct measurement. Free 25OHD levels are calculated from measurements of total 25OHD, DBP, and albumin, plus estimated affinity constants for the latter two. Monoclonal DBP ELISAs underestimate the quantities of the DBP isoform more commonly expressed in AAs. Calculated free 25OHD levels derived from monoclonal DBP ELISA measurement overestimate free 25OHD levels. Calculated free 25OHD levels derived from polyclonal DBP ELISA measurement correlate strongly with directly measured free 25OHD levels.
- AAs were reported to have lower total, but comparable free, 25OHD levels to WAs in earlier studies. These studies may be biased by use of the monoclonal DBP ELISA. Recent studies suggest that in AAs, total and free 25OHD levels are strongly correlated.
- AAs have higher intestinal calcium absorption efficiency and lower urinary calcium excretion compared with WAs. Vitamin D supplementation in AAs with 25OHD levels greater than 10 ng/mL does not enhance intestinal calcium absorption.
- AAs may have skeletal resistance to secondary hyperparathyroidism. The threshold 25OHD level below which PTH secretion increases substantially is generally lower in AAs than in WAs.
- AAs have higher BMD and lower fracture risk. Epidemiologic studies suggest an inverse relation between vitamin D status and BMD in WAs, but not in AAs. Along these lines, randomized controlled trials do not consistently show a benefit to vitamin D supplementation in calcium-replete AA women.

REFERENCES

1. Institute of Medicine & Food and Nutrition Board Institute. Dietary Reference Intakes for Calcium and Vitamin D. 2011.
2. Holick M, Binkley N, Bischoff-Ferrari H, et al. Evaluation, treatment, and prevention of vitamin D deficiency: an Endocrine Society clinical practice guideline. J Clin Endocrinol Metab 2011;96(7):1911–30.
3. Chapuy MC, Schott AM, Garnero P, et al. Healthy elderly French women living at home have secondary hyperparathyroidism and high bone turnover in winter. EPIDOS Study Group. J Clin Endocrinol Metab 1996;81(3):1129–33.

4. Holick MF, Siris ES, Binkley N, et al. Prevalence of vitamin D inadequacy among postmenopausal North American women receiving osteoporosis therapy. J Clin Endocrinol Metab 2005;90(6):3215–24.
5. Steingrimsdottir L, Gunnarsson O, Indridason OS, et al. Relationship between serum parathyroid hormone levels, vitamin D sufficiency, and calcium intake. JAMA 2005;294(18):2336–41.
6. Kritchevsky SB, Tooze JA, Neiberg RH, et al. Hydroxyvitamin D, parathyroid hormone, and mortality in black and white older adults: the health ABC study. J Clin Endocrinol Metab 2012;97(11):4156–65.
7. Hannan MT, Litman HJ, Araujo AB, et al. Serum 25-hydroxyvitamin D and bone mineral density in a racially and ethnically diverse group of men. J Clin Endocrinol Metab 2008;93(1):40–6.
8. Akhter N, Sinnott B, Mahmood K, et al. Effects of vitamin D insufficiency on bone mineral density in African American men. Osteoporos Int 2009;20(5):745–50.
9. Gutierrez OM, Farwell WR, Kermah D, et al. Racial differences in the relationship between vitamin D, bone mineral density, and parathyroid hormone in the National Health and Nutrition Examination Survey. Osteoporos Int 2011;22(6):1745–53.
10. Paik JM, Farwell WR, Taylor EN. Demographic, dietary, and serum factors and parathyroid hormone in the National Health and Nutrition Examination Survey. Osteoporos Int 2012;23(6):1727–36.
11. Chapuy M, Arlot M, Duboeuf F, et al. Vitamin D3 and calcium to prevent hip fractures in elderly women. N Engl J Med 1992;327(23):1637–42.
12. Aloia JF. African Americans, 25-hydroxyvitamin D, and osteoporosis: a paradox. Am J Clin Nutr 2008;88(2):545S–50S.
13. Barrett-Connor E, Siris ES, Wehren LE, et al. Osteoporosis and fracture risk in women of different ethnic groups. J Bone Miner Res 2005;20(2):185–94.
14. Cauley JA, Lui LY, Ensrud KE, et al. Bone mineral density and the risk of incident nonspinal fractures in black and white women. JAMA 2005;293(17):2102–8.
15. Powe C, Ricciardi C, Berg A, et al. Vitamin D–binding protein modifies the vitamin D–bone mineral density relationship. J Bone Miner Res 2011;26(7):1609–16.
16. Aloia J, Mikhail M, Dhaliwal R, et al. Free 25 (OH) D and the vitamin D paradox in African Americans. J Clin Endocrinol Metab 2015;100(9):3356–63.
17. Holick MF, MacLaughlin JA, Clark MB, et al. Photosynthesis of previtamin D3 in human skin and the physiologic consequences. Science 1981;210(4466):203–5.
18. Webb AR, DeCosta BR, Holick MF. Sunlight regulates the cutaneous production of vitamin D3 by causing its photodegradation. J Clin Endocrinol Metab 1989;68(5):882–7.
19. Armas LA, Dowell S, Akhter M, et al. Ultraviolet-B radiation increases serum 25-hydroxyvitamin D levels: the effect of UVB dose and skin color. J Am Acad Dermatol 2007;57(4):588–93.
20. Holick M. Vitamin D deficiency. N Engl J Med 2007;357(3):266–81.
21. Park E. The therapy of rickets. JAMA 1940;115:379.
22. Christensen E, Birn H. Megalin and cubilin: synergistic endocytic receptors in renal proximal tubule. Am J Physiol Renal Physiol 2001;280(4):F5622–73.
23. Adams J, Hewison M. Update in vitamin D. J Clin Endocrinol Metab 2010;95(2):471–8.
24. Heaney RP. Functional indices of vitamin D status and ramifications of vitamin D deficiency. Am J Clin Nutr 2004;80(6):1706–9.
25. Bikle D. Vitamin D metabolism, mechanism of action, and clinical applications. Chem Biol 2014;21(3):319–29.

26. Zehnder D, Bland R, Williams MC, et al. Extrarenal expression of 25-hydroxyvitamin D3-1α-hydroxylase 1. J Clin Endocrinol Metab 2001;86(2):888–94.
27. Hewison M, Burke F, Evans KN, et al. Extra-renal 25-hydroxyvitamin D 3-1α-hydroxylase in human health and disease. J Steroid Biochem Mol Biol 2007; 103(3):316–21.
28. Walters MR. Newly identified actions of the vitamin D endocrine system. Endocr Rev 1992;13(4):719–64.
29. Rosen CJ, Adams JS, Bikle DD, et al. The nonskeletal effects of vitamin D: an Endocrine Society scientific statement. Endocr Rev 2012;33(3):456–92.
30. Chun R, Peercy B, Orwoll E, et al. Vitamin D and DBP: the free hormone hypothesis revisited. J Steroid Biochem Mol Biol 2014;144:132–7.
31. Lundgren S, Carling T, Hjälm G, et al. Tissue distribution of human gp330/megalin, a putative Ca2+-sensing protein. J Histochem Cytochem 1997;445(3): 383–92.
32. Jones K, Assar S, Harnpanich D, et al. 25 (OH) D2 half-life is shorter than 25 (OH) D3 half-life and is influenced by DBP concentration and genotype. J Clin Endocrinol Metab 2014;99(9):3373–81.
33. Cauley JA, Greendale GA, Ruppert K, et al. Serum 25 hydroxyvitamin d, bone mineral density and fracture risk across the menopause. J Clin Endocrinol Metab 2015;100(5):2046–54.
34. Takiar R, Lutsey PL, Zhao D, et al. The associations of 25-hydroxyvitamin D levels, vitamin D binding protein gene polymorphisms, and race with risk of incident fracture-related hospitalization: twenty-year follow-up in a bi-ethnic cohort (the ARIC Study). Bone 2015;78:94–101.
35. Bikle DD, Gee E, Halloran B, et al. Assessment of the free fraction of 25-hydroxyvitamin D in serum and its regulation by albumin and the vitamin D-binding protein. J Clin Endocrinol Metab 1986;63(4):954–9.
36. Mansbach JM, Ginde AA, Camargo CA. Serum 25-hydroxyvitamin D levels among US children aged 1 to 11 years: do children need more vitamin D? Pediatrics 2009;124(5):1404–10.
37. Looker AC, Dawson-Hughes B, Calvo MS, et al. Serum 25-hydroxyvitamin D status of adolescents and adults in two seasonal subpopulations from NHANES III. Bone 2002;30(5):771–7.
38. Moore CE, Murphy MM, Holick MF. Vitamin D intakes by children and adults in the United States differ among ethnic groups. J Nutr 2005;135(10):2478–85.
39. El-Hajj Fuleihan G, Bouillon R, Clarke B, et al. Serum 25-hydroxyvitamin D levels: variability, knowledge gaps, and the concept of a desirable range. J Bone Miner Res 2015;30(7):1119–33.
40. Sempos C, Durazo-Arvizu R, Binkley N, et al. Developing vitamin D dietary guidelines and the lack of 25-hydroxyvitamin D assay standardization: the ever-present past. J Steroid Biochem Mol Biol 2016;164:115–9.
41. Binkley N, Sempos C. Standardizing vitamin D assays: the way forward. J Bone Miner Res 2014;29(8):1709–14.
42. Hirschfeld J. Immune-electrophoretic demonstration of qualitative differences in human sera and their relation to the haptoglobins. Acta Pathol Microbiol Scand 1959;47(2):160–8.
43. Arnaud J, Constans J. Affinity differences for vitamin D metabolites associated with the genetic isoforms of the human serum carrier protein (DBP). Hum Genet 1993;92(2):183–8.
44. Bouillon R, Van Baelen H, De Moor P. Comparative study of the affinity of the serum vitamin D-binding protein. J Steroid Biochem 1980;13(9):1029–34.

45. Powe CE, Evans MK, Wenger J, et al. Vitamin D–binding protein and vitamin D status of black Americans and white Americans. N Engl J Med 2013;369(21):1991–2000.
46. Lauridsen AL, Vestergaard P, Nexo E. Mean serum concentration of vitamin D-binding protein (Gc globulin) is related to the Gc phenotype in women. Clin Chem 2001;47(4):753–6.
47. Safadi FF, Thornton P, Magiera H, et al. Osteopathy and resistance to vitamin D toxicity in mice null for vitamin D binding protein. J Clin Invest 1999;103(2):239–51.
48. Bikle DD, Gee E, Halloran B, et al. Free 1, 25-dihydroxyvitamin D levels in serum from normal subjects, pregnant subjects, and subjects with liver disease. J Clin Invest 1984;74(6):1966–71.
49. Vieth R. Simple method for determining specific binding capacity of vitamin D-binding protein and its use to calculate the concentration of "free" 1, 25-dihydroxyvitamin D. Clin Chem 1994;40(3):435–41.
50. Vermeulen A, Verdonck L, Kaufman JM. A critical evaluation of simple methods for the estimation of free testosterone in serum. J Clin Endocrinol Metab 1999;84(10):3666–72.
51. Schwartz JB, Lai J, Lizaola B, et al. A comparison of measured and calculated free 25 (OH) vitamin D levels in clinical populations. J Clin Endocrinol Metab 2014;99(5):1631–7.
52. Nielson CM, Jones KS, Chun RF, et al. Free 25-hydroxyvitamin D: impact of vitamin D binding protein assays on racial-genotypic associations. J Clin Endocrinol Metab 2016;2023:jc20161104.
53. Denburg MR, Hoofnagle AN, Sayed S, et al. Comparison of two ELISA methods and mass spectrometry for measurement of vitamin D-binding protein: implications for the assessment of bioavailable vitamin D concentrations across genotypes. J Bone Miner Res 2016;31(6):1128–36.
54. Nielson C, Jones K, Chun R, et al. Role of assay type in determining free 25-hydroxyvitamin D levels in diverse populations. N Engl J Med 2016;374(17):1695–6.
55. Alzaman N, Dawson-Hughes B, Nelson J, et al. Vitamin D status of black and white Americans and changes in vitamin D metabolites after varied doses of vitamin D supplementation. Am J Clin Nutr 2016;104(1):205–14.
56. Shieh A, Chun RF, Ma C, et al. Effects of high-dose vitamin D2 versus vitamin D3 on total and free 25-hydroxyvitamin D and markers of calcium balance. J Clin Endocrinol Metab 2016;101(8):3070–8.
57. Wagner D, Hanwell HE, Schnabl K, et al. The ratio of serum 24, 25-dihydroxyvitamin D 3 to 25-hydroxyvitamin D 3 is predictive of 25-hydroxyvitamin D 3 response to vitamin D 3 supplementation. J Steroid Biochem Mol Biol 2011;126(3):72–7.
58. Bosworth CR, Levin G, Robinson-Cohen C, et al. The serum 24, 25-dihydroxyvitamin D concentration, a marker of vitamin D catabolism, is reduced in chronic kidney disease. Kidney Int 2012;82(6):693–700.
59. Kaufmann M, Gallagher JC, Peacock M, et al. Clinical utility of simultaneous quantitation of 25-hydroxyvitamin D and 24, 25-dihydroxyvitamin D by LC-MS/MS involving derivatization with DMEQ-TAD. J Clin Endocrinol Metab 2014;99(7):2567–22574.
60. Berg AH, Powe CE, Evans MK, et al. 24, 25-Dihydroxyvitamin D3 and vitamin D status of community-dwelling black and white Americans. Clin Chem Lab Med 2015;61(6):877–84.

61. Abrams SA, O'Brien KO, Liang LK, et al. Differences in calcium absorption and kinetics between black and white girls aged 5–16 years. J Bone Miner Res 1995;10(5):829–33.
62. Bell NH, Yergey AL, Vieira NE, et al. Demonstration of a difference in urinary calcium, not calcium absorption, in black and white adolescents. J Bone Miner Res 1993;8(9):1111–5.
63. Dawson-Hughes B, Harris S, Kramich C, et al. Calcium retention and hormone levels in black and white women on high-and low-calcium diets. J Bone Miner Res 1993;8(7):779–87.
64. Dawson-Hughes B, Harris SS, Finneran S, et al. Calcium absorption responses to calcitriol in black and white premenopausal women. J Clin Endocrinol Metab 1995;80(10):3068–72.
65. Aloia JF, Chen DG, Yeh JK, et al. Serum vitamin D metabolites and intestinal calcium absorption efficiency in women. Am J Clin Nutr 2010;92(4):835–40.
66. Bryant R, Wastney M, Martin B, et al. Racial differences in bone turnover and calcium metabolism in adolescent females. J Clin Endocrinol Metab 2003;88(3):1043–7.
67. Lau WL, Kalantar-Zadeh K. Why is the association of phosphorus and FGF23 with mortality stronger in African-American hemodialysis patients. Am J Nephrol 2015; 42(1):22–4.
68. Dawson-Hughes B, Harris SS, Finneran S. Calcium absorption on high and low calcium intakes in relation to vitamin D receptor genotype. J Clin Endocrinol Metab 1995;80(12):3657–61.
69. Gallagher JC, Jindal PS, Smith LM. Vitamin D does not increase calcium absorption in young women: a randomized clinical trial. J Bone Miner Res 2014;29(5):1081–7.
70. Sai AJ, Walters RW, Fang X, et al. Relationship between vitamin D, parathyroid hormone, and bone health. J Clin Endocrinol Metab 2010;96(3):E436–46.
71. Need AG, O'Loughlin PD, Morris HA, et al. Vitamin D metabolites and calcium absorption in severe vitamin D deficiency. J Bone Miner Res 2008;23(11):1859–963.
72. Aloia JF, Dhaliwal R, Shieh A, et al. Vitamin D supplementation increases calcium absorption without a threshold effect. Am J Clin Nutr 2014;99(3):624–31.
73. Lewis RD, Laing EM, Hill Gallant KM, et al. A randomized trial of vitamin D3 supplementation in children: dose-response effects on vitamin D metabolites and calcium absorption. J Clin Endocrinol Metab 2013;98(12):4816–25.
74. Ritter CS, Armbrecht HJ, Slatopolsky E, et al. 25-Hydroxyvitamin D3 suppresses PTH synthesis and secretion by bovine parathyroid cells. Kidney Int 2006;70(4): 654–9.
75. Ritter CS, Brown AJ. Direct suppression of PTH gene expression by the vitamin D prohormones doxercalciferol and calcidiol requires the vitamin D receptor. J Mol Endocrinol 2011;46(2):63–6.
76. Harkness L, Cromer B. Low levels of 25-hydroxy vitamin D are associated with elevated parathyroid hormone in healthy adolescent females. Osteoporos Int 2005;16(1):109–13.
77. Aloia JF, Vaswani A, Yeh JK, et al. Risk for osteoporosis in black women. Calcif Tissue Int 1996;59(6):415–23.
78. Cosman F, Morgan DC, Nieves JW, et al. Resistance to bone resorbing effects of PTH in black women. J Bone Miner Res 1997;12(6):958–66.
79. Fuleihan GE, Gundberg CM, Gleason R, et al. Racial differences in parathyroid hormone dynamics. J Clin Endocrinol Metab 1994;79(6):1642–7.
80. Aloia JF, Talwar SA, Pollack S, et al. Optimal vitamin D status and serum parathyroid hormone concentrations in African American women. Am J Clin Nutr 2006; 84(3):602–9.

81. Aloia JF, Chen DG, Chen H. The 25 (OH) D/PTH threshold in black women. J Clin Endocrinol Metab 2010;95(11):5069–73.
82. Wright NC, Chen L, Niu J, et al. Defining physiologically "normal" vitamin D in African Americans. Osteoporos Int 2012;23(9):2283–91.
83. Ryan LM, Teach SJ, Singer SA, et al. Bone mineral density and vitamin D status among African American children with forearm fractures. Pediatrics 2012;130(3):553–60.
84. Greendale GA, Sowers M, Han W, et al. Bone mineral density loss in relation to the final menstrual period in a multiethnic cohort: results from the Study of Women's Health Across the Nation (SWAN). J Bone Miner Res 2012;27(1):111–8.
85. Henry YM, Eastell R. Ethnic and gender differences in bone mineral density and bone turnover in young adults: effect of bone size. Osteoporos Int 2000;11(6):512–7.
86. Aloia JF, Talwar SA, Pollack S, et al. A randomized controlled trial of vitamin D3 supplementation in African American women. Arch Intern Med 2005;165(14):1618–23.
87. Nieves JW, Cosman F, Grubert E, et al. Skeletal effects of vitamin D supplementation in postmenopausal black women. Calcif Tissue Int 2012;91(5):316–24.
88. Warden SJ, Hill KM, Ferira AJ, et al. Racial differences in cortical bone and their relationship to biochemical variables in black and white children in the early stages of puberty. Osteoporos Int 2013;24(6):1869–79.
89. Parisien M, Cosman F, Morgan D, et al. Histomorphometric assessment of bone mass, structure, and remodeling: a comparison between healthy black and white premenopausal women. J Bone Miner Res 1997;12(6):948–57.
90. van Ballegooijen AJ, Robinson-Cohen C, Katz R, et al. Vitamin D metabolites and bone mineral density: the Multi-Ethnic Study of Atherosclerosis. Bone 2015;78:186–93.
91. Barbour KE, Zmuda JM, Horwitz MJ, et al. The association of serum 25-hydroxyvitamin D with indicators of bone quality in men of caucasian and African ancestry. Osteoporos Int 2011;22(9):2475–85.
92. Dong Y, Stallmann-Jorgensen IS, Pollock NK, et al. A 16-week randomized clinical trial of 2000 international units daily vitamin D3 supplementation in black youth: 25-hydroxyvitamin D, adiposity, and arterial stiffness. J Clin Endocrinol Metab 2010;95(10):4584–91.
93. Talwar SA, Aloia JF, Pollack S, et al. Dose response to vitamin D supplementation among postmenopausal African American women. Am J Clin Nutr 2007;86(6):1657–62.
94. Aloia JF, Patel M, DiMaano R, et al. Vitamin D intake to attain a desired serum 25-hydroxyvitamin D concentration. Am J Clin Nutr 2008;87(6):1952–8.
95. Ng K, Scott JB, Drake BF, et al. Dose response to vitamin D supplementation in African Americans: results of a 4-arm, randomized, placebo-controlled trial. Am J Clin Nutr 2014;99(3):587–98.
96. Taylor CL, Carriquiry AL, Bailey RL, et al. Appropriateness of the probability approach with a nutrient status biomarker to assess population inadequacy: a study using vitamin D. Am J Clin Nutr 2013;97(1):72–8.
97. Brannon PM, Mayne ST, Murphy SP, et al. Vitamin D supplementation in African Americans: dose-response. Am J Clin Nutr 2014;100(3):982–4.
98. Dhaliwal R, Mikhail M, Feuerman M, et al. The vitamin D dose response in obesity. Endocr Pract 2014;20(12):1258–64.

Trabecular Bone Score

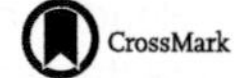

A New DXA–Derived Measurement for Fracture Risk Assessment

Barbara C. Silva, MD, PhD[a,*], William D. Leslie, MD, MSc, FRCPC[b]

KEYWORDS

• Trabecular bone score • FRAX • Osteoporosis • Fracture risk • Bone mineral density

KEY POINTS

- Trabecular bone score (TBS) is a textural index based on evaluating pixel gray-level variations in the lumbar spine dual-energy x-ray absorptiometry (DXA) image.
- TBS predicts the risk of major osteoporotic fracture (MOF) and hip fracture in women and men greater than 40 to 50 years of age.
- TBS can be used to adjust World Health Organization Fracture Risk Assessment Tool (FRAX) probability of fracture in postmenopausal women and older men, assisting in treatment decisions in clinical practice.
- Improvements in TBS due to diverse antiosteoporotic agents tend to be much smaller than those observed in lumbar spine bone mineral density (BMD).

INTRODUCTION

Osteoporosis is characterized by compromised bone strength, predisposing to an increased risk of fracture.[1] An accepted operational definition for osteoporosis in postmenopausal women or in men age 50 years and older is when BMD by DXA is 2.5 or more SDs below the average young reference value (ie, a T score ≤ -2.5).[2,3] Low BMD by DXA is a strong predictor of fracture risk: for each SD decrease in BMD, there is a 1.4-fold to 2.6-fold increase in the risk of fracture.[4,5] Most individuals with fragility fractures have BMD values that do not fall within the osteoporotic range.[6,7] Therefore, the identification of other skeletal and extraskeletal risk factors that contribute to overall fracture risk can be used to better select patients for treatment.

The authors have nothing to disclose.

[a] Department of Medicine, UNI-BH, Santa Casa Hospital, Uberaba, 370/705, Belo Horizonte, MG 30180-010, Brazil; [b] Department of Medicine, University of Manitoba, (C5121) 409 Tache Avenue, Winnipeg, MB R2H 2A6, Canada
* Corresponding author. Rua Uberaba, 370/705, Belo Horizonte, Minas Gerais 30.180-010, Brazil.
E-mail address: barbarasilva2131@gmail.com

Endocrinol Metab Clin N Am 46 (2017) 153–180
http://dx.doi.org/10.1016/j.ecl.2016.09.005
endo.theclinics.com

Readily assessable clinical risk factors, such as age, previous fragility fracture, parental history of hip fracture, smoking, excessive alcohol intake, and prolonged glucocorticoid (GC) use, have all been shown to confer risk independent of BMD measurement. These clinical features gave rise to risk assessment tools, such as the FRAX, which incorporates clinical risk factors with or without femoral neck BMD to estimate 10-year probabilities of hip and MOFs.[8] The ability of FRAX to predict fracture risk has been validated in independent cohorts.[9–11]

In addition, skeletal parameters other than BMD, such as bone geometry, microarchitecture, microdamage, rate of bone turnover, and mineralization, contribute to bone strength and risk of fracture.[12–14] As an example, bone microarchitecture assessed by high-resolution peripheral quantitative CT (HRpQCT) was able to differentiate between women with and without fragility fractures.[15,16] This technology, however, along with several methodologies that evaluate bone strength independent of BMD, are not readily available and are currently used as research tools.

Recently, the TBS was developed, a novel method that assesses skeletal texture from lumbar spine DXA images.[17,18] Longitudinal studies involving multiple cohorts and large numbers of subjects have shown that TBS improves fracture risk prediction beyond that provided by the combination of BMD by DXA and clinical risk factors. TBS is measured by dedicated software (TBS iNsight, Med-Imaps, Pessac, France), which has been cleared for clinical use in the United States to "assist the health care professional in assessment of fracture risk." More recently, a task force of the International Society for Clinical Densitometry (ISCD) developed official positions on how to use TBS in clinical practice.[19] This article reviews technical and clinical aspects of TBS and its potential utility as a clinical tool to predict fracture risk.

TRABECULAR BONE SCORE: TECHNICAL ASPECTS

TBS is a textural index based on evaluating pixel gray-level variations in the lumbar spine (LS) DXA image, providing an indirect index of bone architecture. In general, well-structured bone generates a 2-D DXA image that is more homogeneous, with many gray-level variations of small amplitude. In contrast, deteriorated bone produces a 2-D image with a low number of pixel value variations of high amplitude.[18] TBS is derived from an experimental variogram of those projected images, calculated as the sum of the squared gray-level differences between pixels at a specific distance. The initial slope of the variogram represents the TBS (unitless), with a steeper variogram slope representing a well-structured bone, whereas a lower slope indicates less well-structured architecture. There is no consensus regarding what constitutes "normal" or "abnormal" TBS, but the manufacturer has proposed the following TBS cutoff points: TBS greater than or equal to 1.350 is considered normal; TBS values between 1.200 and 1.350 are consistent with partially degraded bone; and TBS less than or equal to 1.200 is taken to indicate degraded bone.[20]

TBS is typically measured at the LS (from L1 to L4) using the same regions of interest as for conventional BMD measurement, and the result is given for each vertebra and for the overall region of interest. The short-term in vivo precision ranges between 1.1% and 2.1%.[21–26] TBS can be applied to DXA images obtained from current generation fan-beam densitometers (Prodigy and Lunar iDXA, GE Healthcare; Delphi, QDR 4500, and Discovery, Hologic),[27] either at the time of the image acquisition or retrospectively. Similar to BMD derived from DXA, TBS results may not be comparable across different DXA machines or scan modes. A recent in vivo study showed greater TBS values derived from higher-resolution DXA images, as acquired using a Lunar iDXA scan, than those derived from lower-resolution images obtained on a Prodigy densitometer.[25] Similarly, scanning modes that generate higher-resolution images derive greater TBS values.[28,29] Importantly, due to the difference in TBS results across different DXA machines, calibration using a specially constructed phantom should be performed on new installations of the TBS software, allowing the determination of an adjustment factor, which is then incorporated into the software to calibrate the densitometer.[25]

Impact of Abdominal Soft Tissue on Trabecular Bone Score

The excessive amount of abdominal soft tissue can also influence the TBS analysis, degrading the image texture and thus reducing the TBS values. This effect has been shown in both in vitro and in vivo studies.[30–34] The original TBS algorithm had been optimized for women. It has since been updated in version 2.1 to partially address these technical issues and has become applicable to both women and men. In a preliminary study by Leslie and colleagues[35] using Lunar scanners, the tissue effect on TBS seemed to explain the initial findings of a paradoxically greater TBS in women than in men, in whom adiposity tends to be more abdominal, and was corrected under TBS version 2.1.[36]

Using the current version of the TBS software, an effect of body mass index (BMI) and trunk fat mass on TBS is still evident when images are acquired on Hologic DXA systems.[32,37] Using the TBS software version 2.1 and a Hologic DXA system, a TBS evaluation in 7682 US adults from the National Health and Nutrition Examination Survey, 2005 to 2008, revealed that, in certain age groups and ethnic groups, TBS is higher in women than in men.[37] The differences in TBS by gender and ethnicity were small and much lower than BMD differences. In this study, TBS was negatively correlated with BMI, weight, waist circumference, total body fat mass, trunk fat mass, and trunk lean mass. Additional in vivo studies using TBS software version 2.x have consistently found a negative correlation between TBS and waist circumference or visceral fat mass on Hologic scanners.[32–34] The relationship between TBS and volumetric BMD at the LS as measured by QCT seems attenuated in subjects with high BMI.[32]

As a result of this BMI/abdominal adiposity dependence, the manufacturers of the TBS software have not recommended the use of TBS in individuals with BMI lower than 15 kg/m^2 or greater than 37 kg/m^2.

Impact of Osteoarthritis and Other Heterotopic Ossifications on Trabecular Bone Score

In contrast to DXA-derived BMD, osteoarthritic changes of the LS seem to have little effect on TBS.[21,38] In the study by Kolta and colleagues,[38] 1254 postmenopausal women (mean age 66.6 years) had their DXA BMD and TBS evaluated at baseline and at a 6-year time point. Osteoarthritis was assessed on spine lateral radiographs, and its severity was determined by Kellgren and Lawrence (K&L) classification. Although LS BMD was greater in patients with osteoarthritis, and positively correlated with K&L grade in models adjusted for age and BMI, TBS was similar between subjects with and without osteoarthritis and did not correlate with K&L grade. At the 6-year time point, the evaluation of 727 women showed a significant decline in TBS and in hip BMD, whereas the BMD at the LS remained unchanged. The TBS decline over time was independent of K&L grade.

Similarly, TBS may not be affected by the presence of other heterotopic ossifications that typically overestimate LS DXA BMD. In a study of 51 men (mean age 52.2 years) with spondyloarthritis, standard spine radiographs showed lumbar syndesmophytes in 29 participants.[39] Compared with patients without these heterotopic ossifications, patients with syndesmophytes had greater LS BMD T scores

(-1.18 ± 1.16 vs -0.07 ± 1.63; $P = .009$) but lower TBS (1.33 ± 0.11 vs 1.21 ± 0.12; $P = .001$). After controlling for BMI, TBS was marginally reduced ($P = .06$) in patients with syndesmophytes and the difference in LS BMD between the groups was no longer significant. Although these observations suggest that TBS is not affected by osteoarthritis or other heterotopic ossifications in LS, it is unknown if TBS can predict fracture risk in this specific group of patients.

ASSOCIATION OF TRABECULAR BONE SCORE WITH 3-D MEASUREMENTS OF BONE MICROARCHITECTURE AND WITH BONE STRENGTH

In Vitro Studies

Ex vivo studies compared TBS to standard 3-D parameters of bone microarchitecture assessed by micro-CT (μCT) in specimens of human cadaveric bone.[17,18,40,41] In its first description, TBS was derived from simulated 2-D projection of μCT images of human cadaveric bones from different anatomic sites (LS, femoral neck, and distal radius).[18] It was found a significant correlation between TBS of spine samples and direct 3-D measurements of trabecular microarchitecture by μCT, namely, trabecular bone volume to tissue volume (BV/TV), connectivity density (Conn. D), trabecular number (Tb.N), and trabecular separation (Tb.Sp). In a different study, TBS (also derived from 2-D projection μCT images) was significantly correlated with trabecular microarchitecture indices by μCT, independent of the image resolution, up to a simulated pixel size of 1023 μm.[40] At a 93-μm plane resolution, TBS was related to Conn. D ($r^2 = 0.746$; $P<.001$), Tb.N ($r^2 = 0.637$; $P<.001$), and Tb.Sp ($r^2 = 0.430$; $P<.001$) and weakly associated with trabecular thickness (Tb.Th; $r^2 = 0.151$; $P = .034$).

TBS was then derived from DXA images of human cadaver lumbar vertebrae, and significant correlations between trabecular indices by μCT and TBS were confirmed (BV/TV: $r = 0.528$; Tb.Th: $r = -0.553$; Tb.Sp: $r = -0.643$; Tb.N: $r = 0.751$; and Conn.D: $r = 0.821$; all $P<.001$).[17] Surprisingly, TBS was negatively associated with Tb.Th ($r = -0.553$). Roux and colleagues[41] evaluated TBS derived from ex vivo DXA images of lumbar vertebrae (L3) from 16 human donors compared with μCT measures of microarchitecture and mechanically tested bone strength. TBS was significantly associated with BV/TV, structure model index (SMI), and stiffness but not with BMD. The correlation between TBS and stiffness remained significant after adjusting for BMD ($r = 0.62$; $P<.015$). These reported associations between TBS and μCT parameters were not adjusted for age.

Maquer and colleagues[42] used μCT and μCT-derived finite element analyses to assess morphologic indices and the elastic properties of trabecular compartment of 743 bone samples from vertebrae, iliac crest, femur, and radius. TBS was calculated as described by Pothuaud and colleagues.[18] BV/TV and fabric anisotropy were, together, the best determinants of trabecular bone stiffness, whereas TBS and other morphologic indices did not bring any additional contribution. Subsequently, the same group used biomechanical tests to estimate trabecular strength of 62 human vertebrae, and HRpQCT to generate simulated DXA images of the same vertebrae.[43] The initial slope of the variogram, computed using the simulated DXA images based on the same TBS textural principles, was poorly related to bone strength. The initial slope of the variogram, however, as calculated in this study, may not be rigorously equivalent to TBS.

In Vivo Studies

Silva and colleagues[44,45] have examined correlations between TBS with volumetric BMDs and 3-D microarchitecture parameters in vivo. A small study of 22 postmenopausal women with primary hyperparathyroidism revealed moderate correlations between LS TBS and HRpQCT measurements of volumetric densities (r = 0.476–0.507), cortical thickness (r = 0.453), Tb.N (r = 0.505), Tb.Sp (r = −0.492), and whole-bone stiffness (r = 0.442) at the radius (all *P*<.05).[44] TBS was also positively associated with measures of volumetric density (r = 0.471–0.619), cortical thickness (r = 0.515), and whole-bone stiffness (r = 0.516) at the tibia (all *P*<.05). TBS was not associated with Tb.Th or trabecular stiffness at either skeletal site. Subsequently, the same group evaluated 115 Chinese American and white women (71 premenopausal and 44 postmenopausal) and assessed the correlation of TBS with indices of QCT at the LS and femur and indices of HRpQCT at the radius and tibia.[45] TBS was directly associated with QCT parameters of spine trabecular volumetric BMD (r = 0.664) and with trabecular and cortical QCT indices at the femoral neck (r = 0.346–0.651) and total hip (r = 0.491–0.643) (*P*<.001 for all). In a multiple regression model, none of the HRpQCT indices was associated with TBS.

Popp and colleagues[46] have also investigated the correlation of TBS with HRpQCT indices in 72 healthy premenopausal women (mean age 33.8 years). There was a significant association between TBS and trabecular volumetric BMD (r = 0.49–0.57), Tb.N (r = 0.43–0.58), Conn.D (r = 0.43–0.46), and Tb.Sp (r = −0.43 to −0.57) at the radius and tibia (all *P*<.01). TBS was weakly correlated with Tb.Th at the radius (r = 0.37; *P*<.01) but not at the tibia. HRpQCT measures of cortical density, thickness, and porosity were either weakly or not associated with TBS.

Muschitz and colleagues[47] have studied 80 female (median age 39.9 years) and 43 male (median age 42.7 years) patients with idiopathic osteoporosis and low traumatic fractures (60 vertebral, 75 nonvertebral/nonhip, and 8 hip fractures). Patients underwent iliac crest bone biopsies that were analyzed by μCT. TBS was obtained from Lunar iDXA scans. Multiple linear regression models included SMI, Tb.N, Tb.Sp, and BV/TV as the outcome variables, and age, TBS, LS BMD, gender, vertebral fractures, sclerostin, amino-terminal propeptide of type I collagen (P1NP), and cross-linked C-telopeptide of type I collagen (CTX) as the explanatory variables. In these models, TBS was independently associated with SMI (r^2 = 0.302), Tb.Sp (r^2 = 0.274), and BV/TV (r^2 = 0.459).

Finally, in a recent study, 125 postmenopausal women (mean age 63 years) were studied by DXA, including TBS, QCT of LS and femur, and HRpQCT of the radius and tibia.[48] TBS was weakly correlated to trabecular indices of HR-pQCT at the radius and tibia (r = −0.16–0.31, *P*<.01).

In summary, in vivo studies demonstrate that TBS is not associated with HRpQCT indices after multivariable adjustment or explains little of the variance in trabecular microarchitecture. This could be due to variations in trabecular microarchitecture between central (LS) and peripheral (radius and tibia) sites. Alternatively, TBS may primarily assess degradation in skeletal macroarchitecture (eg, trabecular network porosity).[49] As pointed by Bousson and colleagues[27] the best way to test whether TBS reflects trabecular microarchitecture is through the measurement of spine TBS on full cadavers, correlating it with indices of microarchitecture assessed by μCT of the same vertebrae. To date, it is still unknown which bone properties TBS directly measures.

CLINICAL DATA ON TRABECULAR BONE SCORE AND FRACTURE RISK

Cross-sectional Studies

Cross-sectional studies have shown an association between LS TBS and vertebral, hip, and overall osteoporotic fractures in postmenopausal women.[50–60] Data in men, although limited, have confirmed an association between lower TBS and prevalent osteoporotic fractures.[59,61] In general, these retrospective case-control studies have demonstrated that TBS is able to differentiate fractured cases from controls, with odds ratio (OR) for fracture ranging from 1.3 to 3.8 per SD decrease in TBS. In some of these studies, the association between TBS and previous fracture was partially independent of age, BMI and LS BMD. The single study that included exclusively men reported an OR per SD decrease for low-energy fracture of 1.55 (95% CI, 1.09–2.20). A brief report failed to show an association between TBS and fractures in a group of obese (BMI >30 kg/m^2) Lebanese postmenopausal women.[62] Similarly, a recent study of a convenience sample of 825 women, including 390 African Americans and 435 whites, showed that in models adjusted for age, lower BMD T score, and use of GC, TBS was associated with prevalent vertebral fractures in whites (OR 1.54; 95% CI, 1.12–2.13; $P = .008$) but not in African Americans (OR 1.23; 95% CI, 0.89–1.70; $P = .21$).[63] These studies are summarized in **Table 1**, and are reviewed in detail elsewhere.[49,64,65]

Longitudinal Studies

Several longitudinal studies have shown that TBS predicts fracture risk in women and men greater than 40 years old.[22,23,66–72] These studies, summarized in **Table 2**, are described.

A series of retrospective cohort studies from a large clinical DXA registry in the Canadian province of Manitoba was used to assess the relationship between TBS and incident osteoporotic fractures. The first such study included 29,407 women greater than or equal to 50 years old followed for a mean period of 4.7 years[23]; 1668 (5.7%) women had incident MOFs, including 439 (1.5%) clinical vertebral and 293 (1.0%) hip fractures. At baseline, TBS and BMD at all sites were significantly lower in fractured women than in nonfractured subjects (all $P<.0001$). The age-adjusted hazard ratios (HRs) for each SD decline in TBS were 1.35 (95% CI, 1.29–1.42) for MOF, 1.45 (95% CI, 1.32–158) for vertebral fracture, and 1.46 (95% CI, 1.30–1.63) for hip fracture. BMD at the LS, femoral neck, and total hip conferred age-adjusted HRs per SD decrease in BMD of 1.47 to 1.68 for MOFs, 1.72 to 1.76 for vertebral fractures, and 1.31 to 2.60 for hip fractures. There was a small but significant incremental improvement in the area under the receiver operator characteristic curve (AUC) for TBS+BMD compared with BMD alone (LS +0.02, femoral neck +0.01, and total hip +0.01). TBS remained a significant predictor of incident fractures in models adjusted for age, LS BMD, and a combination of clinical risk factors, with HRs per SD decrease in TBS of 1.17 (95% CI, 1.09–1.25) for MOFs, 1.14 (95% CI, 1.03–1.26) for vertebral fractures, and 1.47 (95% CI, 1.30–1.67) for hip fractures.

A subsequent report using the Manitoba database evaluated 33,352 women, ages 40 to 100 years, followed for a mean time of 4.7 years.[69] Over this period, 1872 women sustained at least 1 MOF and 1754 women died. In models adjusted for age and time since baseline, each SD decline in TBS conferred a 36% greater risk of MOF (HR 1.36; 95% CI, 1.30–1.42) and a 32% increase risk of death (HR 1.32; 95% CI, 1.26–1.39). TBS was still a predictor of MOF (HR 1.18; 95% CI, 1.12–1.23) and death (HR 1.20; 95% CI, 1.14–1.26) after controlling for FRAX clinical risk factors and femoral neck BMD T score. As discussed later, this study showed that TBS provides additional information on the 10-year probability of MOF as estimated by the standard FRAX variables.

The ability of TBS to predict fracture risk was also examined in 560 postmenopausal white women from the French Os des Femmes de Lyon (OFELY) cohort.[66] During a mean follow-up of 8.0 $\pm$ 1.1 years, 94 women sustained a low-energy fracture (any site, except the head, toes, and fingers). Fractured women had, at baseline, lower LS BMD (T score: -1.9 ± 1.2 vs -1.4 ± 1.3; $P<.001$) and TBS (1.237 ± 0.098 vs 1.284 ± 0.105; $P<.001$) than women without incident fractures. Fractured subjects were also older and lighter and had a higher prevalence of fractures at baseline. In

Table 1
Summary of cross-sectional studies

Citation	Study Subjects	Mean Age ± SD (y)	Cases	Controls	Trabecular Bone Score Results
Pothuaud et al,[50] 2009	135 White postmenopausal women	66.9 ± 8.0	45 Subjects with vertebral, hip, and other types of osteoporotic Fx (confirmed by radiographs)	90 Age- and LS BMD-matched controls	Unadjusted OR (95% CI): All Fx: 1.95 (1.31–2.89); Vertebral Fx: 2.66 (1.46–4.85)
Winzenrieth et al,[51] 2010	243 White postmenopausal women with osteopenia at LS	63.1 ± 6.7	81 Subjects with morphometric vertebral Fx	162 Age-matched controls	Body weight–adjusted OR (95% CI): 1.97 (1.31–2.96)
Rabier et al,[52] 2010	168 White postmenopausal women with T score <−1.0 at any site	64.1 ± 8.2	42 Subjects with morphometric vertebral Fx	126 Age-matched controls	Body weight–adjusted OR (95% CI): 3.81 (2.17–6.72)
Del Rio et al,[53] 2013	191 White postmenopausal women	66.9 ± 9.1	83 Subjects with osteoporotic femoral neck Fx by self-report	108 Not matched controls	Age-, BMI-, and weight-adjusted OR (95% CI): 1.66 (1.15–2.40)
Krueger et al,[54] 2014	429 White postmenopausal women	71.6 ± 8.0	158 Subjects with low-energy Fx (by self-report) and vertebral Fx (on VFA – n = 91)	271 Age-matched controls	Age, BMI-, and lowest BMD T score–adjusted OR (95% CI): Any Fx: 2.36 (1.8–3.0) Vertebral Fx: 2.44 (1.8–3.3)
Lamy et al,[55] 2012	631 White postmenopausal women	67.4 ± 6.7	164 Subjects with any low-energy Fx (by self-report or VFA for vertebral Fx)	467 Not matched controls	Age, BMI- and LS BMD-adjusted OR (95% CI): Any Fx: 1.3 (1.0–1.7) Vertebral Fx: 1.7 (1.1–2.7) MOF: 1.6 (1.2–2.2)
Leib et al,[57] 2014	2156 White women >40 y old	57.7 ± 7.6	289 Subjects with any low-energy Fx (assessed in medical records)	1876 Not matched controls	Age-, LS BMD-, and family history of osteoporotic fracture-adjusted OR (95% CI): 1.28 (1.13–1.46)

(*continued on next page*)

Table 1
(continued)

Citation	Study Subjects	Mean Age ± SD (y)	Cases	Controls	Trabecular Bone Score Results
Vasic et al,[56] 2014	1031 White women (45–85 y old)	62.9 ± 8.7	271 Any low-energy Fx (hip [7.7%], spine [41.3%], humerus [13.3%], and forearm [42.1%])	760 Not matched controls	Age-, LS BMD-adjusted OR (95% CI): 1.27 (1.07–1.51)
Ayoub et al,[58] 2014	1000 Lebanese postmenopausal women	61.1 ± 11.7	164 Subjects with MOF	836 Not matched controls	TBS was independently associated with Fx ($P = .01$) in a multiple regression analyses using BMI, age, LS BMD, and TBS as explanatory variables
Ayoub et al,[62] 2016	300 Lebanese obese (BMI >30 kg/m^2) postmenopausal women	67.1 ± 8.6	40 Subjects with MOF assessed in medical records	260 Not matched controls	TBS was not associated with Fx using simple logistic regression models
Touvier et al,[60] 2015	255 White postmenopausal women	65.0 ± 12.0	79 Subjects with osteoporotic Fx confirmed by radiographs (forearm, hip, humerus, shoulder, vertebral, and rib)	176 not matched controls	Age, total hip BMD, height, weight, and calcaneus Hurst parameter-adjusted OR (95% CI): 1.83 (1.24–2.77)
Jain et al,[63] 2016	825 Women >40 y old, including 390 African Americans and 435 whites referred for bone densitometry as a part of their routine care	67.1 ± 11.1	130 Subjects (56 African Americans) with vertebral Fx (grades 2 and 3) by VFA; 133 subjects (50 African Americans) with nonvertebral Fx (by self-report)	Not matched controls	Age-, lower BMD T score–, and use of GC-adjusted OR (95% CI): Vertebral Fx - African Americans: 1.23 (0.89–1.70); whites: 1.54 (1.12–2.13) Nonvertebral Fx — African Americans: 1.19 (0.86–1.66); whites: 1.42 (1.06–1.92)
Nassar et al,[59] 2014	362 White men and women >50 y old (77% women) with a low-trauma nonvertebral Fx	74.3 ± 11.7	133 Subjects with both nonvertebral and vertebral Fx by VFA to subjects with nonvertebral Fx only	229 Not matched controls with a low-trauma nonvertebral Fx only	Unadjusted AUC: 0.677
Leib et al,[61] 2014	180 White men >40 y old	63.0 ± 12.1	45 Subjects with low-energy Fx (by self-report)	135 age- and LS BMD-matched controls	Unadjusted: any Fx: 1.55 (1.09–2.20)

Abbreviation: Fx, Fracture.

Table 2
Summary of longitudinal studies

Citation	Study Subjects	Mean Age ± SD (y)	Mean Follow-up (y)	Outcome Measure	Adjustments	Hazard Ratio or Odds Ratio per SD Decrease in Trabecular Bone Score (95% CI)
Manitoba, Hans et al,[23] 2011	29,407 Women $\geq$ 50 y old (98% white)	65.4 $\pm$ 9.5	4.7	1668 MOFs assessed in health service records by fracture codes	Age, LS BMD, and a combination of clinical risk factors[a]	HR 1.17 (1.09–1.25)
				439 Clinical vertebral Fx		HR 1.14 (1.03–1.26)
				239 Hip Fx		HR 1.47 (1.30–1.67)
OFELY, Boutroy et al,[66] 2013	560 Postmenopausal white women	66.2 $\pm$ 7.9	8.0	94 Clinical and radiographic vertebral Fx and fragility Fx at any site (confirmed by radiographs), except head, toes, and fingers	Age, weight, and prevalent fracture at baseline	OR 1.34 (1.04–1.73)
JPOS, Iki et al,[67] 2014	665 Japanese women >50 y old	64.1 $\pm$ 8.1	8.3	92 Vertebral Fx (by VFA)	Age, LS BMD, and prevalent vertebral deformity	OR 1.52 (1.16–2.00)
OPUS, Briot et al,[22] 2013	1007 Postmenopausal white women > 50 y old	65.9 $\pm$ 6.9	6.0	82 Clinical osteoporotic Fx (peripheral and clinical vertebral fractures), by self-report, confirmed by radiographs	None	OR 1.62 (1.30–2.01)
				46 Vertebral Fx (by radiographs)		OR 1.54 (1.17–2.03)

(*continued on next page*)

Table 2
(continued)

Citation	Study Subjects	Mean Age ± SD (y)	Mean Follow-up (y)	Outcome Measure	Adjustments	Hazard Ratio or Odds Ratio per SD Decrease in Trabecular Bone Score (95% CI)
Manitoba, Leslie et al,[69] 2014[c]	33,352 Women ages 40–100 y (98% white)	63.2 ± 10.8	4.7	1872 MOFs assessed in health service records by fracture codes	Clinical risk factors[b] and LS BMD	HR 1.17 (1.11–1.23)
				1754 Deaths		HR 1.26 (1.19–1.32)
SEMOF, Popp et al,[68] 2015	556 Postmenopausal elderly women	76.1 ± 3.0	2.7	52 (9.4%) Clinical fragility fractures (20 forearm, 6 hip, 10 clinical vertebral, 9 humerus, 2 pelvis, 3 ankle, 1 clavicle, and 1 elbow)	Age, BMI, and lowest BMD	HR 1.87 (1.38–2.54)
Manitoba, McCloskey et al,[74] 2015[c]	33,352 Women ages 40–100 y (98% white)	63.2 ± 10.8	4.7	1639 (4.9%) At least 1 MOF, excluding hip Fx (assessed in health service records by fracture codes)	Age, time since baseline, femoral neck BMD, and clinical risk factors (BMI, previous fracture, smoking, GCs, rheumatoid arthritis, secondary osteoporosis and alcohol use)	HR 1.18 (1.12–1.24)
				306 (0.9%) Hip Fx		HR 1.23 (1.09–1.38).
				1754 (5.3%) Deaths		HR 1.20 (1.14–1.26)
Manitoba, Leslie et al,[70] 2014	3620 Men >50 y old (98% white)	67.6 ± 9.8	4.5	183 MOFs assessed in health service records by fracture codes	Clinical FRAX score, osteoporosis treatment, and LS BMD	HR 1.08 (0.92–1.26)
				91 Clinical vertebral Fx		HR 1.02 (0.81–1.27)
				46 Hip Fx		HR 1.44 (1.07–1.94)

FORMEN, Iki et al,[72] 2015	1872 Community-dwelling Japanese men ≥65 y old	73 ± 5.1	4.5 (median)	22 MOFs identified by interviews or mail and telephone surveys	FRAX score	OR 1.76 (1.16–2.67)
MrOS, Schousboe et al,[71] 2016	5863 Community-dwelling men ≥ 65 y old	73.7 ± 5.9	10	448 MOFs identified by mail and confirmed by radiographs	FRAX with BMD 10-year fracture risks and prevalent radiographic vertebral Fx	HR 1.27 (1.17–1.39)
				181 Hip Fx		HR 1.20 (1.05–1.39)
Meta-analysis of international cohorts, McCloskey et al,[73] 2016	17,809 Men and women (59% women) from 14 population-based cohorts	72 (range: 40–90)	6.1	1109 MOFs	Age, time since baseline, and FRAX probability of MOF (with BMD)	HR 1.32 (1.24–1.41)
				298 Hip Fx	Age, time since baseline, and FRAX probability of hip Fx (with BMD)	HR 1.28 (1.13–1.45)

Abbreviations: Fx, fracture; JOPS, the japanese population-based osteoporosis study.

[a] Clinical risk factors: ambulatory diagnostic groups comorbidity score, rheumatoid arthritis, chronic obstructive pulmonary disease, diabetes, substance abuse, BMI, prior osteoporotic fracture, systemic corticosteroid use in the last year, and osteoporosis treatment in the past year.

[b] Clinical risk factors: BMI, previous fracture, chronic obstructive pulmonary disease (smoking proxy), GC use greater than 90 days, rheumatoid arthritis, secondary osteoporosis, and high alcohol use.

[c] These studies included the same study population.

models controlling for these variables (age, body weight, and prevalent fracture), fracture prediction was similar for LS BMD (OR 1.30; 95% CI, 1.06–1.58) and TBS (OR 1.34; 95% CI, 1.04–1.73) but lower than total hip BMD (OR 1.99; 95% CI, 1.52–2.62).

TBS was shown to predict incident morphometric vertebral fractures in a study of 665 Japanese women greater than 50 years old (mean age, 64.1 ± 8.1 years) followed for a median period of 10 years.[67] Incident vertebral fractures (n = 140) were identified by vertebral fracture assessment (VFA) in 92 women. Both LS BDM and TBS were lower in women with vertebral fracture than in those without fractures (BMD 0.729 ± 0.126 vs 0.814 ± 0.141 g/cm^2; TBS 1.132 ± 0.110 vs 1.200 ± 0.095; both P<.0001). After adjusting for confounding variables (age, height, prevalent fractures at baseline, and osteoporosis treatment), the TBS difference was substantially attenuated but still significant (1.175 vs 1.193; P = .0386). Unadjusted models showed ORs for vertebral fracture of 1.69 (95% CI, 1.39–2.05) and 1.98 (95% CI, 1.56–2.51) for each SD decline in LS BMD and TBS, respectively. In models adjusted for age and LS BMD, TBS remained a predictor of vertebral fracture (OR 1.54; 95% CI, 1.17–2.02). The combination of TBS and LS BMD or BMD alone predicted fracture equally well.

TBS and incident fractures were assessed in 1007 postmenopausal women greater than 50 years old from 3 European centers of the Osteoporosis and Ultrasound Study (OPUS).[22] Women were followed, on average, for 6 years. Incident low-energy fractures were reported by 82 (8.1%) participants, whereas incident vertebral fractures were detected on thoracic and LS radiographs in 46 (4.6%) women. Fractured women were older and had lower TBS values and BMD at all sites than nonfractured subjects. Unadjusted models for incident clinical osteoporotic fractures showed an OR of 1.62 (95% CI, 1.30–2.01) for each SD decline in TBS. The ability of TBS to predict clinical osteoporotic fractures was similar to that of BMD at the femoral neck (OR 1.60; 95% CI, 1.26–2.06) and total hip (OR 1.65; 95% CI, 1.30–2.11) but better than LS BMD (OR 1.47; 95% CI, 1.16–1.89). For incident vertebral fractures, the unadjusted OR per SD decrease was 1.54 (95% CI, 1.17–2.03) for TBS, similar to that for femoral neck BMD (OR 1.54; 95% CI, 1.12–2.14) but worse than those for total hip (OR 1.73; 95% CI, 1.26–2.38) and LS BMD (OR 1.75; 95% CI, 1.25–2.48). Age-adjusted models were not reported.

Popp and colleagues[68] studied 556 postmenopausal elderly women (mean age 76.1 ± 3.0 years) who had participated in the prospective Swiss Evaluation of the Methods of Measurement of Osteoporotic Fracture Risk (SEMOF) study as a representative population sample recruited at the study site of Berne, Switzerland. Over the mean follow-up time of 2.7 years, 52 (9.4%) participants sustained a clinical fragility fracture (20 forearm, 6 hip, 10 clinical vertebral, 9 humerus, 2 pelvis, 3 ankle, 1 clavicle, and 1 elbow). Compared with nonfractured subjects, women with an incident fracture were older, had lower TBS values and BMD T scores at all sites, and were more likely to have a positive history of fracture. TBS predicted incident fractures in models adjusted for age and BMI (HR per SD 2.01; 95% CI, 1.54–2.63) and in those further adjusted for the lowest BMD (HR per SD 1.87; 95% CI, 1.38–2.54). The AUC for the combination of LS BMD and TBS (AUC 0.71) was greater than that for LS BMD alone (AUC 0.62; P = .03).

Leslie and colleagues[70] were the first to evaluate TBS and incident fractures in men. This study assessed 3620 men greater than 50 years (mean age 67.7) from the province of Manitoba followed, on average, for 4.5 years. In total, 183 men (5.1%) sustained an incident MOF (hip, clinical spine, forearm, or humerus), including 91 (2.5%) participants with clinical vertebral fractures and 46 (1.3%) with hip fractures. Baseline TBS and BMD T scores at LS and femoral neck were lower, and FRAX probabilities of fracture were higher in men with incident fractures than in those without fractures. Clinical FRAX score and osteoporosis treatment-adjusted HRs per SD were 1.22 (95% CI, 1.05–1.41) for MOF and 1.60 (95% CI, 1.21–2.11) for hip fracture. After further adjustment for femoral neck (HR 1.36; 95% CI, 1.01–1.83) or LS BMD (HR 1.44; 95% CI, 1.07–1.94), TBS remained a predictor of hip fracture but not MOFs. TBS was not a predictor of vertebral clinical fracture in these analyses.

Iki and colleagues[72] assessed TBS and incident fractures in 1872 community-dwelling Japanese men greater than or equal to 65 years of age (mean age 73) from the Fujiwara-kyo Osteoporosis Risk in Men (FORMEN) study. During the median follow-up of 4.5 years, 22 participants sustained 23 MOFs (hip 2, spine 12, radius 7, and humerus 2), identified by interviews or mail and telephone surveys. Baseline TBS was lower in men with MOFs (1.136 ± 0.099) than in those without fractures (1.193 ± 0.083; *P* = .0015). BMD at all sites were also lower, and FRAX scores were higher in men with fractures than in nonfractured subjects. TBS predicted MOFs with an unadjusted OR of 1.89 (95% CI, 1.28, 2.81) for each SD decline in TBS, with AUC of 0.669. The combination of FRAX score and TBS predicted MOFs equally well as FRAX score alone (AUC of 0.684 [95% CI 0.568 – 0.801] vs 0.681 [95% CI 0.586- 0.776], respectively; *P* = .955).

Finally, TBS and incident fractures were assessed in 5863 community-dwelling men greater than or equal to 65 years of age enrolled in the Osteoporotic Fractures in Men (MrOS) study.[71] During a mean follow-up of 10 years, 448 (7.6%) participants experienced an MOF, and 181 (3.1%) men had an incident hip fracture. Fractures were identified by mail and confirmed by radiographs. TBS predicted MOFs and hip fracture in models adjusted for FRAX with BMD 10-year risk score, with HR per SD of 1.31 (95% CI, 1.20–1.43) and 1.24 (95% CI, 1.08–1.49), respectively. TBS remained a predictor of MOF and hip fractures when models were further adjusted for prevalent morphometric vertebral fracture (see **Table 2**).

Finally, a meta-analysis of 14 prospective population-based cohorts from North America, Asia, Australia, and Europe confirmed that TBS provides additional information on the 10-year fracture probabilities as estimated by the standard FRAX variables.[73] The meta-analysis included 17,809 men and women (mean age 72 years old; 59% women), with a mean follow-up of 6.1 years. Over this period, 298 (1.7%) subjects sustained at least 1 hip fracture and 1109 (6.2%) subjects had 1 or more MOFs (hip, spine, humerus, or forearm). FRAX 10-year probabilities of MOF and hip fractures (with femoral neck BMD) were calculated using individual-level data in each cohort based on country-specific models (FRAX v3.8). Gradient of risk (GR), expressed as the HR per SD decrease of TBS, was adjusted for age and time since baseline. TBS predicted both MOF (GR 1.44; 95% CI, 1.35–1.53) and hip fracture (GR 1.44; 95% CI, 1.28–1.62). Although still significant, GRs for TBS decreased on further adjustment for FRAX risk probabilities (see **Table 2**). GRs were similar between men and women (*P*>.10).

In summary, these studies have consistently shown that TBS predicts MOFs and vertebral and hip fractures in postmenopausal women. In men, TBS is associated with incident MOFs and hip fractures. These associations remain even after adjusting for BMD and, in some assessments, for FRAX risk scores or other clinical risk factors. At the time of this review, there were no similar data published in premenopausal women or younger men.

ASSOCIATION OF TRABECULAR BONE SCORE WITH FRAX TO ENHANCE FRACTURE PREDICTION

Recent studies have indicated an incremental improvement in fracture prediction when TBS is used in combination with FRAX. The first such assessment, described previously, examined 33,352 women, ages 40 to 100 years, from the Canadian province of Manitoba, followed for 4.7 years.[69] TBS was able to predict the risk of MOFs and death in models controlled for FRAX clinical risk factors and femoral neck BMD T score. The ability of TBS to predict MOFs remained after accounting for the increased death hazard. A method to adjust FRAX probability of MOF was suggested based on TBS. As such, compared with high TBS (90th percentile), a low TBS (10th percentile) would increase the FRAX risk of MOF by 1.5-fold to 1.6-fold.

Subsequently, McCloskey and colleagues[74] used the same study population described previously to propose models for adjusting FRAX (with BMD) probabilities to account for TBS. The analysis examined interactions of TBS with other risk factors and incorporated competing mortality into the procedure. Among the 33,352 women included (mean age 63.2 years), 1754 (5.3%) women died, 1639 (4.9%) experienced at least 1 MOF excluding hip fracture, and 306 (0.9%) sustained 1 or more hip fracture. In models adjusted for age, time since baseline, femoral neck BMD, and clinical risk factors (BMI, previous fracture, smoking, GCs, rheumatoid arthritis, secondary osteoporosis, and alcohol use), TBS was significantly associated with mortality (HR per SD 1.20; 95% CI, 1.14–1.26), MOF excluding hip fracture (HR per SD 1.18; 95% CI, 1.12–1.24), and hip fracture (HR per SD 1.23; 95% CI, 1.09–1.38). The 10-year probabilities of fracture with and without TBS were calculated based on the associations between TBS and the FRAX risk factors with risks of fracture and death. As an example, in such models, a TBS set at the 10th or the 90th percentile would, respectively, increase or decrease the 10-year probabilities of MOFs and hip fractures calculated without TBS, across a broad range of ages and femoral neck BMD T scores. Given the significant interaction observed between TBS and age, the ability of TBS to enhance the 10-year fracture probability from FRAX was stronger in younger women and less marked in older women. Similarly, there was a lesser effect of TBS in women with lower unadjusted fracture probabilities.

Finally, the adjustment factor derived from the Manitoba study described previously[74] was applied to the meta-analysis cohorts.[73] For MOFs in men and women combined, TBS-adjusted FRAX probability resulted in a slightly greater GR (1.76; 95% CI, 1.65–1.87) than that for unadjusted FRAX probability (GR 1.70; 95% CI, 1.60–1.81). Similar results were seen for hip fracture, with a GR of 2.25 (95% CI, 2.03–2.51) for TBS-adjusted FRAX probability compared with a GR of 2.22 (95% CI, 2.00–2.47) for the standard FRAX probability.

Based on these results, a new feature of the online FRAX risk assessment tool was developed. Using the online calculator on FRAX Web site, following the calculation of fracture probability with the inclusion of BMD, the option to "adjust with TBS" appears. TBS can then be entered, providing a TBS-adjusted 10-year fracture probability of MOF and hip fracture (**Fig. 1**). Recently published ISCD official positions propose that "TBS can be used in association with FRAX and BMD to adjust FRAX-probability of fracture in postmenopausal women and older men."[19] Although the ISCD recommends against the use of TBS as a single measurement to determine treatment recommendations in clinical practice, FRAX probabilities adjusted for TBS could assist in treatment decisions.

EFFECT ON TRABECULAR BONE SCORE OF ANTIOSTEOPOROTIC THERAPY AND BREAST CANCER TREATMENT–INDUCED BONE LOSS

Antiosteoporotic Therapy

The effect of antiosteoporotic agents on TBS was explored in several studies (summarized in **Table 3**). For detailed review, see Silva and colleagues[19] and Harvey and

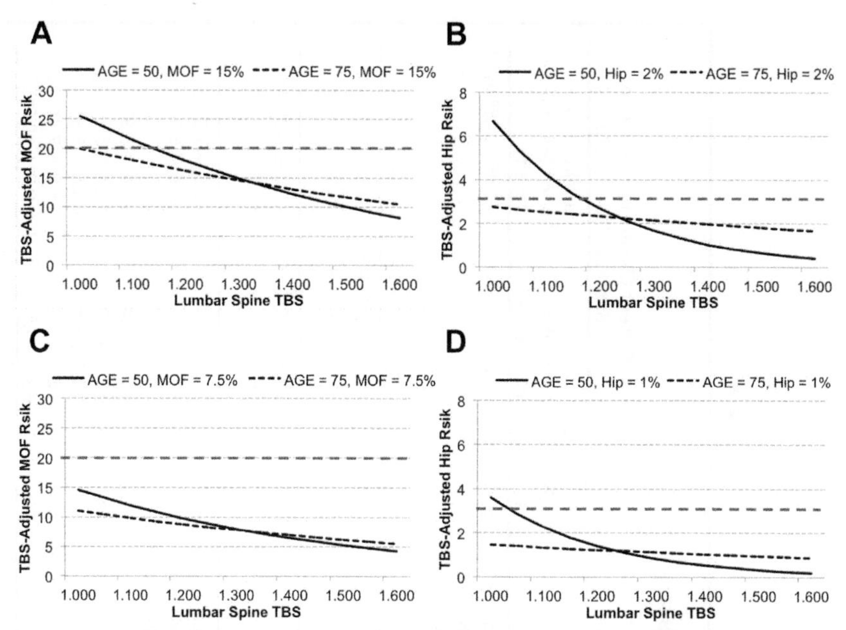

Fig. 1. Magnitude of change in TBS-adjusted FRAX score according to baseline risk, age, and TBS. The dashed gray lines are the National Osteoporosis Foundation treatment thresholds. The black lines represent the TBS-adjusted FRAX risk for a given woman of 50 years of age (*solid lines*) or a woman of 75 years of age (*dashed lines*) according to different TBS values. Notice that TBS has a greater effect in younger (50 years old) than in older (75 years old) women, in those with greater unadjusted fracture probabilities (*A*, *B*), and in hip fracture probability (*B*, *D*) compared with MOF probability (*A*, *C*).

colleagues.[75] In general, changes in TBS due to diverse antiosteoporotic agents tend to be much smaller than those observed in LS BMD. In addition, compared with LS BMD, a lower proportion of patients experience improvements in TBS above the least significant change. Assessments of the use of bisphosphonates for up to approximately 3 to 4 years observed significant but small increases in TBS relative to baseline (see **Table 3**).[24,26,76,77] Similarly, a 12-month treatment with denosumab of 60 postmenopausal women with osteoporosis, including 30 subjects taking GCs, resulted in significant changes in LS BMD in women on GCs (+5.8%) and in those not taking GCs (+6.1%), whereas smaller and not significant improvements in TBS were seen in both groups (see **Table 3**).[78]

It has been suggested that changes in TBS might be a function of the therapeutic class, with greater increases observed with the use of anabolic agents.[26,77] In a nonrandomized study by Senn and colleagues,[26] postmenopausal women were treated with teriparatide (n = 65) or ibandronate (n = 122) for 2 years. There was a significant greater increase in TBS on teriparatide treatment (+4.3%) than with ibandronate (+0.3%). In another open-label trial, changes in TBS in 390 subjects greater than or equal to 40 years old, including 72 men, were compared among various therapies (calcium/vitamin D, alendronate, risedronate, testosterone, denosumab, and teriparatide).[77] Women in the teriparatide group (n = 30) had greater improvements in TBS than subjects on other therapies. Consistent with previous studies, percent changes in LS BMD were greater than those in TBS across all treatment groups (see **Table 3**).

Table 3
Impact of various antiosteoporotic therapies on trabecular bone score and bone mineral density

Citation	Participants	Age (Mean ± SD)	Mean Follow-up Period (y)	Treatment	Number of Subjects per Group	Percent Change in Relative to Baseline (Mean ± SD)	
						Trabecular Bone Score	Lumbar Spine Bone Mineral Density
Krieg et al,[76] 2013 Manitoba	1684 Women ≥50 y old	63.4 ± 7.9	3.7	Antiresorptive agents (86% bisphosphonates, 10% raloxifene, and 4% calcitonin)	534	+0.2 ± 1.9%/y[a,b]	+1.86 ± 1.8%/y[a,b]
				Untreated subjects	1150	−0.31 ± 0.06%/y[a,b]	−0.36 ± 0.05%/y[a,b]
Popp et al,[24] 2013 HORIZON trial	Subset of 107 postmenopausal women	76.8 ± 5.0	3	Zoledronic acid	54	+1.41 ± 0.79%[a,b,c]	+9.58 ± 0.6%[a,b,c]
				Placebo	53	−0.49 ± 0.62%[b,c]	+1.38 ± 0.9%[a,b,c]
Senn et al,[26] 2014	187 Postmenopausal women with osteoporosis	67.9 ± 7.5	2	Teriparatide[d]	65	+4.3 ± 6.6%[a,b]	+7.6 ± 6.3%[a,b]
				Ibandronate	122	+0.3 ± 4.1%[b]	+2.9 ± 3.3%[a,b]
Di Gregorio et al,[77] 2015	390 Subjects ≥40 y old, including 318 women and 72 men	66.1 ± 9.2	1.7 ± 0.5	Untreated subjects	67	−3.1 ± 6.4[a]	+0.5 ± 7.5
				Calcium (2500 mg) and vitamin D_3 (880 IU) daily	87	+1.3 ± 8.1	+1.6 ± 6.2
				Testosterone	36	+1.8 ± 7.4	+4.4 ± 3.8[a]
				Alendronate	88	+1.4 ± 5.5[a]	+4.1 ± 5[a]
				Risedronate	39	+1.4 ± 6.6	+4.8 ± 8.9[a]
				Denosumab	43	+2.8 ± 5.7[a]	+8.8 ± 7.4[a]
				Teriparatide	30	+3.6 ± 6[a]	+8.8 ± 10.6[a]

Petranova et al,[78] 2014	30 Postmenopausal women with BMD T score <−2.5	67.5 ± 9.0	1	Denosumab	30	+0.3[e]	+6.1[a,e]
	30 Postmenopausal women with BMD T score <−2.5 on chronic use of GCs	66.7 ± 7.9			30	+5.0[e]	+5.8[a,e]
Kalder et al,[80] 2015 ProBONE II trial	70 Premenopausal women with hormone-sensitive primary breast cancer on endocrine treatment–induced bone loss	43.0 ± 6.1	2	Placebo (+endocrine treatment–induced bone loss)	36	−2.16± 0.64%[a,b]	−6.4 ± 0.57%[a,b]
				Zoledronic acid, 4 mg, every 3 mo (+endocrine treatment–induced bone loss)	34	+0.75 ± 0.8%[b]	+3.14 ± 0.58%[a,b]
Prasad et al,[81] 2016	109 Postmenopausal women >55 y old, with breast cancer and LS BMD T score between −1 and −2.5, on AIs (anastrozole, letrozole, or exemestane)	63.8 ± 8.1	2	Placebo (+AIs)	54	−2.35% ± 0.77%[a]	−1.7 ± 0.6%[b]
		64.7 ± 7.5		Risedronate (+AIs)	55	−1.3%[e]	+2.3 ± 0.6%[b]

Abbreviations: FU, follow-up; HORIZON, Health Outcomes and Reduced Incidence with Zoledronic Acid Once Yearly.

[a] *P*<.05 compared with baseline within groups.

[b] *P*<.05 between groups.

[c] Mean ± SEM.

[d] One-sixth of the patients in the Teriparatide group were treated for 18 months with teriparatide followed by a single intravenous infusion of zoledronic acid, 5 mg, whereas the remaining subjects in this group were treated with teriparatide during the entire 24-month period.

[e] SD not reported.

Breast Cancer Treatment–Induced Bone Loss

The use of gonadotropin-releasing hormone agonists or aromatase inhibitors (AIs) as adjuvant therapies in women with breast cancer is associated with detrimental effects on DXA BMD and increased fracture risk. Several studies have examined the effect of these estrogen-deprivation therapies on TBS[79–82] (see **Table 3**). A review of these assessments shows that treatment with AIs for approximately 2 years is associated with reductions in LS BMD (−1.7 to −6.4%) and in TBS (−2.1 to −2.35%). Estrogen deprivation due to menopause transition was also associated with decreases in TBS (−4.6%) and LS BMD (−6.8%). Two of these trials examined changes in TBS on zoledronic acid or risedronate treatment in women on estrogen-deprivation therapies. Over 2 years, zoledronic acid in premenopausal women led to a mild, and nonsignificant increase in TBS (+0.75%) and a greater increase in LS BMD (+3.14%).[80] The 2-year use of risedronate in postmenopausal women resulted in a reduction in TBS of 1.3%, and an improvement in LS BMD of 2.3%.

Clinical Use of Trabecular Bone Score to Monitor Osteoporosis Treatment

As reported previously, changes in TBS are, in general, much smaller than changes in LS BMD during antiresorptive treatment. Although few data suggest that TBS improvements in subjects taking teriparatide are greater than in those using antiresorptives, these were small open-label trials and further studies are needed to confirm these observations. In addition, there are no studies that have shown that change in TBS is associated with a change in fracture risk. Accordingly, the ISCD has recommended against use of TBS for monitoring bisphosphonate therapy.[19] The role of TBS for monitoring patients on teriparatide, denosumab, or newer osteoporotic drugs remains uncertain.

ROLE OF TRABECULAR BONE SCORE IN SPECIAL CONDITIONS RELATED TO INCREASED FRACTURE RISK

Diabetes Mellitus

Using the Manitoba database, Leslie and colleagues[83] assessed 29,407 women greater than or equal to 50 years old, of whom 2356 (8.1%) had diabetes mellitus. Compared with controls, diabetic women had higher baseline BMDs at all sites, but lower TBS, even after adjusting for multiple clinical risk factors (age, BMI, GCs, prior major fracture, rheumatoid arthritis, chronic obstructive pulmonary disease as a smoking proxy, alcohol abuse, and osteoporosis therapy). Over 4.7 years of follow-up, 175 (7.4%) women with diabetes sustained at least 1 MOF, which was significantly greater than the incidence of MOFs in nondiabetic women (n = 1493 [5.5%]; *P*<.001). TBS predicted MOF independent of BMD in women with diabetes (HR 1.27; 95% CI, 1.10–1.46) and in those without diabetes (HR 1.31; 95% CI, 1.24–1.38). Based on this study, the ISCD and the European Society for Clinical and Economic Aspects of Osteoporosis and Osteoarthritis recommend that TBS can be used in postmenopausal women with type 2 diabetes mellitus to predict MOF risk.[19,75]

Additional studies have confirmed that diabetics have lower TBS values than nondiabetic controls, despite greater BMD measurements. Kim and colleagues[84] studied 1229 men and 1529 postmenopausal women greater than 50 years old from the Korean Ansung cohort, including 325 (26.4%) men and 370 (24.2%) women with diabetes. TBS was significantly lower in men with than in those without diabetes, even after adjusting for age and BMI (1.287 ± 0.005 vs 1.316 ± 0.003, respectively; *P*<.001). The difference between the groups was attenuated but still significant (1.333 ± 0.004 vs 1.353 ± 0.003, respectively; *P*<.001), when adjusting for age,

BMI, dietary calcium intake, prior major fracture, arthritis, current alcohol abuse, current smokers, regular exercise, and osteoporosis treatment. TBS was also lower in women with diabetes than in those without the disease in unadjusted models. This difference was not significant after controlling for multiple variables. In contrast to TBS, LS BMD was greater in both men and women with diabetes compared with nondiabetic controls in unadjusted and adjusted models. In a different assessment, TBS was lower and LS BMD was higher in 57 women with type 2 diabetes mellitus, mean age of 66 years, than in 43 nondiabetic female controls, even after adjusting for age, BMI, and BMD.[85] In both studies, TBS was inversely associated with hemoglobin A_{1c} (HbA_{1c}).[84,85]

Finally, Zhukouskaya and colleagues[86] assessed 99 postmenopausal women with type 2 diabetes mellitus (mean age 65.7 ± 7.3 and mean HbA_{1c} 6.8%), compared with 107 controls (mean age 64.5 ± 8.2) without the disease. LS and hip BMD were greater in diabetics than in controls, whereas TBS was similar between the groups. Prevalent vertebral fractures (grades 1–3), assessed by radiography, were more frequent in diabetics (34.3%, n = 34) than in controls (18.7%, n = 20; P = .01). BMD and TBS were lower in fractured than in nonfractured subjects, in both groups. TBS and femoral neck BMD were associated with prevalent vertebral fractures (AUC 0.69, P<.0001, and AUC 0.63, P<.004, respectively).

In the single study that assessed TBS in type 1 diabetes mellitus, 119 patients with the disease (59 men and 60 premenopausal women; mean age 43.4 ± 8.9 years) were compared with 68 gender-matched, age-matched, and BMI-matched healthy controls.[87] TBS was similar between the groups (1.357 ± 0.129 in type 1 diabetics vs 1.389 ± 0.085 in controls; P = .075), whereas total hip BMD was lower in diabetics. In the type 1 diabetes mellitus group, 24 (20.2%) subjects had at least 1 prevalent fracture (in total: 15 fractures in forearm/hand and 13 in lower leg/foot, 2 hip fractures, and 4 clinical vertebral fractures). Diabetic patients with prevalent fractures had higher levels of HbA_{1c} and a significantly lower total hip BMD (0.958 ± 0.128 vs 1.023 ± 0.136; P = .04) and TBS (1.309 ± 0.125 vs. 1.370 ± 0.127; P = .04) than healthy controls. In type 1 diabetic subjects, using a multivariate model, TBS (P = .049) and HbA_{1c} (P = .036) were independently associated with prevalent fractures. The AUCs for fracture discrimination were 0.63 (95% CI, 0.51–0.74; P = .048) for TBS and 0.64 (95% CI, 0.51–0.78; P = .032) for total hip BMD.

Long-term Glucocorticoid Exposure

It is well known that long-term GC exposure increases fracture risk, which cannot be fully explained by any decrease in DXA BMD. Several studies have assessed TBS in subjects chronically exposed to exogenous or endogenous GC as an attempt to identify a discriminatory feature between subjects with or without GC exposure or as an additional tool to differentiate between fractured and nonfractured patients.

Paggiosi and colleagues[88] evaluated whether TBS, LS BMD, or a combination of both could discriminate between GC-treated and GC-naive women. They evaluated 484 women (ages 55–79 years), allocated in 1 of 3 groups: women taking prednisolone greater than or equal to 5 mg/d for greater than 3 months (n = 64); a fracture group, comprised of women who had sustained a recent fracture of the distal forearm (n = 46), proximal humerus (n = 37), vertebra (n = 30), or proximal femur (n = 28); or healthy population–based women (n = 279). Both age-adjusted LS BMD and TBS *z* scores were lower in patients with fractures than in healthy controls. In contrast, when compared with healthy controls, women on GCs had similar age-adjusted LS BMD but lower adjusted TBS *z* scores (P<.001). TBS alone (AUC = 0.721), but not LS BMD alone (AUC = 0.572), was able to discriminate between GC-treated and

GC-naive women. The combination of TBS+LS BMD (AUC = 0.721) had no impact on the discriminatory ability of TBS for GC use.

TBS, BMD, and osteoporotic fractures were also assessed in 416 individuals (mean age of 63.4 years; 72 men) taking GCs (prednisone $\geq$5 mg/d for $\geq$3 months) compared with 1104 gender-matched, age-matched, and BMI-matched controls.[89] The prevalence of osteoporotic fractures, assessed in medical records, was not different between cases (16.3%) and controls (13.1%; *P* = .16). Absolute BMD values at the LS and hip sites were also similar between the groups, whereas TBS was lower in the GC group than in healthy subjects (1.267 vs 1.298, *P*<.005). This was also observed when gender stratification was performed. BMD *z* scores at the total hip and femoral neck were lower in GC subjects than in controls. In healthy subjects, but not in individuals on GCs, BMD at the LS and femoral neck were lower in patients with prevalent fractures than in those without fractures. In contrast, compared with nonfractured patients, TBS was lower in fractured subjects in both control and GC-treated groups. In the multivariate model, TBS was associated with the presence of fracture with an OR per SD decrease of 1.51 (95% CI, 1.23–1.86) in TBS and an AUC of 0.648 (95% CI, 0.599–0.693).

TBS was also related to exogenous GC exposure in patients with systemic sclerosis.[90] This study assessed 65 women (mean age 61.6) with systemic sclerosis, compared with 138 age-matched women with rheumatoid arthritis and 227 age-matched female controls. Although daily and cumulative doses of GC were lower in women with systemic sclerosis than in those with rheumatoid arthritis, TBS was similar between these 2 groups. In addition, in both systemic sclerosis and rheumatoid arthritis groups, TBS values were reduced when compared with controls, even in models adjusted for age, BMI, and LS BMD. TBS was significantly lower in systemic sclerosis patients receiving GC greater than or equal to 5 mg/d (n = 29) than in those with GC less than 5 mg/d (*P* = .001). In women with systemic sclerosis, using logistic regression analysis, TBS was independently associated with daily GC dose greater than or equal to 5 mg/d (OR 5.6; 95% CI, 1.7–19.2) and with a T score less than or equal to −2.5 (OR 5.0; 95% CI, 1.5–17.0). In patients with rheumatoid arthritis, associations between GC use and TBS were not seen.

TBS was also assessed in patients with endogenous hypercortisolism.[91,92] In 102 patients (63 women) with adrenal incidentaloma (AI), including 34 with subclinical hypercortisolism (SH), TBS *z* score (-3.18 ± 1.21) was lower in subjects with SH, than in those with AI without SH (-1.70 ± 1.54, *P*<.0001), or 70 matched controls (-1.19 ± 0.99, *P*<.0001).[91] BMD at the LS and total femur was also lower in subjects with SH. A TBS *z* score less than −1.5 was associated with the presence of vertebral fracture, regardless of age, BMI, and gender (OR 4.8 [95% CI, 1.85–12.42]; *P*<.001). In a different study, 182 subjects with Cushing syndrome (149 women; mean age 37.8 years; 152 with Cushing disease, 9 with adrenal adenoma, and 21 with corticotropin ectopic Cushing syndrome) were included.[92] Prevalent clinical fractures (by self-report) and vertebral fractures (by spine radiographs) were confirmed in 81 (44.5%) patients, including 24 patients with nonvertebral and 70 with vertebral fractures. Fracture discrimination as assessed from AUC was 0.548 (0.454–0.641) for TBS, 0.637 (0.545–0.729) for LS BMD, and 0.609 (0.517–0.700) for femoral neck BMD. In binary logistic regression model (that included age, gender, TBS, BMD at all sites, and 24-h urinary-free cortisol levels as independent variables), the only predictor of fracture was the 24 h urinary-free cortisol level (*P* = .001).

Primary Hyperparathyroidism

Two small independent studies found that TBS is lower in patients with primary hyperparathyroidism than in controls.[93,94] In addition, a low TBS was associated with a greater risk of prevalent vertebral fracture in both assessments. In the study of Eller-Vainicher and colleagues,[93] 20 patients with primary hyperparathyroidism underwent parathyroidectomy and were compared with 10 nonsurgically treated cases after 24 months. TBS remained stable in conservatively treated subjects, whereas it improved in patients treated with parathyroidectomy. This finding was also observed in a different study that reported a TBS increase at 1 year after parathyroidectomy in patients with primary hyperparathyroidism.[95]

Other Conditions

Naylor and colleagues[96] evaluated 327 kidney transplant recipients greater than or equal to 18 years (39% men, mean age 45 years, and median time on dialysis 2.1 years) from the Canadian Province of Manitoba, who have had DXA testing after the transplant (median 106 days). For each kidney transplant recipient, 3 controls were selected from the general population, matched for age, gender, and DXA date. At baseline, cases had a lower mean TBS (1.365 $\pm$ 0.129 vs 1.406 $\pm$ 0.125, $P<.001$), were more likely to have recently used GCs (54 vs 16%, $P<.001$), and had higher FRAX probabilities of fracture compared with controls. Participants were followed for 6.6 years, and over this period, 31 kidney transplant recipients sustained at least 1 low-energy incident fracture (excluding hand, foot, and craniofacial). Among kidney transplant recipients, TBS was lower in those with incident fractures than in nonfractured subjects (1.301 $\pm$ 0.144 vs 1.372 $\pm$ 0.125; $P = .003$). TBS was associated with fracture even after adjusting for LS BMD and FRAX score (with femoral neck BMD), with an HR per SD decrease in TBS of 1.55 (95% CI, 1.06–2.27).

TBS was assessed in 185 women with rheumatoid arthritis (mean age 56 $\pm$ 14 years), including 112 patients on chronic use of GCs.[97] Prevalent vertebral fractures were identified by VFA in 33 participants. TBS and BMD T score at all sites were lower in fractured than in nonfractured subjects. A more recent study of 100 Korean women greater than or equal to 50 years old with rheumatoid arthritis evaluated the associations of prevalent vertebral fracture (n = 26) with TBS, FRAX probability of MOF, and LS BMD. The respective AUCs were 0.683, 0.818, and 0.518.[98]

A prospective study evaluated the effect of a 2-year growth hormone (GH) replacement on TBS in 147 subjects with GH deficiency (mean age 35.1 years; 84 men).[99] Over this period, there were significant improvements in LS BMD (+14%), total femur BMD (+7%), and TBS (+4% in a subgroup of 32 subjects). TBS was recorded at the level of L4 only, limiting this analysis. In another report,[100] GH replacement for 7 years in 18 adult subjects with GH deficiency resulted in a nonsignificant decrease in TBS of −0.86%, despite the significant increase in LS BMD of +4.73% ($P = .01$).

BMD at all sites and TBS were also significantly lower in adult patients with thalassemia major (n = 124; 73 women; mean age 36.1) than in 65 nonthalassemic older women (mean age 45.71).[101] In patients with Ehlers-Danlos syndrome, TBS is also reduced and it is associated with prevalent vertebral fractures.[102] Recently, it was shown that TBS is inversely related to free T4 levels ($\beta = -0.111$; $P = .002$) in a group of 648 postmenopausal euthyroid women.[103] Finally, low TBS values were also described in patients with acromegaly,[104] anorexia nervosa,[105] and on hemodialysis.[106]

In general, these data suggest that TBS may play a role in the evaluation of fracture risk in diverse conditions. Nevertheless, besides the study that evaluated TBS and incident MOF in a large number of women with diabetes, those reports enrolled a small number of individuals or fractured cases or have not assessed incident fractures. Thus, additional studies are required to evaluate the use of TBS in a broad variety of conditions related to increased bone fragility.

SUMMARY

TBS is a textural index from spine DXA images that predicts fracture risk independent of DXA-derived BMD and clinical risk factors. TBS is associated with incident vertebral, hip, and MOFs in postmenopausal women and with hip and MOFs in men greater than 50 years of age. TBS can be used to adjust FRAX probabilities of fracture, directing treatment recommendations in clinical practice. Although TBS improves on diverse antiosteoporotic treatments, these changes are usually smaller than improvements in LS BMD and many times do not exceed the least significant change. Finally, TBS may play a role in the evaluation of fracture risk in diverse conditions, such as diabetes or chronic GC exposure.

REFERENCES

1. Osteoporosis prevention, diagnosis, and therapy. NIH Consensus Statement 2000;17(1):1–45.
2. WHO. Assessment of fracture risk and its application to screening for postmenopausal osteoporosis. Report of a WHO Study Group. World Health Organ Tech Rep Ser 1994;843:1–129.
3. Schousboe JT, Shepherd JA, Bilezikian JP, et al. Executive summary of the 2013 International Society for Clinical Densitometry Position Development Conference on bone densitometry. J Clin Densitom 2013;16(4):455–66.
4. Johnell O, Kanis JA, Oden A, et al. Predictive value of BMD for hip and other fractures. J Bone Miner Res 2005;20(7):1185–94.
5. Kanis JA, Borgstrom F, De Laet C, et al. Assessment of fracture risk. Osteoporos Int 2005;16(6):581–9.
6. Siris ES, Miller PD, Barrett-Connor E, et al. Identification and fracture outcomes of undiagnosed low bone mineral density in postmenopausal women: results from the National Osteoporosis Risk Assessment. JAMA 2001;286(22):2815–22.
7. Miller PD, Siris ES, Barrett-Connor E, et al. Prediction of fracture risk in postmenopausal white women with peripheral bone densitometry: evidence from the National Osteoporosis Risk Assessment. J Bone Miner Res 2002;17(12):2222–30.
8. Kanis JA, Oden A, Johnell O, et al. The use of clinical risk factors enhances the performance of BMD in the prediction of hip and osteoporotic fractures in men and women. Osteoporos Int 2007;18(8):1033–46.
9. Leslie WD, Lix LM, Johansson H, et al. Independent clinical validation of a Canadian FRAX tool: fracture prediction and model calibration. J Bone Miner Res 2010;25(11):2350–8.
10. Tamaki J, Iki M, Kadowaki E, et al. Fracture risk prediction using FRAX(R): a 10-year follow-up survey of the Japanese Population-Based Osteoporosis (JPOS) Cohort Study. Osteoporos Int 2011;22(12):3037–45.
11. Hillier TA, Cauley JA, Rizzo JH, et al. WHO absolute fracture risk models (FRAX): do clinical risk factors improve fracture prediction in older women without osteoporosis? J Bone Miner Res 2011;26(8):1774–82.
12. Wang J, Stein EM, Zhou B, et al. Deterioration of trabecular plate-rod and cortical microarchitecture and reduced bone stiffness at distal radius and tibia in postmenopausal women with vertebral fractures. Bone 2016;88:39–46.
13. Sroga GE, Vashishth D. Effects of bone matrix proteins on fracture and fragility in osteoporosis. Curr Osteoporos Rep 2012;10(2):141–50.
14. Garnero P, Hausherr E, Chapuy MC, et al. Markers of bone resorption predict hip fracture in elderly women: the EPIDOS Prospective Study. J Bone Miner Res 1996;11(10):1531–8.

15. Stein EM, Liu XS, Nickolas TL, et al. Microarchitectural abnormalities are more severe in postmenopausal women with vertebral compared to nonvertebral fractures. J Clin Endocrinol Metab 2012;97(10):E1918–26.
16. Nishiyama KK, Macdonald HM, Hanley DA, et al. Women with previous fragility fractures can be classified based on bone microarchitecture and finite element analysis measured with HR-pQCT. Osteoporos Int 2013;24(5):1733–40.
17. Hans D, Barthe N, Boutroy S, et al. Correlations between trabecular bone score, measured using anteroposterior dual-energy X-ray absorptiometry acquisition, and 3-dimensional parameters of bone microarchitecture: an experimental study on human cadaver vertebrae. J Clin Densitom 2011;14(3):302–12.
18. Pothuaud L, Carceller P, Hans D. Correlations between grey-level variations in 2D projection images (TBS) and 3D microarchitecture: applications in the study of human trabecular bone microarchitecture. Bone 2008;42(4):775–87.
19. Silva BC, Broy SB, Boutroy S, et al. Fracture Risk Prediction by Non-BMD DXA Measures: the 2015 ISCD Official Positions Part 2: Trabecular Bone Score. J Clin Densitom 2015;18(3):309–30.
20. Cormier C, Lamy O, Poriau S. TBS in routine clinial practice: proposals of use. Medimaps Group; 2012. Available at: http://www.medimapsgroup.com/upload/MEDIMAPS-UK-WEB.pdf. Accessed November 2, 2016.
21. Dufour R, Winzenrieth R, Heraud A, et al. Generation and validation of a normative, age-specific reference curve for lumbar spine trabecular bone score (TBS) in French women. Osteoporos Int 2013;24(11):2837–46.
22. Briot K, Paternotte S, Kolta S, et al. Added value of trabecular bone score to bone mineral density for prediction of osteoporotic fractures in postmenopausal women: the OPUS study. Bone 2013;57(1):232–6.
23. Hans D, Goertzen AL, Krieg MA, et al. Bone microarchitecture assessed by TBS predicts osteoporotic fractures independent of bone density: the Manitoba study. J Bone Miner Res 2011;26(11):2762–9.
24. Popp AW, Guler S, Lamy O, et al. Effects of zoledronate versus placebo on spine bone mineral density and microarchitecture assessed by the trabecular bone score in postmenopausal women with osteoporosis: a three-year study. J Bone Miner Res 2013;28(3):449–54.
25. Krueger D, Libber J, Binkley N. Spine trabecular bone score precision, a comparison between GE lunar standard and high-resolution densitometers. J Clin Densitom 2015;18(2):226–32.
26. Senn C, Gunther B, Popp AW, et al. Comparative effects of teriparatide and ibandronate on spine bone mineral density (BMD) and microarchitecture (TBS) in postmenopausal women with osteoporosis: a 2-year open-label study. Osteoporos Int 2014;25(7):1945–51.
27. Bousson V, Bergot C, Sutter B, et al. Trabecular bone score (TBS): available knowledge, clinical relevance, and future prospects. Osteoporos Int 2012; 23(5):1489–501.
28. Bandirali M, Di Leo G, Messina C, et al. Reproducibility of trabecular bone score with different scan modes using dual-energy X-ray absorptiometry: a phantom study. Skeletal Radiol 2015;44(4):573–6.
29. Chen W, Slattery A, Center J, et al. The effect of changing scan mode on trabecular bone score using lunar prodigy. J Clin Densitom 2016. [Epub ahead of print].
30. Amnuaywattakorn S, Sritara C, Utamakul C, et al. Simulated increased soft tissue thickness artefactually decreases trabecular bone score: a phantom study. BMC Musculoskelet Disord 2016;17:17.

31. Kim JH, Choi HJ, Ku EJ, et al. Regional body fat depots differently affect bone microarchitecture in postmenopausal Korean women. Osteoporos Int 2016; 27(3):1161–8.
32. Langsetmo L, Vo TN, Ensrud KE, et al. The association between trabecular bone score and lumbar spine volumetric bmd is attenuated among older men with high body mass index. J Bone Miner Res 2016;31(10):1820–6.
33. Lv S, Zhang A, Di W, et al. Assessment of Fat distribution and Bone quality with Trabecular Bone Score (TBS) in Healthy Chinese Men. Sci Rep 2016;6:24935.
34. Romagnoli E, Lubrano C, Carnevale V, et al. Assessment of trabecular bone score (TBS) in overweight/obese men: effect of metabolic and anthropometric factors. Endocrine 2016;54(2):342–7.
35. Leslie WD, Lix L, Morin S, et al. Difference in spine TBS between men and women: real or technical? [abstract]. J Clin Densitom 2014;17(3):406–7. Available at: http://www.clinicaldensitometry.com/article/S1094-6950(14)00079-1/abstract. Accessed November 2, 2016.
36. Leslie WD, Winzenrieth R, Majumdar S, et al. Clinical performance of an updated version of trabecular bone score in men and women: the manitoba BMD cohort [abstract]. J Bone Miner Res 2014;29(1):S97. Avalialable at: http://www.asbmr.org/education/AbstractDetail?aid=87225632-8722552 1c-87224347-a87225667b-bd87225636ee87790990c. Accessed November 2, 2016.
37. Looker AC, Sarafrazi Isfahani N, Fan B, et al. Trabecular bone scores and lumbar spine bone mineral density of US adults: comparison of relationships with demographic and body size variables. Osteoporos Int 2016;27(8):2467–75.
38. Kolta S, Briot K, Fechtenbaum J, et al. TBS result is not affected by lumbar spine osteoarthritis. Osteoporos Int 2014;25(6):1759–64.
39. Wildberger L, Boyadzhieva V, Hans D, et al. Impact of lumbar syndesmophyte on bone health as assessed by bone density (BMD) and bone texture (TBS) in men with axial spondyloarthritis. Joint Bone Spine 2016. [Epub ahead of print].
40. Winzenrieth R, Michelet F, Hans D. Three-dimensional (3D) microarchitecture correlations with 2D projection image gray-level variations assessed by trabecular bone score using high-resolution computed tomographic acquisitions: effects of resolution and noise. J Clin Densitom 2013;16(3):287–96.
41. Roux JP, Wegrzyn J, Boutroy S, et al. The predictive value of trabecular bone score (TBS) on whole lumbar vertebrae mechanics: an ex vivo study. Osteoporos Int 2013;24(9):2455–60.
42. Maquer G, Musy SN, Wandel J, et al. Bone volume fraction and fabric anisotropy are better determinants of trabecular bone stiffness than other morphological variables. J Bone Miner Res 2015;30(6):1000–8.
43. Maquer G, Lu Y, Dall'Ara E, et al. The initial slope of the variogram, foundation of the trabecular bone score, is not or is poorly associated with vertebral strength. J Bone Miner Res 2016;31(2):341–6.
44. Silva BC, Boutroy S, Zhang C, et al. Trabecular bone score (TBS)–a novel method to evaluate bone microarchitectural texture in patients with primary hyperparathyroidism. J Clin Endocrinol Metab 2013;98(5):1963–70.
45. Silva BC, Walker MD, Abraham A, et al. Trabecular bone score is associated with volumetric bone density and microarchitecture as assessed by central QCT and HRpQCT in Chinese American and white women. J Clin Densitom 2013;16(4):554–61.
46. Popp AW, Buffat H, Eberli U, et al. Microstructural parameters of bone evaluated using HR-pQCT correlate with the DXA-derived cortical index and the trabecular

bone score in a cohort of randomly selected premenopausal women. PLoS One 2014;9(2):e88946.
47. Muschitz C, Kocijan R, Haschka J, et al. TBS reflects trabecular microarchitecture in premenopausal women and men with idiopathic osteoporosis and low-traumatic fractures. Bone 2015;79:259–66.
48. Amstrup AK, Jakobsen NF, Moser E, et al. Association between bone indices assessed by DXA, HR-pQCT and QCT scans in post-menopausal women. J Bone Miner Metab 2016;34(6):638–45.
49. Leslie WD, Binkley N. Spine bone texture and the trabecular bone score (TBS). In: Patel VB, Preedy VR, editors. Biomarkers in disease: methods, discoveries and applications. biomarkers in bone disease: Springer; in press.
50. Pothuaud L, Barthe N, Krieg MA, et al. Evaluation of the potential use of trabecular bone score to complement bone mineral density in the diagnosis of osteoporosis: a preliminary spine BMD-matched, case-control study. J Clin Densitom 2009;12(2):170–6.
51. Winzenrieth R, Dufour R, Pothuaud L, et al. A retrospective case-control study assessing the role of trabecular bone score in postmenopausal Caucasian women with osteopenia: analyzing the odds of vertebral fracture. Calcif Tissue Int 2010;86(2):104–9.
52. Rabier B, Heraud A, Grand-Lenoir C, et al. A multicentre, retrospective case-control study assessing the role of trabecular bone score (TBS) in menopausal Caucasian women with low areal bone mineral density (BMDa): Analysing the odds of vertebral fracture. Bone 2010;46(1):176–81.
53. Del Rio LM, Winzenrieth R, Cormier C, et al. Is bone microarchitecture status of the lumbar spine assessed by TBS related to femoral neck fracture? A Spanish case-control study. Osteoporos Int 2013;24(3):991–8.
54. Krueger D, Fidler E, Libber J, et al. Spine trabecular bone score subsequent to bone mineral density improves fracture discrimination in women. J Clin Densitom 2014;17(1):60–5.
55. Lamy O, Krieg MA, Stoll D, et al. The OsteoLaus Cohort Study: Bone mineral density, micro-architecture score and vertebral fracture assessment extracted from a single DXA device in combination with clinical risk factors improve significantly the identification of women at high risk of fracture. Osteologie 2012;21: 77–82.
56. Vasic J, Petranova T, Povoroznyuk V, et al. Evaluating spine micro-architectural texture (via TBS) discriminates major osteoporotic fractures from controls both as well as and independent of site matched BMD: the Eastern European TBS study. J Bone Miner Metab 2014;32(5):556–62.
57. Leib E, Winzenrieth R, Lamy O, et al. Comparing bone microarchitecture by trabecular bone score (TBS) in Caucasian American women with and without osteoporotic fractures. Calcif Tissue Int 2014;95(3):201–8.
58. Ayoub ML, Maalouf G, Bachour F, et al. DXA-based variables and osteoporotic fractures in Lebanese postmenopausal women. Orthop Traumatol Surg Res 2014;100(8):855–8.
59. Nassar K, Paternotte S, Kolta S, et al. Added value of trabecular bone score over bone mineral density for identification of vertebral fractures in patients with areal bone mineral density in the non-osteoporotic range. Osteoporos Int 2014;25(1):243–9.
60. Touvier J, Winzenrieth R, Johansson H, et al. Fracture discrimination by combined bone mineral density (BMD) and microarchitectural texture analysis. Calcif Tissue Int 2015;96(4):274–83.

61. Leib E, Winzenrieth R, Aubry-Rozier B, et al. Vertebral microarchitecture and fragility fracture in men: a TBS study. Bone 2014;62:51–5.
62. Ayoub ML, Maalouf G, Cortet B, et al. Trabecular bone score and osteoporotic fractures in obese postmenopausal women. J Clin Densitom 2016. [Epub ahead of print].
63. Jain RK, Narang DK, Hans D, et al. Ethnic differences in trabecular bone score. J Clin Densitom 2016. [Epub ahead of print].
64. Silva BC, Leslie WD, Resch H, et al. Trabecular bone score: a noninvasive analytical method based upon the DXA image. J Bone Miner Res 2014;29(3): 518–30.
65. Bousson V, Bergot C, Sutter B, et al. Trabecular bone score: where are we now? Joint Bone Spine 2015;82(5):320–5.
66. Boutroy S, Hans D, Sornay-Rendu E, et al. Trabecular bone score improves fracture risk prediction in non-osteoporotic women: the OFELY study. Osteoporos Int 2013;24(1):77–85.
67. Iki M, Tamaki J, Kadowaki E, et al. Trabecular bone score (TBS) predicts vertebral fractures in Japanese women over 10 years independently of bone density and prevalent vertebral deformity: the Japanese Population-Based Osteoporosis (JPOS) cohort study. J Bone Miner Res 2014;29(2):399–407.
68. Popp AW, Meer S, Krieg MA, et al. Bone mineral density (BMD) and vertebral trabecular bone score (TBS) for the identification of elderly women at high risk for fracture: the SEMOF cohort study. Eur Spine J 2016;25(11):3432–8.
69. Leslie WD, Johansson H, Kanis JA, et al. Lumbar spine texture enhances 10-year fracture probability assessment. Osteoporos Int 2014;25(9):2271–7.
70. Leslie WD, Aubry-Rozier B, Lix LM, et al. Spine bone texture assessed by trabecular bone score (TBS) predicts osteoporotic fractures in men: the Manitoba Bone Density Program. Bone 2014;67:10–4.
71. Schousboe JT, Vo T, Taylor BC, et al. Prediction of incident major osteoporotic and hip fractures by trabecular bone score (TBS) and prevalent radiographic vertebral fracture in older men. J Bone Miner Res 2016;31(3):690–7.
72. Iki M, Fujita Y, Tamaki J, et al. Trabecular bone score may improve FRAX(R) prediction accuracy for major osteoporotic fractures in elderly Japanese men: the Fujiwara-kyo Osteoporosis Risk in Men (FORMEN) Cohort Study. Osteoporos Int 2015;26(6):1841–8.
73. McCloskey EV, Oden A, Harvey NC, et al. A meta-analysis of trabecular bone score in fracture risk prediction and its relationship to FRAX. J Bone Miner Res 2016;31(5):940–8.
74. McCloskey EV, Oden A, Harvey NC, et al. Adjusting fracture probability by trabecular bone score. Calcif Tissue Int 2015;96(6):500–9.
75. Harvey NC, Gluer CC, Binkley N, et al. Trabecular bone score (TBS) as a new complementary approach for osteoporosis evaluation in clinical practice. Bone 2015;78:216–24.
76. Krieg MA, Aubry-Rozier B, Hans D, et al. Effects of anti-resorptive agents on trabecular bone score (TBS) in older women. Osteoporos Int 2013;24(3): 1073–8.
77. Di Gregorio S, Del Rio L, Rodriguez-Tolra J, et al. Comparison between different bone treatments on areal bone mineral density (aBMD) and bone microarchitectural texture as assessed by the trabecular bone score (TBS). Bone 2015;75: 138–43.
78. Petranova T, Sheytanov I, Monov S, et al. Denosumab improves bone mineral density and microarchitecture and reduces bone pain in women with

osteoporosis with and without glucocorticoid treatment. Biotechnol Biotechnol Equip 2014;28(6):1127–37.
79. Kalder M, Hans D, Kyvernitakis I, et al. Effects of Exemestane and Tamoxifen treatment on bone texture analysis assessed by TBS in comparison with bone mineral density assessed by DXA in women with breast cancer. J Clin Densitom 2014;17(1):66–71.
80. Kalder M, Kyvernitakis I, Albert US, et al. Effects of zoledronic acid versus placebo on bone mineral density and bone texture analysis assessed by the trabecular bone score in premenopausal women with breast cancer treatment-induced bone loss: results of the ProBONE II substudy. Osteoporos Int 2015;26(1):353–60.
81. Prasad C, Greenspan SL, Vujevich KT, et al. Risedronate may preserve bone microarchitecture in breast cancer survivors on aromatase inhibitors: a randomized, controlled clinical trial. Bone 2016;90:123–6.
82. Pedrazzoni M, Casola A, Verzicco I, et al. Longitudinal changes of trabecular bone score after estrogen deprivation: effect of menopause and aromatase inhibition. J Endocrinol Invest 2014;37(9):871–4.
83. Leslie WD, Aubry-Rozier B, Lamy O, et al. TBS (Trabecular Bone Score) and diabetes-related fracture risk. J Clin Endocrinol Metab 2013;98(2):602–9.
84. Kim JH, Choi HJ, Ku EJ, et al. Trabecular bone score as an indicator for skeletal deterioration in diabetes. J Clin Endocrinol Metab 2015;100(2):475–82.
85. Dhaliwal R, Cibula D, Ghosh C, et al. Bone quality assessment in type 2 diabetes mellitus. Osteoporos Int 2014;25(7):1969–73.
86. Zhukouskaya VV, Eller-Vainicher C, Gaudio A, et al. The utility of lumbar spine trabecular bone score and femoral neck bone mineral density for identifying asymptomatic vertebral fractures in well-compensated type 2 diabetic patients. Osteoporos Int 2016;27(1):49–56.
87. Neumann T, Lodes S, Kastner B, et al. Trabecular bone score in type 1 diabetes–a cross-sectional study. Osteoporos Int 2016;27(1):127–33.
88. Paggiosi MA, Peel NF, Eastell R. The impact of glucocorticoid therapy on trabecular bone score in older women. Osteoporos Int 2015;26(6):1773–80.
89. Leib ES, Winzenrieth R. Bone status in glucocorticoid-treated men and women. Osteoporos Int 2016;27(1):39–48.
90. Koumakis E, Avouac J, Winzenrieth R, et al. Trabecular bone score in female patients with systemic sclerosis: comparison with rheumatoid arthritis and influence of glucocorticoid exposure. J Rheumatol 2015;42(2):228–35.
91. Eller-Vainicher C, Morelli V, Ulivieri FM, et al. Bone quality, as measured by trabecular bone score in patients with adrenal incidentalomas with and without subclinical hypercortisolism. J Bone Miner Res 2012;27(10):2223–30.
92. Belaya ZE, Hans D, Rozhinskaya LY, et al. The risk factors for fractures and trabecular bone-score value in patients with endogenous Cushing's syndrome. Arch Osteoporos 2015;10:44.
93. Eller-Vainicher C, Filopanti M, Palmieri S, et al. Bone quality, as measured by trabecular bone score, in patients with primary hyperparathyroidism. Eur J Endocrinol 2013;169(2):155–62.
94. Romagnoli E, Cipriani C, Nofroni I, et al. "Trabecular Bone Score" (TBS): An indirect measure of bone micro-architecture in postmenopausal patients with primary hyperparathyroidism. Bone 2013;53(1):154–9.
95. Rolighed L, Rejnmark L, Sikjaer T, et al. Vitamin D treatment in primary hyperparathyroidism: a randomized placebo controlled trial. J Clin Endocrinol Metab 2014;99(3):1072–80.

96. Naylor KL, Lix LM, Hans D, et al. Trabecular bone score in kidney transplant recipients. Osteoporos Int 2016;27(3):1115–21.
97. Breban S, Briot K, Kolta S, et al. Identification of rheumatoid arthritis patients with vertebral fractures using bone mineral density and trabecular bone score. J Clin Densitom 2012;15(3):260–6.
98. Kim D, Cho SK, Kim JY, et al. Association between trabecular bone score and risk factors for fractures in Korean female patients with rheumatoid arthritis. Mod Rheumatol 2016;26(4):540–5.
99. Kuzma M, Kuzmova Z, Zelinkova Z, et al. Impact of the growth hormone replacement on bone status in growth hormone deficient adults. Growth Horm IGF Res 2014;24(1):22–8.
100. Allo Miguel G, Serraclara Pla A, Partida Munoz ML, et al. Seven years of follow up of trabecular bone score, bone mineral density, body composition and quality of life in adults with growth hormone deficiency treated with rhGH replacement in a single center. Ther Adv Endocrinol Metab 2016;7(3):93–100.
101. Baldini M, Ulivieri FM, Forti S, et al. Spine bone texture assessed by trabecular bone score (TBS) to evaluate bone health in thalassemia major. Calcif Tissue Int 2014;95(6):540–6.
102. Eller-Vainicher C, Bassotti A, Imeraj A, et al. Bone involvement in adult patients affected with Ehlers-Danlos syndrome. Osteoporos Int 2016;27(8):2525–31.
103. Hwangbo Y, Kim JH, Kim SW, et al. High-normal free thyroxine levels are associated with low trabecular bone scores in euthyroid postmenopausal women. Osteoporos Int 2016;27(2):457–62.
104. Hong AR, Kim JH, Kim SW, et al. Trabecular bone score as a skeletal fragility index in acromegaly patients. Osteoporos Int 2016;27(3):1123–9.
105. Donaldson AA, Feldman HA, O'Donnell JM, et al. Spinal bone texture assessed by trabecular bone score in adolescent girls with anorexia nervosa. J Clin Endocrinol Metab 2015;100(9):3436–42.
106. Brunerova L, Ronova P, Veresova J, et al. Osteoporosis and impaired trabecular bone score in hemodialysis patients. Kidney Blood Press Res 2016;41(3):345–54.

Drug-Related Adverse Events of Osteoporosis Therapy

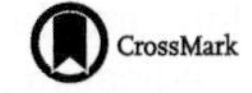

Moin Khan, MD, MSc, FRCSC[a,1], Angela M. Cheung, MD, PhD, FRCPC[b,1], Aliya A. Khan, MD, FRCPC[a,*,1]

KEYWORDS

- Bisphosphonates • Denosumab • Raloxifene • Teriparatide
- Atypical femoral fractures • Osteonecrosis of the jaw

KEY POINTS

- Bisphosphonates and denosumab are effective in reducing the risk of vertebral, nonvertebral, and hip fracture and are well tolerated with only minor side effects with short-term use.
- Long-term use of bisphosphonates and denosumab is associated with a small increased risk of atypical femoral fracture and rarely osteonecrosis of the jaw; these uncommon adverse events can be prevented or identified early with close monitoring and patient education.
- Teriparatide, an anabolic agent, is effective in reducing the risk of vertebral and nonvertebral fracture and is well tolerated with minor side effects.
- Raloxifene and bazedoxifene are effective in lowering the risk of vertebral fracture only and are associated with hot flashes and an increased risk of thromboembolic events.
- Pharmacologic intervention requires careful review of fracture risk and in the absence of contraindications the benefits are far greater than the potential risk of therapy.

INTRODUCTION

Postmenopausal osteoporosis is associated with microarchitectural deterioration and an increased risk of fracture.[1] Osteoporosis therapy has been demonstrated to effectively reduce the risk of vertebral, nonvertebral, and hip fracture and also has been associated with increased survival.[1] Currently approved treatments for osteoporosis include bisphosphonates, denosumab, selective estrogen receptor modulators, and

Disclosures: Dr Moin Khan reports no disclosures; Dr Angela Cheung reports honoria from Amgen, Lilly, and Merck for consultation and/or CMEs; Dr Aliya A. Khan reports research grants from Amgen, Meck, and Shire.

[a] McMaster University, 1200 Main Street West, Hamilton, ON L8N 3Z5, Canada; [b] University of Toronto, 200 Elizabeth Street, 7 Eaton North Room 221, Toronto, ON M5G 2C4, Canada
[1] Present address: #223, 3075 Hospital Gate, Oakville, Ontario, Canada.
* Corresponding author.
E-mail address: Aliya@mcmaster.ca

Endocrinol Metab Clin N Am 46 (2017) 181–192
http://dx.doi.org/10.1016/j.ecl.2016.09.009 endo.theclinics.com
0889-8529/17/

teriparatide.[1] This article reviews the adverse events of therapy associated with these medical interventions. Hormone replacement therapy is not included, because it is no longer indicated as first line therapy for the treatment of osteoporosis in all countries. Calcitonin and strontium ranelate also are not included, because their indication for osteoporosis has recently been limited or withdrawn.

BISPHOSPHONATES

Amino-bisphosphonates (aBPs) have been demonstrated to be effective in reducing the risk of fragility fracture in postmenopausal osteoporosis, osteoporosis in men, and glucocorticoid-induced osteoporosis as noted in pivotal fracture trials.[1] Currently, alendronate, risedronate, ibandronate, and zoledronate are approved for the treatment of postmenopausal osteoporosis. These compounds are not metabolized by any organ system and have few systemic side effects. They are cleared through the kidney and are contraindicated in stages 4 and 5 chronic kidney disease (estimated glomerular filtration rate is <30–35 mL/min).

Dosing and Administration

Alendronate is administered orally 70 mg weekly or 10 mg daily. Risedronate is administered orally 5 mg daily or 35 mg weekly or 150 mg monthly. Zoledronate is administered intravenously 5 mg over 15 to 30 minutes annually.[1]

Side Effects

Gastroesophageal adverse events

Oral aBPs have been associated with gastrointestinal side effects, including nausea, epigastric pain, esophagitis, and gastric ulcer.[2] Oral aBPs may impair the healing of esophageal acid–induced injury and are contraindicated in the presence of gastroesophageal reflux.[3] These side effects may be more pronounced with the use of generic oral bisphosphonates.[4]

Acute phase response

Intravenous zoledronic acid administration may be associated with an acute phase response usually observed after the first infusion and occurs in approximately 30% of patients.[5] This response is characterized by myalgias, arthralgias, low-grade fever, headache, and bone pain.[5] It usually resolves in 3 to 4 days and is less common with subsequent infusions. The acute phase response appears to be mediated by the release of cytokines (interleukin-6 and tumor necrosis factor-a) by activated T cells, resulting in an inflammatory response.[6,7]

Atrial fibrillation

An association between atrial fibrillation and the use of bisphosphonates was suggested in the phase 3 trial for zoledronic acid in comparison with placebo[8] (1.3% vs 0.5%, $P<.001$).[8] An increased risk of atrial fibrillation was observed, as well, in a small case control study with alendronate use.[9] A subsequent meta-analysis confirmed no association between the use of bisphosphonates and the development of atrial fibrillation.[10,11]

Esophageal cancer

The possible association between oral bisphosphonate use and esophageal cancer has been evaluated in the UK General Practice Research Database Cohort and an increase in the risk of esophageal cancer from 1 case per 1000 to 2 cases per 1000 patients with 5 years of use was reported.[12] A reanalysis of the same data did not confirm an association between oral bisphosphonate use and esophageal cancer risk.[13] Other investigators have also not identified an association between oral bisphosphonate use and the development of esophageal cancer in a Danish open cohort registry–based study.[14]

Uveitis, scleritis, and conjunctivitis

Ocular side effects can rarely occur with intravenous as well as oral aBP use and reports of uveitis, scleritis, and orbital inflammatory disease have been published.[15–17] A retrospective review suggests an incidence of 0.8% for the development of acute uveitis.[18] A recent prospective study evaluated the incidence of ocular side effects occurring within 3 months of receiving intravenous zoledronate 5 mg or placebo in 1054 postmenopausal women.[19] Fourteen individuals developed ocular symptoms following the infusion. The incidence of acute anterior uveitis and episcleritis was 1.1% (95% confidence interval [CI] 0.5–2.1) and 0.1% (95% CI 0.0–0.7), respectively, for the zoledronate group with no cases in the placebo group. The mean time for the development of symptoms was 3 days (range 2–4) Topical treatment with cyclopentolate and corticosteroids was initiated with no long-term sequelae. None of the individuals lost vision.[19] It is recommended to inform patients about the possibility of ocular side effects with intravenous zoledronate infusion.

Atypical femoral fractures

Incidence and risk factors Epidemiologic studies have confirmed an increased risk of femoral shaft and subtrochanteric fractures with prolonged use of bisphosphonates.[20–22] Randomized control trials of bisphosphonates in comparison with placebo have not demonstrated an increased risk of atypical femoral fractures (AFFs) and this may be a reflection of the relatively small number of individuals enrolled in the randomized control trials.[23–25] A systematic review and meta-analysis of published studies evaluating the association of bisphosphonates with subtrochanteric femoral shaft fractures and AFFs included 11 studies, 5 of which were case control and 6 were cohort studies.[26] Bisphosphonate exposure was associated with an increased risk of subtrochanteric femoral shaft fractures and AFFs with an adjusted relative risk of 1.70 (95% CI 1.22–2.37).[26] The risk of AFFs during and after bisphosphonate use was evaluated in Sweden in a nationwide cohort study.[27] Radiographs of 5342 Swedish women and men ages 55 and older who had experienced a femoral shaft fracture between 2008 and 2010 were reviewed, and 172 patients had AFFs.[27] The age-adjusted relative risk of atypical fracture with bisphosphonate use was 55 (95% CI 39–79) in women and 54 (CI 15–192) in men.[27] Women had a threefold higher risk of AFF in comparison with men. The risk of an AFF decreased by 70% per year following cessation of bisphosphonate use.[27]

AFFs appear to be more common in Asian women in comparison with white women.[28] A greater proportion of Asian women were noted to have AFFs in association with long-term bisphosphonate use in comparison with white women on long-term bisphosphonate therapy.[28] The risk of AFF increases with duration of bisphosphonate use and rises after 3 to 4 years with even greater increases in risk after 6 to 20 years of use.[27,29]

Other risk factors that have been identified for AFF include a slightly higher body mass index (26.2 ± 5.1 kg/m^2 vs 23.6 ± 6.2 kg/m^2).[30] Associations with oral glucocorticoid use, statins and proton pump inhibitor use have also been described.[30,31] Prodromal symptoms have been reported in 51.6% of patients.[30] Other investigators have found prodromal symptoms with thigh pain in 69% of patients.[29]

Pathophysiology The pathophysiology resulting in AFF is not clearly understood. Prolonged suppression of bone remodeling may result in accumulation of microcracks that may not be repaired.[32] Bisphosphonate therapy increases bone mineralization and may result in a uniform or homogeneous pattern of mineralization enabling crack propagation and may increase the risk of stress fracrtures.[33] Bone biopsy data are currently not conclusive and the underlying pathophysiology leading to AFF remains unclear.

The proximal femur geometry may also impact the likelihood of developing an AFF.[30] The presence of proximal femoral varus and a narrow femoral neck width was seen more frequently in individuals with AFF in comparison with controls.[30] Thicker lateral and medial bone cortices were also seen more frequently in patients with AFF in comparison with controls.[30] There may be a correlation between the lateral bowing angle of the femur and the location of the AFF.[34] These geometric risk factors also need to be further evaluated in large prospective studies.[35]

Osteonecrosis of the jaw

Definition Osteonecrosis of the jaw (ONJ) was first described in association with bisphosphonate use in oncology patients.[36] The definition of ONJ was clarified by the American Society for Bone and Mineral Research.[37] ONJ is defined as an area of exposed bone in the maxillofacial region that does not heal within 8 weeks in an individual who has been exposed to an antiresorptive agent and has not had radiation therapy.[37] Other risk factors for ONJ include chemotherapy, major oral surgery, periodontal disease, antiangiogenic drugs, diabetes, and glucocorticoid therapy. ONJ has significant morbidity and requires careful follow-up by an oral surgeon.[38]

ONJ lesions can remain asymptomatic for weeks or several months. They subsequently become symptomatic with inflammation in the surrounding tissues and can present with pain, swelling, ulceration, paresthesias, and tooth mobility.[39–41]

Incidence The incidence of ONJ is estimated largely from case series, retrospective observational data, and retrospective cohort data, because very limited prospective data evaluating the true incidence of ONJ in patients with osteoporosis are currently available. The incidence of ONJ in patients with osteoporosis is approximately 0.01% to 0.001%.[42–53]

Postmarketing of alendronate, Merck (New Jersey) estimated the incidence of ONJ to be less than 1 in 100,000 following exposure to alendronate. In the HORIZON study with 7765 postmenopausal women randomized to zoledronic acid in comparison with placebo, there were 2 cases of ONJ identified.[49] One was in a patient with a dental abscess and receiving zoledronic acid, the other occurred in a patient receiving placebo and prednisone therapy. Both of these cases resolved with antibiotics and debridement. Four additional clinical trials with zoledronic acid were reviewed and no additional cases of ONJ were identified. The incidence of adjudicated ONJ in 5903 patients treated with zoledronic acid in the 5 clinical trials was less than 1 in 14,200 patient treatment-years.[49]

In the oncology patient population receiving high doses of intravenous aBPs, the incidence of ONJ is higher and is estimated to be approximately 1% to 15%. The quality of evidence in the oncology patient population is much greater with both prospective and retrospective published studies. The oncology patient population is exposed to other risk factors associated with ONJ, including glucocorticoid therapy, chemotherapy, antiangiogenic agents, and radiotherapy. High-dose aBP therapy is associated with greater osteoclast inhibition. In patients with cancer, the incidence of ONJ appears to be related to the dose and duration of bisphosphonate therapy.[54–57]

The first large prospective evaluation of ONJ was in 5723 oncology patients with metastatic bone disease. These individuals were enrolled in 3 registration trials comparing denosumab 120 mg with zoledronic acid 4 mg given monthly. Oral examinations were conducted every 6 months, and 89 adjudicated cases of ONJ were identified. The incidence of ONJ with zoledronic acid and denosumab was not statistically different in this 36-month study.[54] The ONJ resolution rate appeared to be greater in individuals receiving denosumab in comparison with zoledronic acid; however, this requires further evaluation. Skeletal-related events were significantly decreased and the benefit of therapy greatly outweighed the risk of ONJ by a factor of 17.[54] In the oncology patients being prospectively evaluated, most individuals with ONJ developed ONJ in association with an oral event, such as a tooth extraction, in two-thirds of patients. Coinciding oral infection was seen in one-half of the patients and patients also had other risk factors for ONJ, such as the use of glucocorticoid therapy, which was seen in 73% of patients with ONJ in comparison with 62.3% without ONJ. Antiangiogenic agents were used in 15.7% of patients with ONJ and only 8% without ONJ.[54]

In the oncology patient population, risk factors for ONJ include intravenous bisphosphonate use, denosumab exposure, dental extractions, chemotherapy, periodontal disease, glucocorticoid therapy, diabetes, denture use, smoking, hyperthyroidism, dialysis, antiangiogenic agents, and being of older age.[57–67]

Pathophysiology Decreases in bone remodeling and osteocyte death appear to be factors in the development of ONJ. Infection also plays a key role in the development of ONJ and can contribute to and result from destruction of the oral mucosa. Infection may precede or follow necrosis and bacteria and polymorphonuclear leukocytes are usually seen in ONJ tissue.[68,69] Bacteria stimulate bone resorption and may contribute to the development bone necrosis.

Bisphosphonates can impact the immune response by having an impact on gamma-delta T cells and lead to macrophage dysfunction.

Bisphosphonates can activate the gamma-delta T cells and impact the immune response to infeca T cells and impact the immune response to infection.[70–72] Suppression of bone remodeling appears to play a role in the development of ONJ.[73,74]

Bisphosphonates have been demonstrated to have antiangiogenic effects[71,75] and may contribute to the development of ONJ. Antiangiogenic agents also may play a key role in the development of ONJ.

Prevention of osteonecrosis of the jaw The risk of ONJ appears to decrease with conservative therapy, including antimicrobial mouth rinses[38] and antibiotics before and after oral surgery.[38] Maintaining good oral hygiene is of key importance in preventing the development of ONJ.[38] It is recommended that oral surgery be completed before initiation of high-dose antiresorptive therapy in oncology patients. In this population, dental radiographs also should be obtained before initiation of high-dose antiresorptive therapy with identification of dental disease before initiation of antiresorptive therapy.[38] Any necessary dental procedures, including dental extraction or implants should be completed before initiation of therapy. Nonurgent procedures may be delayed if necessary. If they are urgently required, then they can be performed and the oncology doses of bisphosphonate or denosumab may be withheld until soft tissue closure is achieved. Currently, there is no evidence that interrupting drug therapy for patients requiring dental surgery will reduce the risk of ONJ or the progression of the disease. Delaying antiresorptive therapy until the surgical site heals in individuals at a high risk of ONJ may be of value of reducing the probability of ONJ.[38] In determining the suitability of drug interruption, the risk of ONJ must be weighed with the risk of skeletal-related events in oncology patients as well as the risk of fracture in individuals with osteoporosis.[38] In individuals with osteoporosis receiving low doses of bisphosphonate or denosumab therapy, antiresorptive treatment may be continued in the absence of significant comorbidity. The management decisions regarding interruption of drug therapy are ideally made by the dental and medical team managing patient care.

DENOSUMAB

Denosumab, an inhibitor of RANKL (receptor activator of nuclear factor KB), is a potent antiresorptive agent and is generally well tolerated. It is effective in lowering the risk of vertebral, hip, and nonvertebral fracture in postmenopausal osteoporosis.[76]

Dosing and Administration

Denosumab is administered subcutaneously in doses of 60 mg every 6 months.

Side Effects

In comparison with placebo, serious side effects were observed in 24.9% of individuals in comparison with 23.8% of controls.[77] In the FREEDOM study, there were no significant differences reported for side effects evaluated separately.[76] Arthralgias have been reported more frequently with denosumab in comparison with placebo (16.6% vs 14.3%); however, this difference has not been a statistically significant difference.[77] Symptomatic hypocalcemia occurred in 0.01% of individuals in the denosumab group in comparison with 0.05% of individuals in the placebo group. As denosumab is a potent antiresorptive agent, it is essential to ensure that serum calcium is normal before starting denosumab and also to ensure that patients are vitamin D replete, as vitamin D insufficiency can contribute to the development of hypocalcemia with denosumab therapy.

Dermatitis can be seen as an uncommon side effect.

Following introduction of denosumab in the market, several case reports have been published of AFF in individuals treated with denosumab.[78] In the FREEDOM study evaluating denosumab in comparison with placebo, 2 AFFs have been observed. One was in the cross-over arm, with 6 doses of denosumab use and one occurred in the long-term arm with 14 doses of exposure (Amgen, personal communication, 2015). The number needed to harm for denosumab has been estimated to be 1 in 10,000.

In the population of patients with osteoporosis receiving denosumab therapy, ONJ cases have been identified. The incidence appears to be very low and appears to be only slightly greater than that seen in the general population.

In the FREEDOM clinical trial of denosumab versus placebo involving almost 8000 postmenopausal osteoporotic women over 3 years, there were no cases of ONJ. In the extension of the FREEDOM study to 7 to 10 years of exposure, 13 cases of ONJ were identified.[79]

The postmarketing exposure to denosumab has been estimated to be 1,960,405 patient-years in 2,427,475 patients as of May 2014.[80] Following this exposure, 47 cases of adjudicated ONJ (based on the American Association of Oral and Maxillofacial Surgeons criteria) have been confirmed. All of these individuals had at least one other risk factor for ONJ. These included concurrent glucocorticoid use, concurrent chemotherapy, prior bisphosphonate use, or invasive dental procedures. The ONJ lesions resolved in a third of the cases and are ongoing in another third. The status of the remaining one-third is not known.[80]

TERIPARATIDE

Teriparatide is the only anabolic agent currently approved for the treatment of post-menopausal osteoporosis. It has been demonstrated to effectively reduce the risk of vertebral and nonvertebral fracture.[81] The pivotal fracture trial was terminated early and only 5 hip fractures were observed in the study. There were 4 hip fractures in the placebo group and 1 in the teriparatide group and the CI crossed 1.[1]

Dosing and Administration

Teriparatide is administrated subcutaneously in doses of 20 μg daily for up to 2 years.

Side Effects

This drug is also well tolerated. Adverse events observed in patients include nausea, headache, dizziness, and leg cramps.[81]

In carcinogenicity studies with rats, near lifetime treatment with systemic exposure ranging from 3 to 60 times the exposure in humans was associated with osteosarcoma in rats.[82] Osteosarcoma, however, has not been observed in humans, and the incidence of osteosarcoma in individuals treated with teriparatide is no different from the incidence seen in the general population. In the US postmarketing surveillance study of adult osteosarcoma and teriparatide, there was no association between teriparatide treatment and osteosarcoma in humans.[83]

SELECTIVE ESTROGEN RECEPTOR MODULATORS

Raloxifene and bazedoxifene have been demonstrated to reduce the risk of vertebral fracture in comparison with placebo.[1] A reduction in the risk of nonvertebral or hip fracture risk has not been observed in studies completed to date.

Dosing and Administration

Raloxifene is administered orally 60 mg daily.

Side Effects

Raloxifene has been evaluated in comparison with placebo,[84] as well as in comparison with tamoxifen in a head-to-head trial.[85] The drug is well tolerated with side effects limited to hot flashes, vaginal dryness, and a small increase in the risk of thromboembolic events.[84] In comparison with tamoxifen, raloxifene had a better safety profile, with 36% fewer uterine cancers and 29% fewer deep vein thromboses.[85]

In the RUTH study conducted in 10,101 postmenopausal women assigned to raloxifene 60 mg daily versus placebo for a median of 5.6 years, raloxifene was associated with a 50% decrease in the risk of invasive breast cancer.[86] The risk of vertebral fractures decreased by 35%.[86] There was a 50% increase in the risk of venous thromboembolic events and an increase in the risk of fatal stroke by 49%.[86]

SUMMARY/FUTURE CONSIDERATIONS

Osteoporosis therapy is safe and generally well tolerated. The benefits of therapy greatly outweigh potential harm. Selecting the best drug for each patient requires a review of the fracture risk for each patient as well as their suitability for the drug with respect to potential adverse effects. The risk for long-term adverse effects can be minimized by close follow-up of patients and advising patients to report the development of prodromal symptoms of an AFF. Interruption of bisphosphonate therapy after 3 to 5 years is also of value in reducing the potential risk of AFF.

Sequential use of anabolic therapy following prolonged antiresorptive therapy appears to be a valuable strategy in reducing both fracture risk and the risk of long-term adverse events in association with prolonged suppression of bone remodeling. The risk of ONJ also can be minimized by advising patients to ensure good oral hygiene is maintained in addition to regular dental care. Patient education is key to minimizing the actual and perceived adverse events of therapy while ensuring compliance with the available treatment options today.

Future directions for research include development of new anabolic molecules and the development of sequential therapy strategies designed to lower the risk of fracture while minimizing the potential risks of oversuppression of bone remodeling. Advances in imaging will also be of value in the early detection of AFF and ONJ. Identification of individuals with genetic predisposition for the development of AFF or ONJ will also be of value in selecting the best treatment option for each individual patient.

REFERENCES

1. Khan A, Fortier M, Reid R, et al. Osteoporosis in menopause. SOGC Clinical Practice Guideline 2014;36(9):839–43.
2. Adami S, Zamberlan N. Adverse effects of bisphosphonates. A comparative review. Drug Saf 1996;14:158–70.
3. Cadarette SM, Katz JN, Brookhart MA, et al. Comparative gastrointestinal safety of weekly oral bisphosphonates. Osteoporos Int 2009;20:1735–47.
4. Kanis JA, Reginster JY, Kaufman JM, et al. A reappraisal of generic bisphosphonates in osteoporosis. Osteoporos Int 2012;23:213–21.
5. Adami S, Bhalla AK, Dorizzi R, et al. The acute phase response after bisphosphonate administration. Calcif Tissue Int 1987;41:326–31.
6. Sauty A, Pecherstorfer M, Zimmer-Roth I, et al. Interleukin-6 and tumour necrosis factor alpha levels after bisphosphonates treatment in vitro and in patients with malignancy. Bone 1996;18:133–9.
7. Kunzmann V, Bauer E, Wilhelm M. Gamma/delta T cell stimulation by pamidronate. N Engl J Med 1999;340:737–8.
8. Black DM, Delmas PD, Eastell R, et al. Once-yearly zoledronic acid for treatment of postmenopausal osteoporosis. N Engl J Med 2007;356:1809–22.
9. Heckbert SR, Li G, Cummings SR, et al. Use of alendronate and risk of incident atrial fibrillation in women. Arch Intern Med 2008;168(8):826–31.
10. Rhee CW, Lee J, Oh S, et al. Use of bisphosphonate and risk of atrial fibrillation in older women with osteoporosis. Osteoporos Int 2012;23:247–54.
11. Barrett-Connor E, Swern AS, Hustad CM, et al. Alendronate and atrial fibrillation: a meta-analysis of randomized placebo-controlled clinical trials. Osteoporos Int 2012;23(1):233–45.
12. Green J, Czanner G, Reeves G, et al. Oral bisphosphonates and risk of cancer of esophagus, stomach, and colorectum: case-control analysis within a UK primary care cohort. BMJ 2012;34:c4444.
13. Cradwell CR, Abnet CC, Cantwell MM, et al. Exposure to oral bisphosphonates and risk of esophageal cancer. JAMA 2010;304:657–63.
14. Abrahamsen B, Pazianas M, Eiken P, et al. Esophageal and gastric cancer incidence and mortality in alendronate users. J Bone Miner Res 2012;27:679–86.
15. Durnian JM, Olujohungbe A, Kyle G. Bilateral acute uveitis and conjunctivitis after zoledronic acid therapy. Eye 2005;19:221–2.
16. Woo TCS, Joseph DJ, Wilkinson R. Serious ocular complications of zoledronate. Clin Oncol (R Coll Radiol) 2006;18:545–6.

17. Kaur H, Uy C, Kelly J, et al. Orbital inflammatory disease in a patient treated with zoledronate. Endocr Pract 2011;17:e101–3.
18. Patel DV, Horne A, House M, et al. The incidence of acute anterior uveitis after intravenous zoledronate. Ophthalmology 2013;120:773–6.
19. Patel V, Bolland M, Nisa Z, et al. Incidence of ocular side effects with intravenous zoledronate: secondary analysis of a randomized controlled trial. Osteoporos Int 2015;26:499–503.
20. Park-Wyllie LY, Mamdani MM, Juurlink DN, et al. Bisphosphonate use and the risk of subtrochanteric or femoral shaft fractures in older women. JAMA 2011;305: 783–9.
21. Schilcher J, Michaelsson K, Aspenberg P. Bisphosphonate use and atypical fractures of the femoral shaft. N Engl J Med 2011;364:1728–37.
22. Vestergaard P, Schwartz F, Rejnmark L, et al. Risk of femoral shaft and subtrochanteric fractures among users of bisphosphonates and raloxifene. Osteoporos Int 2011;22:993–1001.
23. Black DM, Kelly MP, Genant HK, et al. Bisphosphonate and fractures of the subtrochanteric or diaphyseal femur. N Engl J Med 2010;362(19):1761–71.
24. Kim SY, Schneeweiss S, Katz JN, et al. Oral bisphosphonates and risk of subtrochanteric or diaphyseal femur fractures in a population-based cohort. J Bone Miner Res 2011;26(5):993–1001.
25. Hsiao FY, Huang WF, Chen YM, et al. Hip and subtrochanteric or diaphyseal femoral fractures in alendronate users: a 10-year, nationwide retrospective cohort study in Taiwanese women. Clin Ther 2011;33(11):1659–67.
26. Gedmintas L, Solomon D, Kim SC. Bisphosphonates and risk of subtrochanteric, femoral shaft, and atypical femur fracture: a systematic review and meta-analysis. J Bone Miner Res 2013;28(8):1729–37.
27. Schilcher J, Koeppen V, Aspenberg P, et al. Risk of atypical femoral fracture during and after bisphosphonate use. Acta Orthop 2015;86(10):100–7.
28. Marcano A, Taormina D, Egol KA, et al. Are race and sex associated with the occurrence of atypical femoral fractures? Clin Orthop Relat Res 2014;427: 1020–7.
29. Dell RM, Adams AL, Greene DF, et al. Incidence of atypical nontraumatic diaphyseal fractures of the femur. J Bone Miner Res 2012;27(12):2544–50.
30. Mahjoub Z, Jean S, Leclerc JT, et al. Incidence and characteristics of atypical femoral fractures: clinical and geometrical data. J Bone Miner Res 2016;31(4): 767–76.
31. Giusti A, Hamdy NA, Papapoulos SE. Atypical fractures of the femur and bisphosphonate therapy: a systematic review of case/case series studies. Bone 2010;47(2):169–80.
32. Allen MR, Burr DB. Three years of alendronate treatment results in similar levels of vertebral microdamage as after one year of treatment. J Bone Miner Res 2007;22: 1759–65.
33. Turner CH, Burr DB. Principles of bone biomechanics. In: Lane NE, Sambrook PN, editors. Osteoporosis and the osteoporosis of rheumatic disease. Philadelphia: Mosby Elsevier; 2006.
34. Chen LP, Chang TK, Huang TY, et al. The correlation between lateral bowing angle of the femur and the location of atypical femur fractures. Calcif Tissue Int 2014;95(3):240–7.
35. Khan AA, Leslie WD, Lentle B, et al. Atypical femoral fractures: a teaching perspective. Can Assoc Radiol J 2014;66(2):102–7.

36. Khan AA, Sandor GK, Dore E, et al. Bisphosphonate associated osteonecrosis of the jaw. J Rheumatol 2009;36:478–90.
37. Khosla S, Burr D, Cauley J, et al. Bisphosphonate-associated osteonecrosis of the jaw: report of a task force of the American Society for Bone and Mineral Research. J Bone Miner Res 2007;22:1479–91.
38. Khan A, Morrison A, Hanley D, et al. Diagnosis and management of osteonecrosis of the jaw: a systematic review and international consensus. J Bone Miner Res 2014;29:1–21.
39. Khan AA, Sandor GK, Dore E, et al. Canadian consensus practice guidelines for bisphosphonate associated osteonecrosis of the jaw. J Rheumatol 2008;35: 1391–7.
40. Ruggiero SL, Dodson TB, Fantasia J, et al. Medication-related osteonecrosis of the jaw—2014 update. 2014.
41. Ruggiero SL, Dodson TB, Fantasia J, et al, American Association of Oral and Maxillofacial Surgeons. American Association of Oral and Maxillofacial Surgeons position paper on medication-related osteonecrosis of the jaw—2014 update. J Oral Maxillofac Surg 2014;72(10):1938–56.
42. Mavrokokki T, Cheng A, Stein B, et al. Nature and frequency of bisphosphonate-associated osteonecrosis of the jaws in Australia. J Oral Maxillofac Surg 2007;65: 415–23.
43. Powell D, Bowler C, Roberts T, et al. Incidence of serious side effects with intravenous bisphosphonate: a clinical audit. QJM 2012;105:965–71.
44. Khan AA, Rios LP, Sandor GK, et al. Bisphosphonate-associated osteonecrosis of the jaw in Ontario: a survey of oral and maxillofacial surgeons. J Rheumatol 2011; 38:1396–402.
45. Etminan M, Aminzadeh K, Matthew IR, et al. Use of oral bisphosphonates and the risk of aseptic osteonecrosis: a nested case-control study. J Rheumatol 2008;35: 691–5.
46. Tennis P, Rothman KJ, Bohn RL, et al. Incidence of osteonecrosis of the jaw among users of bisphosphonates with selected cancers or osteoporosis. Pharmacoepidemiol Drug Saf 2012;21:810–7.
47. Ulmner M, Jarnbring F, Torring O. Osteonecrosis of the jaw in Sweden associated with the oral use of bisphosphonate. J Oral Maxillofac Surg 2014;72:76–82.
48. Fedele S, Porter SR, D'Aiuto F, et al. Nonexposed variant of bisphosphonate-associated osteonecrosis of the jaw: a case series. Am J Med 2010;123:1060–4.
49. Grbic JT, Landesberg R, Lin SQ, et al. Incidence of osteonecrosis of the jaw in women with postmenopausal osteoporosis in the health outcomes and reduced incidence with zoledronic acid once yearly pivotal fracture trial. J Am Dent Assoc 2008;139:32–40.
50. Devogelaer JP, Brown JP, Burckhardt P, et al. Zoledronic acid efficacy and safety over five years in postmenopausal osteoporosis. Osteoporos Int 2007;18:1211–8.
51. Papapoulos S, Chapurlat R, Libanati C, et al. Five years of denosumab exposure in women with postmenopausal osteoporosis: results from the first two years of the FREEDOM extension. J Bone Miner Res 2012;27:694–701.
52. Zavras AI, Zhu S. Bisphosphonates are associated with increased risk for jaw surgery in medical claims data: is it osteonecrosis? J Oral Maxillofac Surg 2006;64: 917–23.
53. Pazianas M, Blumentals WA, Miller PD. Lack of association between oral bisphosphonates and osteonecrosis using jaw surgery as a surrogate marker. Osteoporos Int 2008;19:773–9.

54. Saad F, Brown JE, Van PC, et al. Incidence, risk factors, and outcomes of osteonecrosis of the jaw: integrated analysis from three blinded active-controlled phase III trials in cancer patients with bone metastases. Ann Oncol 2012;23:1341–7.
55. Cartsos VM, Zhu S, Zavras AI. Bisphosphonate use and the risk of adverse jaw outcomes: a medical claims study of 714,217 people. J Am Dent Assoc 2008;139:23–30.
56. Durie BG, Katz M, Crowley J. Osteonecrosis of the jaw and bisphosphonates. N Engl J Med 2005;353:99–102.
57. Vahtsevanos K, Kyrgidis A, Verrou E, et al. Longitudinal cohort study of risk factors in cancer patients of bisphosphonate-related osteonecrosis of the jaw. J Clin Oncol 2009;27:5356–62.
58. Barasch A, Cunha-Cruz J, Curro FA, et al. Risk factors for osteonecrosis of the jaws: a case-control study from the CONDOR dental PBRN. J Dent Res 2011;90:439–44.
59. Cafro AM, Barbarano L, Nosari AM, et al. Osteonecrosis of the jaw in patients with multiple myeloma treated with bisphosphonates: definition and management of the risk related to zoledronic acid. Clin Lymphoma Myeloma 2008;8:111–6.
60. Zervas K, Verrou E, Teleioudis Z, et al. Incidence, risk factors and management of osteonecrosis of the jaw in patients with multiple myeloma: a single-centre experience in 303 patients. Br J Haematol 2006;134:620–3.
61. Hoff AO, Toth BB, Altundag K, et al. Frequency and risk factors associated with osteonecrosis of the jaw in cancer patients treated with intravenous bisphosphonates. J Bone Miner Res 2008;23:826–36.
62. Badros A, Weikel D, Salama A, et al. Osteonecrosis of the jaw in multiple myeloma patients: clinical features and risk factors. J Clin Oncol 2006;24:945–52.
63. Wessel JH, Dodson TB, Zavras AI. Zoledronate, smoking, and obesity are strong risk factors for osteonecrosis of the jaw: a case-control study. J Oral Maxillofac Surg 2008;66:625–31.
64. Kyrgidis A, Vahtsevanos K, Koloutsos G, et al. Bisphosphonate-related osteonecrosis of the jaws: a case-control study of risk factors in breast cancer patients. J Clin Oncol 2008;26:4634–8.
65. Tsao C, Darby I, Ebeling PR, et al. Oral health risk factors for bisphosphonate-associated jaw osteonecrosis. J Oral Maxillofac Surg 2013;71:1360–6.
66. Jadu F, Lee L, Pharoah M, et al. A retrospective study assessing the incidence, risk factors and comorbidities of pamidronate-related necrosis of the jaws in multiple myeloma patients. Ann Oncol 2007;18:2015–9.
67. Thumbigere-Math V, Tu L, Huckabay S, et al. A retrospective study evaluating frequency and risk factors of osteonecrosis of the jaw in 576 cancer patients receiving intravenous bisphosphonates. Am J Clin Oncol 2012;35:386–92.
68. Sedghizadeh PP, Kumar SK, Gorur A, et al. Microbial biofilms in osteomyelitis of the jaw and osteonecrosis of the jaw secondary to bisphosphonate therapy. J Am Dent Assoc 2009;140:1259–65.
69. Lesclous P, Abi NS, Carrel JP, et al. Bisphosphonate-associated osteonecrosis of the jaw: a key role of inflammation? Bone 2009;45:843–52.
70. Santini D, Vincenzi B, Dicuonzo G, et al. Zoledronic acid induces significant and long-lasting modifications of circulating angiogenic factors in cancer patients. Clin Cancer Res 2003;9:2893–7.
71. Vincenzi B, Santini D, Dicuonzo G, et al. Zoledronic acid-related angiogenesis modifications and survival in advanced breast cancer patients. J Interferon Cytokine Res 2005;25:144–51.

72. Brunello A, Saia G, Bedogni A, et al. Worsening of osteonecrosis of the jaw during treatment with sunitinib in a patient with metastatic renal cell carcinoma. Bone 2009;44:173–5.
73. Allen MR. Animal models of osteonecrosis of the jaw. J Musculoskelet Neuronal Interact 2007;7:358–60.
74. Allen MR. Bisphosphonates and osteonecrosis of the jaw: moving from the bedside to the bench. Cells Tissues Organs 2009;189:289–94.
75. Fournier P, Boissier S, Filleur S, et al. Bisphosphonates inhibit angiogenesis in vitro and testosterone-stimulated vascular regrowth in the ventral prostate in castrated rats. Cancer Res 2002;62:6538–44.
76. Cummings SR, SanMartin J, McClung MR, et al. Denosumab for prevention of fractures in postmenopausal women with osteoporosis. N Engl J Med 2009; 361:756–65.
77. Diédhiou D, Cuny T, Sarr A, et al. Efficacy and safety of denosumab for the treatment of osteoporosis: a systematic review. Ann Endocrinol (Paris) 2015;76:650–7.
78. Aspenberg P. Denosumab and atypical femoral fractures. Acta Orthop 2014; 85(1):1.
79. Watts NB, Grbic JT, McClung MR, et al. Evaluation of invasive oral procedures and events in women with postmenopausal osteoporosis treated with denosumab: results from the pivotal phase 3 fracture study extension. J Bone Miner Res 2014;29(S1).
80. Geller ML, Wagman RB, Ho P-R, et al. Findings from denosumab (Prolia®) postmarketing safety surveillance for atypical femoral fracture, osteonecrosis of the jaw, severe symptomatic hypocalcemia, and anaphylaxis. J Bone Miner Res 2014;29(S1).
81. Neer RM, Arnaud CD, Zanchetta JR, et al. Effect of parathyroid hormone (1–34) on fractures and bone mineral density in postmenopausal women with osteoporosis. N Engl J Med 2001;344:1434–41.
82. Vahle JL, Sato M, Long GG, et al. Skeletal changes in rats given daily subcutaneous injections—a recombinant human PTH 1-34 for 2 years and relevance to human safety. Toxicol Pathol 2002;30:312–21.
83. Andrews EB, Gilsenan AW, Midkiff K, et al. 2012 The US postmarketing surveillance study of adult osteosarcoma and teriparatide: study design and findings from the first 7 years. J Bone Miner Res 2012;27(12):2429–37.
84. Delmas PD, Ensrud KE, Adachi JD, et al, Multiple Outcomes of Raloxifene Evaluation Investigators. Efficacy of raloxifene on vertebral fracture risk reduction in postmenopausal women with osteoporosis: four-year results from randomized clinical trial. J Clin Endocrinol Metab 2002;87:3609–17.
85. Vogel VG, Costantino JP, Wickerham DL, et al, National Surgical Adjuvant Breast and Bowel Project. Effects of tamoxifen vs raloxifene on the risk of developing invasive breast cancer and other disease outcomes: the NSABP Study of Tamoxifen and Raloxifene (STAR) P-2 trial. JAMA 2006;295:2727–41.
86. Barrett-Connor E, Mosca L, Collins P, et al, Raloxifene Use for The Heart (RUTH) Trial Investigators. Effects of raloxifene on cardiovascular events and breast cancer in postmenopausal women. N Engl J Med 2006;355:125–37.

Combined Pharmacologic Therapy in Postmenopausal Osteoporosis

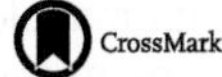

Yang Shen, MD[a], Dona L. Gray, MD[b], Dorothy S. Martinez, MD[c,*]

KEYWORDS

• Postmenopausal osteoporosis • Antiresorptive agent • Anabolic agent
• Teriparatide • Combination therapy

KEY POINTS

- Clinical guidelines recommend initiating pharmacologic treatment of patients with a history of hip or vertebral fracture, with a T score in osteoporotic range, or patients with significantly elevated fracture risks.
- Current pharmacologic treatments can be classified into antiresorptive and anabolic agents based on their mechanism of action; antiresorptive agents include raloxifene (selective estrogen receptor modulator [SERM]), bisphosphonates, and denosumab (receptor activator of nuclear factor κβ ligand inhibitor).
- Teriparatide is the only Food and Drug Administration–approved anabolic agent for osteoporosis treatment; synergistic effects of combining teriparatide with an antiresorptive agent have been proposed and studied in multiple clinical studies.
- Small increases of bone density were observed in the combination therapy for teriparatide and estrogen/SERM and that of teriparatide and denosumab; however, those studies were limited by small sample sizes and lack of fracture outcomes.
- Results of the combination therapy for teriparatide and bisphosphonates were mixed; heterogeneity of the pharmacologic characteristics of antiresorptive agents as well as trial designs may be significant contributors of inconsistent results.

INTRODUCTION

Osteoporosis is a common skeletal disease characterized by low bone density and increased bone fragility and, therefore, is associated with significant fracture risks. A clinical guideline from the National Osteoporosis Foundation recommends initiating

Disclosure Statement: The authors have nothing to disclose.

[a] Endocrinology Clinic, Huntington Health Physicians, 10 Congress Street, Suite 408, Pasadena, CA 91105, USA; [b] Endocrinology Clinic, Indiana University Health Arnett, 2600 Ferry Street, Lafayette, IN 47904, USA; [c] Divisions of Endocrinology, Diabetes and Metabolism, David Geffen School of Medicine, University of California, Los Angeles, 200 UCLA Medical Plaza, Suite 530, Los Angeles, CA 90095, USA
* Corresponding author.
E-mail address: dmartinez@mednet.ucla.edu

Endocrinol Metab Clin N Am 46 (2017) 193–206
http://dx.doi.org/10.1016/j.ecl.2016.09.008
endo.theclinics.com
0889-8529/17/

pharmacologic treatment of patients with a hip or vertebral fracture or who have a bone mineral density (BMD) T score of −2.5 or less or who have a BMD T score between 1.0 and 2.5 and a 10-year probability of a hip fracture 3% or greater or a 10-year probability of a major osteoporosis-related fracture of 20% or greater based on the Fracture Risk Assessment Tool algorithm.[1] Depending on their mechanism of action, pharmacologic treatments for osteoporosis can be classified into either antiresorptive agents or anabolic agents.[2] This classification is based on the phase of the bone remodeling process: if the main action of a drug is to inhibit the resorption process and/or shorten the life span of osteoclasts, then the agent is thought to be antiresorptive. On the other hand, if the main action of a drug is to stimulate osteoblast function and promote bone formation, then the agent is anabolic. **Table 1** lists the major pharmacologic agents that have been approved by the Food and Drug Administration (FDA) for the treatment of postmenopausal osteoporosis.

MECHANISMS OF ACTION FOR TREATMENT OF POSTMENOPAUSAL OSTEOPOROSIS

Many research efforts on the pathogenesis of osteoporosis were focused on postmenopausal women because estrogen plays a central role in bone remodeling.[3] Estrogen, mediated by estrogen receptor α, directly and indirectly attenuates resorption of trabecular bone.[4] In the postmenopausal state, estrogen deficiency results in an increase of bone resorption and remodeling. Binding of receptor activator of nuclear factor $\kappa\beta$ ligand (RANKL) to RANK also plays an essential role in this process: estrogen deficiency increased the expression of RANKL in B lymphocytes, which leads to more binding of RANKL to RANK that eventually gives rise to the initiation and differentiation of osteoclasts.[4,5] Postmenopausal bone change is a continuum. The aging process plays a significant role in bone loss.[6] Osteoporosis may develop in women in their 50s, 60s, 70s, or 80s, suggesting individual heterogeneity in pathogenesis.

Estrogen replacement therapy in postmenopausal women is known to prevent bone loss and vertebral and hip fractures.[7] Estrogen replacement is no longer routinely used because of increased risks of breast cancer and cardiovascular adverse effects. Raloxifene, a selective estrogen receptor modulator (SERM) that mimics estrogen's effects on bone remodeling, has been approved for treatment of postmenopausal osteoporosis. Clinical trial data of raloxifene showed that it inhibits bone turnover and increases BMD. It reduced the fracture risk in vertebrae but not in hip or nonvertebral sites.[8,9] Use of raloxifene is also associated with a reduced risk for breast cancer but has increased thromboembolic events.

Bones are woven structures of type I collagen strengthened with crystals of calcium hydroxyapatite. Bisphosphonates are nitrogen-containing analogues to pyrophosphates that actively bind to hydroxyapatite crystals in bone and, thus, interfere with isoprenylation of small guanosine triphosphatases in osteoclasts in a process that eventually causes reduced bone resorption and apoptosis of osteoclasts.[5] There are several bisphosphonates approved for osteoporosis treatment; differences in their side chain structure determine their binding strength to the bone as well as their distribution within the bone and dosing frequencies. Major clinical trials for alendronate, risedronate, and zoledronic acid demonstrated significant fracture risk reduction in vertebral, nonvertebral, and hip areas.[10–12] Increases in bone density were observed after 6 months of initiating use of bisphosphonates.[10–14] Common adverse events for oral bisphosphonates are gastrointestinal irritation and symptoms of esophagitis. Atypical femur fractures and osteonecrosis of the jaw are rare adverse events associated with this drug class. An acute phase reaction with flulike symptoms can occur in

Table 1
Major treatments approved by the Food and Drug Administration for postmenopausal osteoporosis

			Fracture Risk Reduction[b]			BMD Improvement[c] (%)		Side Effects	
Drug Class	**Drug Name**	**Dose/Frequency[a]**	**Vertebrae**	**Hip**	**Nonvertebral**	**Lumbar Spine**	**Total Hip**	**Common**	**Rare**
Antiresorptive agent									
SERM	Raloxifene	Oral: 60 mg/d	Yes			2.1	1.7	Hot flashes, nausea	VTE
Bisphosphonate	Alendronate	Oral: 70 mg/wk	Yes	Yes	Yes	5.7	4.0	Esophagitis, MK symptom	ONJ, atypical fractures
	Risedronate	Oral: 35 mg/wk or 150 mg/mo or 75 mg × 2 consecutive day	Yes	Yes	Yes	4.0	2.7	Esophagitis, MK symptom	ONJ, atypical fractures
	Ibandronate	Oral: 150 mg/mo or IV: 3 mg every 3 mo	Yes			Oral: 5.3	Oral: 3.6	ONJ, atypical fractures	ONJ, atypical fractures
	Zoledronic acid	IV: 5 mg/y	Yes	Yes	Yes	6.2	4.3	Acute-phase response, MK symptom	ONJ, atypical fractures
RANKL inhibitor	Denosumab	Subc: 60 mg every 6 mo	Yes	Yes	Yes	7.1	4.5	Cellulitis, skin reactions	ONJ, atypical fractures
Anabolic agent	Teriparatide	Subc: 20 μg/d	Yes		Yes	9.7	3.2	Nausea, leg cramps	Hypercalcemia, osteosarcoma

Calcitonin is approved for treatment of postmenopausal osteoporosis but not commonly used in clinical practice and, therefore, is not included.

Abbreviations: IV, intravenous; MK, musculoskeletal; ONJ, osteonecrosis of the jaw; RANKL, receptor activator of nuclear factor κβ ligand; SERM, selective estrogen receptor modulator; Subc, subcutaneous; VET, venous thromboembolism.

[a] Only the treatment doses and frequencies of postmenopausal osteoporosis are listed.

[b] Only the sites demonstrated significant fracture risk reduction in pivotal trials are listed as *Yes*.

[c] Predicted difference from placebo in percent BMD change from baseline at 24 months using data from a meta-analysis and modeling.[34]

up to one third of patients who received the intravenous zoledronic acid for the first time, but zoledronic acid is much better tolerated in subsequent doses.

Denosumab is a monoclonal antibody that binds to RANKL and prevents its interaction to RANK. As a result, the formation of osteoclasts is blocked. Denosumab inhibits the resorption process, prevents bone loss, and reduces the risk of vertebral and hip fractures. It is available as a subcutaneous injection with the dosage of 60 mg every 6 months. Denosumab is a potent antiresorptive agent: it has been shown to rapidly reduce C-telopeptide of type I collagen (CTX) and serum procollagen type I N-terminal propeptide (PINP) and reduce resorption by 86% at 1 month.[15] It is overall well tolerated in the treatment dose for postmenopausal osteoporosis; the most common side effects include local reactions, such as cellulitis and eczema. Case reports of osteonecrosis of the jaw and atypical femur fractures have been reported. It is administered concomitantly with calcium and vitamin D supplements to prevent hypocalcemia.

Teriparatide, a recombinant hormone containing a 34 amino acid sequence of the N-terminal of parathyroid hormone (PTH 1–34), is the only anabolic agent approved in the United States for osteoporosis. PTH, acting directly and indirectly and through multiple signaling pathways, regulates osteoblast lineage cell function and increases osteoblast production. PTH is short acting. Intermittent low doses of PTH have been found to increase bone density, especially for cancellous bones.[16] Compared with placebo, teriparatide, given 20 mcg daily, increased vertebral BMD by approximately 9% and femoral BMD by approximately 3% over a 21-month period.[17] Those measurements were taken by dual-energy x-ray absorptiometry. Because the anabolic effect on bone strength is most present in bone microarchitecture, some have argued that measurement of BMD, if assessed in volumetric density (grams per cubic centimeter) by quantitative computed tomography (CT), will be greater in scale for bone strength changes on teriparatide. Teriparatide lowers the risks of vertebral and hip fractures. For patients with increased baseline risks of osteosarcoma, such as Paget disease, elevated alkaline phosphate, young adults with open epiphyses, or history of radiation to the skeleton, teriparatide should not be used. Teriparatide administration increases the risk of hypercalcemia; therefore, it should not be used in patients with hypercalcemia or hyperparathyroidism.

Although combining more than one antiresorptive agents is not logical for increasing bone strength, there has been much interest in combining an anabolic agent (in this case, teriparatide) with another antiresorptive agent. Combining an anabolic agent with an antiresorptive agent may achieve superior results than monotherapy because of their potential synergistic effects. However, clinical results have been mixed. **Table 2** tabulates major randomized clinical trials studying combination therapy for anabolic and antiresorptive agents. The authors also examine those results based on the drug class of the antiresorptive agent.

TERIPARATIDE PLUS ESTROGEN OR SELECTIVE ESTROGEN RECEPTOR MODULATOR

Lindsay and colleagues[18] conducted a randomized placebo controlled trial in 1990 to 1992 of adding teriparatide 20 mcg daily injection to postmenopausal women with osteoporosis taking hormone replacement therapy (HRT). Thirty-four women who had been on HRT for 1 year were randomized into treatment groups of teriparatide (n = 17) or placebo (n = 17). The HRT (most participants take oral estrogen 0.625 mg daily) was continued during the study period of 3 years. Biomarkers of serum osteocalcin (OC) and urine cross-linked n-telopeptide (NTx) increased by 6 months for teriparatide-treated patients on estrogen, with serum OC increasing more rapidly and in greater magnitude at 1 month. The increase of biomarkers was observed until

Table 2
Effects of combination therapy for antiresorptive agents and teriparatide in major randomized clinical trials for postmenopausal women

					Biomarker		BMD			
Trial	Sample Size	Randomization	Treatment	Duration	Bone Formation	Bone Resorption	Lumbar	Total Hip	Total Body	Fracture
TPTD + estrogen/SERM										
Lindsay et al,[18] 1997	34	1:1	TPTD + HRT vs placebo + HRT	36 mo	OC: early elevation at 1 mo, converge at 3 y	NTx: elevation at 6 mo, converge at 3 y	13% vs NS	2.7% vs NS	7.8% vs NS	↓[a]
Cosman et al,[19] 2001	52	1:1	TPTD + HRT vs placebo + HRT	36 mo	BSAP: elevation at 6 mo, converge at 3 y	NTx: elevated at 6 mo, converge at 3 y	13% vs NS	4.4% vs NS	3.7% vs NS	↓[a]
Ste-Marie et al,[21] 2006	247	1:1:1:1	TPTD + HRT vs placebo + HRT (pre-HRT treated and not pretreated)	12 mo	BSAP: early elevation at 1 mo, elevation at 12 mo	NTx: early elevation at 1 mo, elevation at 12 mo	14% vs 3%	4.7% vs 1.7%	1.4% vs NS	N/A
Deal et al,[22] 2005	137	1:1	TPTD + RAL vs TPTD + placebo	6 mo	PINP: elevation in both groups, higher with TPTD + pla	CTX: both elevated from baseline; higher elevation in TPTD + pla	6% vs 5%	2% vs NS	—	N/A

(continued on next page)

Table 2
(continued)

Trial	Sample Size	Randomization	Treatment	Duration	Biomarker: Bone Formation	Biomarker: Bone Resorption	BMD: Lumbar	BMD: Total Hip	BMD: Total Body	Fracture
TPTD + bisphosphonate										
Finkelstein et al,[23] 2010	93	1:1:1	TPTD + ALN (I) vs TPTD (II) vs ALN (III)	30 mo	OC & PINP: mirrors ALN group more than TPTD	NTx: mirrors ALN group more than TPTD	11.9% (I) vs 17.8% (II) vs 6.8% (III)	2.9% (I) vs 8.1% (II) vs 3.1% (III)	4.0% (I) vs 3.6% (II) vs 4.8% (III)	N/A
Cosman et al,[26] 2011	412	1:1:1	TPTD + ZOL (I) vs TPTD (II) vs ZOL (III)	12 mo	PINP: decline early but progressively increase after 8 wk	CTX: decline early but progressive increase after 8 wk	7.5% (I) vs 7.0% (II) vs 4.4% (III)	2.3% (I) vs 1.1% (II) vs 2.2% (III)	—	↓[b]
Muschitz et al,[27] 2013	125	9 mo of TPTD then 1:1:1	TPTD + ALN (I) vs TPTD + RAL (II) vs TPTD alone (III)	Additional 12 mo	PINP: decline in both combination groups (I & II)	CTX: decline in both combination groups (I & II)	9.2% (I) vs 10.0% (II) vs 6.0%	7.0% (I) vs 4.2% (II) vs 4.4% (III)	—	N/A

Cosman et al,[28] 2009	102	18 mo of ALN then 1:1	TPTD + ALN vs TPTD	18 mo	PINP & BSAP: increased but less than TPTD alone	CTX: no change	8% vs 4%	3.2% (I) vs NS	—	↓[b]
	96	18 mo of RAL then 1:1	TPTD + RAL vs TPTD	18 mo	PINP & BSAP: increased but less than TPTD alone	CTX: increased but less than TPTD alone	Similar 6%–8%	Similar 1%–2%	—	↓[b]
TPTD + denosumab										
Tsai et al,[30] 2013	100	1:1:1	TPTD + DMAB (I) vs TPTD alone (II) vs DMAB alone (III)	12 mo + extension	OC & PINP: mirrors DMAB group with decline from baseline	CTX: mirrors DMAB group with decline from baseline	9.1% (I) vs 6.2% (II) vs 5.5% (III)	4.9% (I) vs 0.7% (II) vs 2.5% (III)	—	N/A

Abbreviations: ALN, alendronate; BSAP, bone-specific alkaline phosphatase; CTX, carboxy-terminal collagen crosslinks; DMAB, denosumab; HRT, hormone replacement therapy; N/A, not available; NS, not significant (not reported); NTx, cross-linked N-terminal telopeptide of type I collagen; OC, osteocalcin; pla, placebo; RAL, raloxifene; TPTD, teriparatide; ZOL, zoledronic acid.

[a] Vertebral fracture only; measured as vertebral height reduced by 15%.

[b] Fractures reported as adverse events.

approximately 30 months of treatment; by that time they converge to baseline. Patients treated with estrogen + teriparatide, compared with patients treated with estrogen + placebo, had significantly increased BMD in vertebral, hip, and total body sites. The vertebral deformity rate was also noted as being lower in the teriparatide-treated group compared with that of the placebo group.

Cosman and colleagues[19] compared the efficacy and safety of treating osteoporosis in postmenopausal women with teriparatide + estrogen (n = 27) versus placebo + estrogen (n = 25) in a randomized clinical trial. The dosage of teriparatide was 25 mcg daily, slightly higher than the FDA-approved dosage. The lead time of estrogen therapy was 2 years. Similar to Lindsay and colleagues' finding, the bone formation biomarker (serum bone-specific alkaline phosphatase in this study) increased first and was followed by the increase of urine NTx during the first 6 months; the early phase of this period when the augmentation of bone formation exceeds the stimulation of bone resorption has been referred to as anabolic window, hypothesized as the most efficient bone-building period for teriparatide.[20] BMD continued to improve during the 36-month study period, with a mean increase of 14% in the lumbar spine and 4% in the hip and total body for women on teriparatide + estrogen treatment. The placebo group did not show significant changes from baseline. Occurrence of vertebral deformity was reduced in the group treated with teriparatide + estrogen, compared with group treated with placebo + estrogen.

Ste-Marie and colleagues'[21] study on teriparatide and HRT further characterized their synergistic effects on the increase of BMD. The study enrolled 247 postmenopausal patients who had low bone mass. Among them, 122 patients were treated with HRT (pretreated HRT) and 125 patients were not treated with HRT (not pretreated) in the 12 months before study. Within each group, the patients were randomized into receiving HRT alone or HRT + teriparatide 40 mcg daily. At 12 months, women who was not pretreated with HRT and received HRT + teriparatide had the greatest increase in BMD at all bone sites (lumbar spine, total hip, femoral neck, ultradistal radius and whole body); the increases were greater than patients who were previously treated with HRT and then added teriparatide to the HRT. The two groups of patients treated with teriparatide + HRT (pretreated or non-pretreated) had significantly higher BMD than patients who were treated with HRT alone. Interestingly, the increase of biomarker activities, including both bone-specific alkaline phosphatase as a bone formation marker and the urine NTx as a bone resorption marker, were less pronounced within the patients treated with teriparatide + HRT who were not pretreated, in comparison with those who were pretreated and on teriparatide + HRT therapy. This finding supports that teriparatide can increase BMD, even with the suppressive effects of estrogen on bone formation and bone reabsorption. This study used a higher dose of teriparatide than the 20 mcg daily dose approved by the FDA. Overall teriparatide and HRT were well tolerated, with nausea and leg cramps reported more frequently in the patients who received combination therapy.

Deal and colleagues'[22] randomized placebo controlled study directly compared teriparatide + raloxifene versus teriparatide alone for 6 months (n = 137). PINP was elevated in both treatment groups at 1 month, and the elevations were continued at 3 and 6 months. CTX, a bone resorption marker, was not significantly increased from baseline at 1 month in either treatment group. At 3 months, CTX was significantly increased from baseline in the teriparatide-alone group but not in the teriparatide + raloxifene group. At 6 months, CTX had significantly increased in both treatment groups; but the increase in the teriparatide + raloxifene group was much less. Six-month treatment of teriparatide alone significantly increased BMD only at the lumbar spine, whereas 6-month treatment of teriparatide + raloxifene significantly increased BMD at the lumbar spine, femoral neck, and total hip area. Those findings suggest the combination of raloxifene with teriparatide may enhance the bone-forming effects of teriparatide by reducing the bone resorption during the anabolic window period and enhance the bone density at the femoral neck area by mitigating the teriparatide-induced increase in cortical porosity. Hypercalcemia was observed in 5.8% of patients in this study.

TERIPARATIDE PLUS BISPHOSPHONATE

Clinical research data on combination therapy for teriparatide with bisphosphonate have had mixed outcomes.[23–25] Finkelstein and colleagues[23] randomized 93 postmenopausal women with low bone density who have never received osteoporosis treatment to alendronate 10 mg daily, teriparatide 40 mcg daily, or both for 30 months. In the 2 groups taking teriparatide, teriparatide was started 6 months after alendronate and continued for 24 months. More than one-third of patients randomized to receive teriparatide (alone or in combination) discontinued the study early, mostly due to discomfort or inconvenience associated with daily injection. The dose of teriparatide used in this study was higher than the FDA-approved dose, and 25% to 50% of patients on teriparatide required dose adjustments. After 24-month treatment of teriparatide, the combination therapy for teriparatide + alendronate did not improve the BMD in the lumbar spine or femoral neck more than teriparatide alone. Biomarkers, including PINP, OC, and serum NTx, were attenuated in the combination therapy compared with teriparatide alone. Alendronate is, therefore, thought to attenuate teriparatide-induced bone turnover; coadministration of alendronate and teriparatide reduce the ability of teriparatide to increase BMD.

Concomitant initiation of teriparatide 20 mcg daily and one dose of 5 mg intravenous zoledronic acid has shown positive effect on BMD with the combination therapy. Cosman and colleagues[26] had randomized 412 postmenopausal women with osteoporosis at a ratio of 1:1:1 to teriparatide + zoledronic acid, teriparatide + placebo, and zoledronic acid only treatment arms. Patients who received combination therapy demonstrated significantly higher BMD increments in the lumbar spine and hip area as early as week 13 and maintained a BMD increase to the end point of this 52-week study. At 52 weeks, combination therapy had a 7.3% increase in lumbar spine BMD from baseline, similar to the increase observed in the teriparatide arm and much higher than the 4.4% increase in the zoledronic acid arm. In the total hip, the 2.3% increase in BMD in the combination arm is close to the 2.2% BMD increase with zoledronic acid, both were significantly higher than the 1.1% increase in the teriparatide-alone arm. Serum CTX and PINP levels were remarkably low in the first 8 weeks but increased steadily afterward and remained significantly elevated at week 52, though the increase of those biomarkers started early and ended higher in the teriparatide-alone arm. No significant changes from baseline with the biomarkers were observed in the zoledronic acid arm. This study also had fracture data (recorded as adverse events): 2.9%, 5.8%, and 9.5% of patients in the teriparatide + zoledronic acid, teriparatide-alone, and zoledronic acid–alone arms had reported clinical fractures. Serum calcium level abnormality rates were similar between the combination group and teriparatide-alone group.

Was the mitigating effect on BMD with the combination of alendronate and teriparatide subject to the timing of introducing teriparatide to alendronate? During the initial start of teriparatide, it is known to have moderate elevation of biomarkers accompanied by an increase of bone formation. The initial phase of the anabolic window is characterized by moderate bone resorption activities and a high level of the bone formation process. If patients were pretreated with a potent antiresorptive agent, such as alendronate, then it would be difficult for the teriparatide-induced bone remodeling to take hold. What would happen if starting teriparatide first and then adding bisphosphonate into the treatment regimen with teriparatide – would inhibiting the antiresorptive process in the late phase of teriparatide treatment prolong its anabolic effect? Muschitz and colleagues[27] enrolled 125 postmenopausal women who received teriparatide treatment for 9 months and then randomize them to stay on teriparatide alone or initiate combination therapy with alendronate or raloxifene. At 6 months and 12 months after adding antiresorptive therapy, the PINP and CTX concentrations were reduced in the combination treatment arms. But significantly higher increases in BMD lumbar spine and total hip were observed in the teriparatide + alendronate arm compared with the teriparatide-alone arm (9.2% vs 6.0% and 7.0% vs 4.4%, respectively). Significant increases in BMD lumbar spine were observed in the teriparatide + raloxifene arm but not in hip region. Volumetric BMP (vBMP) using dedicated CT scanner and Quantitative computed tomography (QCT) pro bone densitometry software (Mindways Software, Inc., Austin, USA) was also used. The vBMP increase in the combination therapy was significantly superior to the other two groups in the L2 vertebra, total hip region, and the integral femoral neck. There was no significant difference of fractures (recorded as adverse effects) among the treatment groups.

For patients who were treated with antiresorptive therapy, does teriparatide work better with the continuation or discontinuation of the prior therapy? Cosman and colleagues[28] enrolled 102 postmenopausal women with osteoporosis who were on alendronate and 96 patients who were on raloxifene for at least 18 months before the start of the randomized study into continuation of their baseline therapy plus teriparatide or switching into teriparatide alone. In this 18-month study, patients who were on alendronate and added teriparatide treatment to alendronate had less of an increase of biomarkers (PINP, bone-specific alkaline phosphatase) and experienced more BMD increases in lumbar spine and total hip than those patients who switched to teriparatide alone. In the raloxifene stratum, the increase of biomarkers was also less pronounced in the teriparatide + raloxifene arm than in the teriparatide-alone group; BMD increase at multiple sites was not statistically significant at the end of the 18-month study between the two arms.

A cyclic treatment of teriparatide with bisphosphonate was studied. One hundred and twenty-six women who have been taking alendronate for at least one year then randomized to receive teriparatide 25 mcg daily with alendronate, alendronate alone, or 3-month-on, 3-month-off teriparatide treatment for 15 months.[29] Bone formation markers increased in the 2 teriparatide treatment arms; a cyclic pattern was observed with the cyclic teriparatide treatment, and the decline of biomarker activities was observed during the off cycle. BMD in the lumbar spine increased 6.1% in the continuous teriparatide treatment and 5.4% in the cyclic treatment group, whereas there was no significant change from baseline in the alendronate-alone group. There was no difference in the hip BMD among the groups. One woman in the continuous teriparatide + alendronate group, 2 in the cyclic teriparatide + alendronate group, and 4 in the alendronate group had new or worsening vertebral deformities. Musculoskeletal symptoms, gastrointestinal effects, and elevated urinary calcium/creatinine ratio were significantly higher in the teriparatide-treated group.

TERIPARATIDE PLUS DENOSUMAB

The DATA (The Denosumab and Teriparatide Administration) trial conducted by Tsai and colleagues[30] is the largest trial to evaluate the combination therapy for teriparatide with denosumab. In this trial, 100 postmenopausal women with high fracture risks were randomized in a 1:1:1 ratio to receive 20 mcg teriparatide daily, 60 mg denosumab every 6 months, or both teriparatide and denosumab. At 12 months, the combination group had more BMD increases in lumbar spine, femoral neck, and total hip than either teriparatide or denosumab alone. All the biomarkers of bone turnover, including OC, PINP, and CTX, were significantly increased from baseline in the teriparatide-alone group. The changes of biomarkers from baseline in the combination group resembles those in the denosumab-alone group in that a steady decrease was observed in nearly all measured time points (3 months, 6 months, 9 months, 12 months). These trends persisted at the end of 24 months.[31] The vBMD at the radius and tibia using HR-pQCT (High-resolution quantitative computed tomography) techniques was calculated and reported in this study. Total vBMP at the radius and tibia, cortical vBMD at the tibia, as well as trabecular vBMD at the radius were increased more in the combination group than the monotherapy group,[32] suggesting teriparatide's action to increase bone formation may be enhanced by denosumab-induced suppression of bone resorption. A preplanned switch study, in which patients in the combination arm changed into denosumab, patients in the denosumab arm switched to teriparatide, and patients in the teriparatide arm switched to denosumab, was continued for an additional 2 years after completing the original DATA trial.[31] Continued increase of BMD levels in lumbar spine, total hip, and femoral neck was observed among patients switching from teriparatide or combination therapy to denosumab, whereas a progressive or transient decrease in BMD was observed among patients who switched from denosumab to teriparatide. The marked differences observed in the DATA and DATA-switch trials advocate the importance of choosing the sequential treatment of osteoporosis because of the critical role of the temporal unlinking of bone formation and resorption in bone remodeling.

DISCUSSIONS

The mixed results of combination therapy partially reflect the challenges of treating osteoporosis. Bone remodeling is a temporally regulated process involving the coordinated efforts of osteoclasts and osteoblasts within the microscopic basic multicellular units (BMUs). For adult bones, bone sites that have microdamages or have renewal needs attract osteoclasts to start bone resorption process; after the bone surface is resorbed then come the osteoblasts which start to form new bone matrix. The bone resorption process takes 3 to 5 weeks and the subsequent action of osteoblasts in bone formation can take 3 to 5 months.[16] Bone interactions and durations of remodeling process differ between trabecular bone and cortical bone, vary from one region to another, and subject to changes from external forces. The signaling process of initiation, maintaining, and completion of remodeling are still under intense research and not yet entirely illustrated. When configuring combination therapy, the timing and duration of teriparatide treatment to a specific antiresorptive agent may play critical roles in the outcomes of the trial. Although it is impossible to observe momentous changes in BMUs, knowing the patterns of biomarker changes may help in understanding the changes at the microarchitectural level. When teriparatide is combined with estrogen or SERM, the biomarker changes follow the pattern of teriparatide as a monotherapy. Similar to what is observed in teriparatide monotherapy, the increase of biomarker activities of teriparatide with estrogen/SERM occur early in the treatment course and peak around 6 months and then gradually converge to baseline in about 3 years, suggesting the maintenance of the anabolic window effect. When teriparatide is combined with bisphosphonate or denosumab, the activities of biomarkers tend to follow the patterns of the antiresorptive agent. BMD results from a couple of trials suggest those subdued activities of biomarkers may be beneficial in increasing BMD, as seen in combination of teriparatide with bisphosphonate following a pretreatment of teriparatide or combining teriparatide with a potent antiresorptive agent like denosumab.[27,33]

The effects of combination therapy seem to depend on the type of the antiresorptive agent, its mode of action, the timing of administration, or pharmacodynamic aspect of the medications. Overall the trials for combination therapy have a short duration of study time. BMD changes following treatment take months to years to reach maximal effects. It was estimated that 8.8 months, 9.6 months, and 10.2 months are needed for bisphosphonates, teriparatide, and denosumab treatment to achieve 50% of maximal effects on lumbar spine, respectively; and 20.0 months, 27.9 months, and 20.1 months are needed to have 50% of maximal effects on total hip for the aforementioned 3 drug classes, respectively.[34] The current evidence from clinical trials falls short of seeing the full effects of treatment.

In terms of measurements, BMD scores, especially when measured in 2 dimensions, is imperfect but a practical and efficient test for assessment of bone quality. The vBMD measurements are not widely available and may be cost prohibitive. Rarely bone biopsies are performed. Ultimately it is the reduction of fracture risks that determines the efficacy of treatment. Although most trials have compared BMD results from different combination therapies, few have systemically collected fracture data. To demonstrate fracture benefits, much larger and longitudinal studies of combination therapies are needed.

In practice, the clinicians often face the challenges of finding the best treatment in situations that are not always delineated in clinical guidelines. Should a patient with a recent hip fracture be treated the same as a patient who had a vertebral fracture? What should be done if osteoporosis progresses after bisphosphonate treatment: change into teriparatide or denosumab or combination of both and for how long? Although current evidence does not yet support a change in clinical practice, the combination of teriparatide with antiresorptive agents such as denosumab is promising in offering additive effects. Those benefits can be very important in treating severe osteoporosis and osteoporosis-associated bone fractures; however, additional costs, adverse effects, pill burden as well as patient's likelihood of adherence to therapy have to be weighted into the individualized medical decision process.

REFERENCES

1. Cosman F, de Beur SJ, LeBoff MS, et al. Clinician's guide to prevention and treatment of osteoporosis. Osteoporos Int 2014;25(10):2359–81.
2. Black DM, Rosen CJ. Clinical practice. postmenopausal osteoporosis. N Engl J Med 2016;374(3):254–62.
3. Raisz LG. Pathogenesis of osteoporosis: concepts, conflicts, and prospects. J Clin Invest 2005;115(12):3318–25.
4. Manolagas SC, O'Brien CA, Almeida M. The role of estrogen and androgen receptors in bone health and disease. Nat Rev Endocrinol 2013;9(12):699–712.
5. Favus MJ. Bisphosphonates for osteoporosis. N Engl J Med 2010;363(21): 2027–35.
6. Seeman E, Delmas PD. Bone quality–the material and structural basis of bone strength and fragility. N Engl J Med 2006;354(21):2250–61.
7. Belchetz PE. Hormonal treatment of postmenopausal women. N Engl J Med 1994;330(15):1062–71.
8. Ettinger B, Black DM, Mitlak BH, et al. Reduction of vertebral fracture risk in postmenopausal women with osteoporosis treated with raloxifene: results from

a 3-year randomized clinical trial. Multiple Outcomes of Raloxifene Evaluation (MORE) Investigators. JAMA 1999;282(7):637–45.
9. Crandall CJ, Newberry SJ, Diamant A, et al. Comparative effectiveness of pharmacologic treatments to prevent fractures: an updated systematic review. Ann Intern Med 2014;161(10):711–23.
10. Black DM, Cummings SR, Karpf DB, et al. Randomised trial of effect of alendronate on risk of fracture in women with existing vertebral fractures. Fracture Intervention Trial Research Group. Lancet 1996;348(9041):1535–41.
11. Black DM, Delmas PD, Eastell R, et al. Once-yearly zoledronic acid for treatment of postmenopausal osteoporosis. N Engl J Med 2007;356(18):1809–22.
12. McClung MR, Geusens P, Miller PD, et al. Effect of risedronate on the risk of hip fracture in elderly women. Hip Intervention Program Study Group. N Engl J Med 2001;344(5):333–40.
13. Chesnut CH 3rd, Skag A, Christiansen C, et al. Effects of oral ibandronate administered daily or intermittently on fracture risk in postmenopausal osteoporosis. J Bone Miner Res 2004;19(8):1241–9.
14. Harris ST, Watts NB, Genant HK, et al. Effects of risedronate treatment on vertebral and nonvertebral fractures in women with postmenopausal osteoporosis: a randomized controlled trial. Vertebral Efficacy With Risedronate Therapy (VERT) Study Group. JAMA 1999;282(14):1344–52.
15. Cummings SR, San Martin J, McClung MR, et al. Denosumab for prevention of fractures in postmenopausal women with osteoporosis. N Engl J Med 2009;361(8):756–65.
16. Canalis E, Giustina A, Bilezikian JP. Mechanisms of anabolic therapies for osteoporosis. N Engl J Med 2007;357(9):905–16.
17. Neer RM, Arnaud CD, Zanchetta JR, et al. Effect of parathyroid hormone (1-34) on fractures and bone mineral density in postmenopausal women with osteoporosis. N Engl J Med 2001;344(19):1434–41.
18. Lindsay R, Nieves J, Formica C, et al. Randomised controlled study of effect of parathyroid hormone on vertebral-bone mass and fracture incidence among postmenopausal women on oestrogen with osteoporosis. Lancet 1997;350(9077):550–5.
19. Cosman F, Nieves J, Woelfert L, et al. Parathyroid hormone added to established hormone therapy: effects on vertebral fracture and maintenance of bone mass after parathyroid hormone withdrawal. J Bone Miner Res 2001;16(5):925–31.
20. Cosman F. Combination therapy for osteoporosis: a reappraisal. Bonekey Rep 2014;3:518.
21. Ste-Marie LG, Schwartz SL, Hossain A, et al. Effect of teriparatide [rhPTH(1-34)] on BMD when given to postmenopausal women receiving hormone replacement therapy. J Bone Miner Res 2006;21(2):283–91.
22. Deal C, Omizo M, Schwartz EN, et al. Combination teriparatide and raloxifene therapy for postmenopausal osteoporosis: results from a 6-month double-blind placebo-controlled trial. J Bone Miner Res 2005;20(11):1905–11.
23. Finkelstein JS, Wyland JJ, Lee H, et al. Effects of teriparatide, alendronate, or both in women with postmenopausal osteoporosis. J Clin Endocrinol Metab 2010;95(4):1838–45.
24. Finkelstein JS, Hayes A, Hunzelman JL, et al. The effects of parathyroid hormone, alendronate, or both in men with osteoporosis. N Engl J Med 2003;349(13):1216–26.

25. Black DM, Greenspan SL, Ensrud KE, et al. The effects of parathyroid hormone and alendronate alone or in combination in postmenopausal osteoporosis. N Engl J Med 2003;349(13):1207–15.
26. Cosman F, Eriksen EF, Recknor C, et al. Effects of intravenous zoledronic acid plus subcutaneous teriparatide [rhPTH(1-34)] in postmenopausal osteoporosis. J Bone Miner Res 2011;26(3):503–11.
27. Muschitz C, Kocijan R, Fahrleitner-Pammer A, et al. Antiresorptives overlapping ongoing teriparatide treatment result in additional increases in bone mineral density. J Bone Miner Res 2013;28(1):196–205.
28. Cosman F, Wermers RA, Recknor C, et al. Effects of teriparatide in postmenopausal women with osteoporosis on prior alendronate or raloxifene: differences between stopping and continuing the antiresorptive agent. J Clin Endocrinol Metab 2009;94(10):3772–80.
29. Cosman F, Nieves J, Zion M, et al. Daily and cyclic parathyroid hormone in women receiving alendronate. N Engl J Med 2005;353(6):566–75.
30. Tsai JN, Uihlein AV, Lee H, et al. Teriparatide and denosumab, alone or combined, in women with postmenopausal osteoporosis: the DATA study randomised trial. Lancet 2013;382(9886):50–6.
31. Leder BZ, Tsai JN, Uihlein AV, et al. Denosumab and teriparatide transitions in postmenopausal osteoporosis (the DATA-Switch study): extension of a randomised controlled trial. Lancet 2015;386(9999):1147–55.
32. Tsai JN, Uihlein AV, Burnett-Bowie SM, et al. Effects of two years of teriparatide, denosumab, or both on bone microarchitecture and strength (DATA-HRpQCT study). J Clin Endocrinol Metab 2016;101(5):2023–30.
33. Tsai JN, Zhu Y, Foley K, et al. Comparative resistance to teriparatide-induced bone resorption with denosumab or alendronate. J Clin Endocrinol Metab 2015;100(7):2718–23.
34. Mandema JW, Zheng J, Libanati C, et al. Time course of bone mineral density changes with denosumab compared with other drugs in postmenopausal osteoporosis: a dose-response-based meta-analysis. J Clin Endocrinol Metab 2014;99(10):3746–55.

Novel Therapies for Postmenopausal Osteoporosis

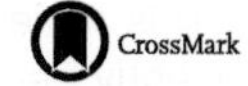

Leonardo Bandeira, MD, John P. Bilezikian, MD*

KEYWORDS

• Osteoporosis • Postmenopausal • Antiresorptive • Osteoanabolic • Therapeutics

KEY POINTS

- Recently discovered mechanisms in the regulation of mineral metabolism have led to the development of new therapies for osteoporosis.
- These developments have led to new classes of drugs for the treatment of osteoporosis.
- Despite numerous advances over the past 2 decades, the search for newer therapies continues.

INTRODUCTION

Osteoporosis, the most common metabolic bone disorder, is characterized by low bone mass and microarchitectural deterioration, both of which lead to reduced bone strength and increased fracture risk.[1,2] With millions of postmenopausal women at risk for an osteoporotic fracture, osteoporosis is a major public health issue. Data from the National Health and Nutrition Examination Survey, 2005 to 2010, show a 15.4% prevalence of osteoporosis in women over 50 years old in the United States.[3]

Over the past 2 decades, an impressive array of pharmacologic therapies for postmenopausal osteoporosis has been introduced and shown to be efficacious. Nevertheless, the search for newer therapeutics continues for 3 reasons. First, none of the therapeutic classes available at this time eliminates osteoporotic fracture risk. Second, all classes of drugs have side effects, some of which, although rare, have engendered reluctance on the part of both practitioners and patients. Third, the perfect drug would be one that restores the microarchitectural deterioration that is characteristic of the disease. The latter continues to be an elusive goal.

The authors have nothing to disclose.
Department of Medicine, College of Physicians and Surgeons, Columbia University, 630 West 168th Street, PH8W-864, New York, NY 10032, USA
* Corresponding author.
E-mail address: jpb2@columbia.edu

Endocrinol Metab Clin N Am 46 (2017) 207–219
http://dx.doi.org/10.1016/j.ecl.2016.11.001 endo.theclinics.com
0889-8529/17/

This review summarizes the data regarding therapies for osteoporosis that have recently been introduced or that are in development. Newly discovered mechanisms that form the basis for these new developments are focused on.

ANTIRESORPTIVE AGENTS

Denosumab

The drug denosumab has taken advantage of the discovery of a key activator of osteoclast function and development. Receptor activator of nuclear factor κB (RANK) ligand (RANKL) is a product of the osteocyte and a member of the tumor necrosis factor cytokine family. It binds to its cognate receptor, RANK, promoting both the activation of mature osteoclasts and the development of preosteoclasts. Recognition that RANKL has a natural inhibitor, known as osteoprotegerin, led to the development of the drug known as denosumab. This is a fully human antibody that binds to and inhibits RANKL's actions.[4–7]

The pivotal clinical trial leading to the approval of denosumab as a treatment of osteoporosis is known as Fracture Reduction Evaluation of Denosumab in Osteoporosis Every 6 Months (FREEDOM). In this study, 7868 postmenopausal women with osteoporosis were randomly assigned to receive denosumab, 60 mg, by subcutaneous injection, or placebo injection every 6 months for 3 years. In the denosumab group, there was a 68% reduction in risk of new vertebral fractures (VFs) ($P<.001$), a 40% reduction in risk of hip fractures ($P = .04$), and a 20% reduction in risk of nonvertebral fractures ($P = .01$) compared with placebo.[8]

The bone turnover markers (BTMs), C-telopeptide of type I collagen (CTX) and procollagen type 1 amino-terminal propeptide (P1NP), reflecting bone resorption and bone formation, respectively, showed similar and highly significant reductions of 72% and 76% ($P<.001$ for both). Denosumab was associated with a 9.2% gain at lumbar spine (LS) bone mineral density (BMD) and a 6% gain at total hip (TH) BMD ($P<.005$ for both compared with placebo). BMD also increased at the femoral neck (FN), trochanter, 1/3 radius, and total body ($P<.005$ for all compared with placebo).[8,9] In subjects who underwent quantitative CT (QCT), there was an increase in volumetric BMD (vBMD) at all sites in the denosumab group (21.8% at LS, 7.8% at TH, and 5.9% at FN; $P\leq.0001$ for all compared with placebo).[10]

The drug was shown to be safe and well tolerated. Because RANKL is also expressed in lymphocytes, infection risk was a theoretic concern. Superficial skin infections were a common adverse event (AE). In terms of serious AEs, 0.3% of patients in the denosumab group developed cellulitis compared with less than 0.1% in the placebo group ($P = .002$). The cellulitis was amenable to effective treatment. There were no cases of osteonecrosis of the jaw (ONJ) or atypical femur fracture (AFF).[8,11,12] Extension of this trial has not sustained the apparent imbalance in superficial skin infections that was seen in the first 3 years of the trial. Most experts have discounted the theoretic risk of infection as a major concern.[13]

In another multicenter phase 3 study, 1189 postmenopausal women with low bone mass were studied in a 1-year trial comparing denosumab and alendronate. In the denosumab group, there was a significantly greater increase in BMD compared with alendronate at all sites (3.5% vs 2.6% at TH, 2.4% vs 1.8% at FN, 5.3% vs 4.2% at LS, 1.1% vs 0.6% at 1/3 radius, and 4.5% vs 3.4% at trochanter; $P\leq.0001$ for all). BMD gains were greater for the denosumab group as early as month 6, the earliest time point measured. By the end of the trial, both groups showed major reductions in CTX (−74% denosumab vs −76% alendronate; $P = .52$), but the denosumab group had a greater reduction from month 1 to month 9 ($P\leq.0001$ compared with the alendronate group). Throughout the trial, P1NP showed greater suppression by denosumab (−72% vs −65%; *P*<.0001 compared with alendronate). AEs were similar between the groups.[14] The simultaneous combined use of denosumab and teriparatide improved BMD and also cortical microarchitecture and bone stiffness by high-resolution peripheral QCT to a greater extent than either drug alone.[15,16] When the group receiving teriparatide was switched to denosumab, gains in BMD continued at all sites. When the group receiving denosumab was switched to teriparatide, however, bone loss ensued for 6 to 12 months, followed by bone gains at the LS and hip sites. At the 1/3 radius, BMD continued to decrease progressively during the 2-year observation period after switching from denosumab to teriparatide.[17]

The FREEDOM study has been extended in an open-label design for up to 10 years. Subjects who took the medication for 8 years continued to show sustained reduction of BTMs. BMD increased progressively, reaching cumulative gains of 18.4% at LS, 8.3% at TH, and 7.8% at FN (*P*<.05 for all compared with both FREEDOM baseline and extension baseline) after 8 years. The risk of new fractures remained low in these patients, with a cumulative incidence of 5.5% for VFs, 6.6% for nonvertebral fractures, and 0.7% for hip fractures during the 5-year extension. There was a tendency for nonvertebral fractures to show greater reductions over time. AEs were similar to the original study but, as discussed previously, the apparent increase in skin infections was no longer seen with the prolonged use of denosumab. There was 1 case of AFF, which occurred in the fourth extension year, and 5 cases of ONJ in the long-term group.[13]

The study design of FREEDOM, long term, called for a crossover of those in placebo for the first 3 years to denosumab thereafter. The crossover group showed BTM suppression, BMD gains, and fracture risk reduction similar to the long-term group during their first 5 years of denosumab exposure. AEs rates confirmed those reported for the corresponding time period in the long-term group. There were 1 case of AFF and 3 cases of ONJ during the 5 years in the crossover group.[13]

These long-term data have been substantiated further with the 10-year experience in which BMD continued to increase, reaching cumulative gains of 21.6% and a 9.1% at the LS and TH, respectively (*P*<.0001 for both from study baseline). The crossover group experienced cumulative gains of 16.3% at LS and 7.3% at TH during the 7 years of denosumab exposure (*P*<.0001 for both from baseline). Sustained reduction in BTMs was observed in both groups and rates of new vertebral and nonvertebral fractures remained low. There was no increase in AEs incidence.[18]

As is true for all drug classes, except the bisphosphonates, discontinuance is associated with returns of BTMs toward baseline and a reduction in BMD. A phase 2 trial[19] with denosumab showed even a transient overshoot of BTMs to values higher than baseline along with rapid declines in BMD. This disposition to show rapid reversibility has been substantiated by a cohort from FREEDOM and its extension in which drug was discontinued. Not only was there an increase in BTMs and a reduction in BMD but also there was an increase in VF incidence to levels compared with placebo after 6 months. Subjects who had a new VF after drug cessation had a higher risk of multiple fractures than the placebo group. Those with a history of prior VF were at greater risk. These data bring into question whether patients on denosumab should ever be given a drug holiday, as recommended for many patients who have been exposed to long-term continuous bisphosphonate therapy. If therapy is to be discontinued after chronic denosumab use, current recommendations are to smoothly transition to another therapy.[20–22]

Cathepsin K Inhibitors

Cathepsin K is an important osteoclast enzyme that degrades type 1 collagen and thus helps create the bone remodeling unit. It is a lysosomal cysteine protease. Other cathepsins (eg, B, L, and S) are not specific to bone but degrade collagen in other tissues, such as skin and lung.[23,24] There is a certain degree of overlap with regard to tissue specificity for all cathepsins. The idea of developing a cathepsin K antagonist arose from the knowledge of a rare autosomal recessive disease called pycnodysostosis. Patients with this disorder have increased bone mass due to an inactivating mutation of the cathepsin K gene.[25] The search for a cathepsin K inhibitor took into account the need to be as specific for bone type 1 collagen as possible to not risk adverse effects on other collagens in lung, skin, and elsewhere.

One result of this search is odanacatib, a highly selective cathepsin K inhibitor that blocks this specific osteoclast function. Different from other classes, such as the bisphosphonates and the RANKL inhibitor, denosumab, odanacatib does not seem to interfere with other functions of the osteoclast, such as its osteoblast signaling mechanisms. Thus, the concomitant reduction in bone formation, seen commonly with an antiresorptive agent, is not expected to be as great in the presence of odanacatib. At an oral dosage of 50 mg weekly, a 2-year phase 2 study showed, in postmenopausal women with low bone mass, gains of 5.7% at LS, 4.1% at TH, 4.7% at FN, 5.1% at trochanter, and 2.9% at 1/3 radius ($P<.05$ for all compared with placebo). Urinary N-telopeptide of type I collagen (NTX) fell by 51.8% ($P\leq.001$ compared with placebo). CTX also fell in the first weeks and then increased gradually toward the baseline but still remained lower than the control group at month 24 ($P\leq.001$). Bone formation markers (P1NP and bone alkaline phosphatase) followed a similar pattern, namely, initial reduction followed by progressive increase after 6 months. At the end of 24 months, both were still below baseline ($P\leq.011$ compared with placebo). As discussed previously, odanacatib did not reduce bone formation markers to the extent that it reduced bone resorption markers. After 2 years, bone formation markers had returned to levels close to baseline.[26]

In extensions of this phase 2 trial, BMD continued to increase in patients receiving odanacatib for 3 and 5 years.[27,28] By the fifth year, the cumulative gains were 11.9% at LS, 8.5% at TH, 9.8% at FN, and 10.9% at trochanter. Bone resorption markers (CTX and NTX) remained approximately 55% below baseline. In contrast, discontinuance of drug after 2 year of exposure led to reductions in BMD to values that were lower than baseline after the fifth year. Also similar to the experience with denosumab, bone resorption markers increased as early as 1 month to levels above baseline. By 2 years, bone formation markers were no longer markedly reduced and, when drug was discontinued, further reversibility was evident.

Phase 3 trials gave confirmation of these effects in which fracture efficacy was demonstrated. Not only were there the expected increases in BMD at all sites and effects on BTMs but also effects by bone biopsy were appreciated, as noted by increased trabecular thickness and number.[29]

By QCT, odanacatib was associated with increases in trabecular vBMD at the LS, and cortical, subcortical and trabecular vBMD at all hip sites. Cortical volume, thickness, area, and bone mineral content (BMC) were also increased at the hip.[29,30]

The definitive phase 3 trial, Long-Term Odanacatib Fracture Trial (LOFT), enrolled more than 16.000 postmenopausal osteoporotic women. This randomized, double-blind, placebo-controlled trial is the largest ever performed in this field. Results showed a 52% decrease in VFs, 48% decrease in hip fractures, 26% decrease in nonvertebral fractures, and 67% decrease on clinical VFs in the odanacatib group after 5 years ($P<.001$ for all compared with placebo). In addition, odanacatib led to improvements in BMD (10.9% at LS and 10.3% at TH; $P<.001$ for both compared with placebo).[31,32]

Odanacatib was well tolerated and seemed safe. The most common AEs were mild cutaneous reactions and urinary infection.[26–29] In LOFT, AFF and morphea-like skin lesions in the odanacatib group were seen. The imbalance in numbers of subjects who were adjudicated to have experienced AFF (10 vs none in the placebo group) was noteworthy. No case of ONJ was observed.[33] During the first 3 years of the LOFT trial, an imbalance was observed in several cardiovascular endpoints, the most important one of which was stroke. To investigate this association further, an extensive analysis of this and other major adverse cardiac events endpoints was conducted by an impartial panel. The results became known in September, 2016, and were presented at the Annual Meeting of the American Society for Bone and Mineral Research.[34] The imbalance in death due to strokes was further substantiated. As a result, the drug company announced that it would no longer develop odanacatib nor seek regulatory approval for the treatment of osteoporosis.[35,36]

Another cathepsin K inhibitor, known as ONO-5334, is under development in Japan. Studies have shown that, like odanacatib, ONO-5334 reduces bone resorption markers to a greater extent than bone formation markers. Bone mineral density increased at LS and hip sites. Improvements in trabecular and cortical BMD at the spine and the hip by QCT were also observed. The effects on BMD, bone microarchitecture and resorption markers were similar to alendronate. There were no safety concerns. After drug cessation, BTMs rapidly increased.[37–40] Data regarding fracture risk are not yet available.

OSTEOANABOLIC AGENTS

Parathyroid Hormone and Analogs

In a series of historic insights into mechanisms of parathyroid hormone (PTH) action, this hormone has been successfully developed as an efficacious therapy for osteoporosis. Although this article focuses on newer drugs, it is worth reviewing the important observation made 2 decades ago that the way PTH is administered governs the manner in which it influences skeletal metabolism. Dobnig and Turner[41] showed in rats that continuous administration of PTH led to bone resorption, whereas intermittent, daily, low-dose, administration of PTH unmasked latent osteoanabolic properties. This observation not only helped explain the catabolic actions of PTH in the classic disease, primary hyperparathyroidism, in which the skeleton is exposed to continuous excessive PTH, but also led the way to the development of a biologically active fragment of PTH, known as teriparatide, for the treatment of osteoporosis. Teriparatide is a 34–amino acid fragment that is identical in primary sequence to residue 34 of the full-length 84–amino acid peptide. As shown by Neer and colleagues,[42] teriparatide reduces vertebral and nonvertebral fractures along with increasing BMD at the lumbar spine and the hip. The drug is associated with the occurrence of osteosarcoma in rats exposed to high dose PTH over a period of 2 years. Two years of a rat's life is equivalent to 75 years of a human life. Nevertheless, this observation was of concern. Surveillance studies over the past 14 years have not revealed any signal in human subjects, exposed to teriparatide, that osteosarcoma is a risk for patients receiving drug. Nevertheless, the drug was approved with and continues to carry a black box warning regarding this rat toxicity.[43–45]

Teriparatide is used for 2 years, by which time bone resorption markers increase and match the earlier increase in bone formation markers. The kinetics by which teriparatide first stimulates bone formation followed by bone resorption has given rise to the concept that teriparatide is creating an anabolic window, during which time the osteoanabolic properties of PTH are optimal.[46,47] This information led to the quest for a PTH analog that would demonstrate greater effects on bone formation than bone resorption, thus maximizing the anabolic window. The first studies using amino-terminal PTH-related protein (PTHrP[1–36]) were promising.[48–50] Another insight became important, namely, appreciation that the PTH/PTHrP receptor has 2 configurations: a prolonged state of ligand-receptor interaction and a more transient state of ligand-receptor interaction (Rg). The experiments of Dobnig and Turner,[41] in which the fleeting exposure of PTH and analogs was associated with an anabolic effect, could be explained by a preferential affinity for the transient Rg state of the PTH/PTHrP receptor. To this end, a search followed for a PTHrP analog that would favor the Rg state of the PTH/PTHrP receptor. The molecule, now known as abaloparatide, was discovered to show such a proclivity to the Rg state of the PTH/PTHrP receptor. Abaloparatide shares with PTHrP a primary sequence that is identical to PTHrP through residue 22. Thereafter, to residue 34, there are several substitutions that alter the property of PTHrP to be more favorable with regard to the Rg configuration.[51]

Abaloparatide has been studied in a multinational, phase 3 trial, the results of which have recently been published. This placebo-controlled protocol used a subcutaneous, daily dosage of abaloparatide of 80 μg per day—4 times the dose of teriparatide. The protocol included an open-label arm of teriparatide in which subjects were evenly matched to the abaloparatide and placebo groups. With regard to BTMs, the results showed that, as expected, abaloparatide is associated with a wider differential effect to stimulate bone formation than to stimulate bone resorption. VF incidence is markedly reduced by more than 80%, similar to the results of the teriparatide arm. Nonvertebral fractures were also reduced significantly, a result in this study that was not seen in those receiving teriparatide. Time to effect vis-à-vis clinical and nonvertebral fractures showed a much earlier effect of abaloparatide than teriparatide. The side-effect profile showed fewer hypercalcemic events than with teriparatide.[52]

This drug shows great promise. Further information about its development and potential availability is awaited, pending Food and Drug Administration review, which is ongoing.

Antisclerostin Antibodies

One of the main mediators of bone formation is the Wnt signaling pathway. The family of Wnt comprises 19 glycoproteins, which are involved in growth, differentiation, proliferation, function, and death of many cell lineages. Related to bone, the canonical Wnt pathway governs a system that leads for bone formation. Activation of this pathway occurs by an interaction between Wnt and its receptor, known as LRP5/6, and its coreceptor, known as Frizzled. This binding step on the plasma membrane of the cell leads to the activation of Disheveled, an intracellular protein that inhibits glycogen synthase kinase 3β. By virtue of the inactivation of this enzyme, cytoplasmic β-catenin survives to be translocated to the nucleus and to facilitate gene transcription. The activation leads to differentiation, maturation, and proliferation of cells, such as osteoblasts and chondrocytes. Other actions related to the activation of this canonical Wnt signaling pathway are inhibition of osteoblast and osteocyte apoptosis, inhibition of osteoclastogenesis, and increase in osteoprotegerin expression.[53–55] These further actions serve to limit, at least in part, the effects of uncontrolled stimulation of this pathway.

At the initial step in the activation of the canonical Wnt signaling pathway, there is another regulatory mechanism. Similar to osteoprotegerin limiting the effects of RANKL, sclerostin limits Wnt signaling by impairing the interaction between Wnt and LRP5/6. Sclerostin, a 190-kDa glycoprotein encoded by the SOST gene, is produced primarily by osteocytes. The inhibition of Wnt signaling by sclerostin seems specific to bone, even though the SOST gene is expressed in many other cells.[53,56]

Similarly to the development of odanacatib, the idea of developing a sclerostin antagonist arose from the knowledge of 2 rare autosomal recessive diseases associated with an inactive SOST gene product. Found as rare autosomal recessive disorders among the Dutch, sclerosteosis and van Buchem disease are both characterized by mutations in the SOST gene, leading to loss of an active sclerostin. As a result, the Wnt signaling pathway is not controlled and a high bone mass phenotype develops. Patients with sclerosteosis and van Buchem disease have elevated bone mass, decreased risk of fractures, and increased BTMs (pointing to an increase in bone formation).[53,57–60] The homozygous forms of these diseases are not benign because the bone overgrowth leads, in time, to serious neurologic sequellae because neuronal foramina are compromised. The clue to appreciating a safe approach to interfering with sclerostin came from heterozygous carriers of these diseases in which patients are protected from fractures, because of high bone mass, but this more mild form of the disease is not associated with neurologic complications.

Knowledge of the role of sclerostin in this signaling pathway, along with the rare human diseases of sclerostin deficiency, led to the development of an antisclerotin human monoclonal antibody, romosozumab. By binding sclerostin, Romosozumab facilitates the activation of Wnt signaling by the Wnt-LRP5/6 interaction. Without significant opposition, the activated canonical Wnt signaling cascade has the potential to be powerfully osteoanabolic.[54,61]

The initial actions of romosozumab, administered as a subcutaneous injection, leads to increases in bone formation markers and reductions in bone resorption markers. These actions suggest that the drug does not depend on an initial remodeling event to stimulate bone formation but rather that it directly stimulates bone formation. An effect to stimulate bone formation on quiescent bone surfaces is compatible with a modeling mechanism, as shown by Ominksy and colleagues.[62] The resulting anabolic window is large in the early period of romosozumab actions.

The kinetics by which romosozumab stimulates bone metabolism is unique. After an early, 2-fold increase in P1NP, levels return to baseline at around month 6. Simultaneously, CTX levels decline by approximately 50% within the first week and remain below baseline at year 1. These actions are to be contrasted with teriparatide in which there is a more sustained increase in P1NP followed by a marked increase in CTX.[63,64]

After 1 year of exposure to romosozumab, BMD increases by a remarkable 11.3% at LS, 4.1% at TH, and 3.7% at FN ($P<.001$ for all compared with placebo, alendronate, and teriparatide). Gains in BMD were observed as early as 6 months at all sites ($P<.02$ for all compared with placebo, alendronate, and teriparatide). No changes were observed at 1/3 radius.[63] As assessed by QCT, romosozumab was also associated with increases in vBMD, BMC, trabecular vBMD, and cortical BMC at LS and TH as well as increases in cortical vBMD and cortical thickness at the LS. Most of the microarchitecture improvements were greater than observed with teriparatide.[65]

The results of the definitive phase 3 clinical trial, known as Fracture Study in Postmenopausal Women with Osteoporosis (FRAME), were recently published.[66] This study evaluated risk of fractures in 7180 postmenopausal osteoporotic women, randomized to romosozumab, 210 mg monthly, or placebo for 1 year, followed by denosumab in year 2 for both groups. After only 1 year, the active group was associated with a 73% reduction in new VFs (0.5% vs 1.8%; $P<.001$) and a 36% reduction in clinical fractures (1.6% vs 2.5%; $P = .008$) compared with placebo. After the second year, the cumulative incidence of new VFs was 75% lower in the romosozumab/denosumab group (0.6% vs 2.5%; *P*<.001, compared with the placebo/denosumab group), whereas there was no difference in risk of clinical fractures.

No difference was observed in nonvertebral fractures at any point of the study. The preplanned test for geographic heterogeneity was positive. This observation was followed by a post hoc analysis of geographic differences among study sites. When study subjects from Latin America, which comprised 46% of the study cohort, were excluded, a 42% reduction in nonvertebral fractures was found in the romosozumab group compared with placebo at month 12 (1.6% vs 2.7%; *P* = .04).[66] The Latin American cohort showed no effect of drug on nonvertebral fractures. To account for these geographic differences, further analysis revealed that fracture risk among the Latin American enrollees was substantially lower than subjects from the rest of the world. This reduced fracture risk was substantiated by baseline FRAX 10-year risk of major osteoporotic fractures that was much lower than those from other parts of the world (8.7% vs 17%).[66]

Romosozumab led to gains in BMD after 1 year (13.3% at LS, 6.9% at TH, and 5.9% at FN; *P*<.001 for all compared with placebo). After transition to denosumab, BMD increased in both groups but continued to be higher in the group that had taken romosozumab in the first year (*P*<.001 compared with placebo/denosumab group at month 24). Romosozumab was associated with a rapid increase in P1NP (approximately 150% peak at day 14; *P*<.001) followed by a return to baseline at month 9. CTX fell, reaching an approximately 50% nadir after 14 days (*P*<.001), and remained below baseline at the end of 12 months. Sequential treatment with denosumab, in year 2, led to suppression of both BTMs.[66]

Romosozumab was well tolerated and AEs were mild. The most common AEs were constipation, headache, back pain, nasopharyngitis, and injection-site reactions. The latter were usually mild, improved without intervention, and did not recur even with continued drug administration.[63,66–68] In FRAME, there were 2 (<0.1%) cases of ONJ and 1 (<0.1%) case of AFF in the romosozumab group. Despite theoretic concerns regarding malignancy risk due to the drug mechanism of action (activation of Wnt signaling pathway), there was no difference in cancer incidence between the groups.[66]

Results from another phase 3 study, not yet reported in complete form, showed that postmenopausal osteoporotic women transitioning from bisphosphonate to romosozumab had significant increases at LS and TH BMD and also in hip strength compared with another group transitioning from bisphosphonate to teriparatide after 1 year.[69]

Another representative of the antisclerostin antibodies class is blosozumab. Phases 1 and 2 studies showed dose-dependent response in BTMs and BMD in subjects who took the medication. These effects were not affected by prior bisphosphonate use. In postmenopausal women with low bone mass, blosozumab led to gains at LS and hip sites BMD. Similar to romosozumab, the drug induced an increase in bone formation and decrease in bone resorption markers. One year after drug discontinuation, BTMs returned to baseline and BMD decreased but remained greater than the placebo group. Mild injection-site reactions were more common in the blosozumab group; however, the drug was usually well tolerated with no noteworthy safety concerns.[70–72] Recently, the drug company developing blosozumab announced that it was scaling back its development program to phase 1 because of difficulties in finding a formulation that could be given by subcutaneous injection.[73,74]

SUMMARY

This review highlights recent insights in the development of new classes of drugs for the treatment of postmenopausal osteoporosis. It is likely that some of these drugs, based on knowledge of new pathways of bone biology, will become clinically useful.

REFERENCES

1. Kanis JA, Melton J III, Christiansen C, et al. The diagnosis of osteoporosis. J Bone Miner Res 1994;9(8):1137–41.
2. NIH Consensus Development Panel on Osteoporosis Prevention, Diagnosis, and Therapy. Osteoporosis prevention, diagnosis, and therapy. JAMA 2001;285(6): 785–95.
3. Wright NC, Looker AC, Saag KG, et al. The recent prevalence of osteoporosis and low bone mass in the United States based on bone mineral density at the femoral neck or lumbar spine. J Bone Miner Res 2014;29(11):2520–6.
4. Chan CK, Mason A, Cooper C, et al. Novel advances in the treatment of osteoporosis. Br Med Bull 2016;119(1):129–42.
5. Silva BC, Costa AG, Cusano NE, et al. Osteoporosis: what's new and on the horizon. Clin Obstet Gynecol 2013;56(4):730–8.
6. Darnay BG, Haridas V, Ni J, et al. Characterization of the intracellular domain of receptor activator of NF-kappaB (RANK). Interaction with tumor necrosis factor receptor-associated factors and activation of NF-kappab and c-Jun N-terminal kinase. J Biol Chem 1998;273(32):20551–5.
7. Galibert L, Tometsko ME, Anderson DM, et al. The involvement of multiple tumor necrosis factor receptor (TNFR)-associated factors in the signaling mechanisms of receptor activator of NF-kappaB, a member of the TNFR superfamily. J Biol Chem 1998;273(51):34120–7.
8. Cummings SR, San Martin J, McClung MR, et al. Denosumab for prevention of fractures in postmenopausal women with osteoporosis. N Engl J Med 2009; 361(8):756–65.
9. Bolognese MA, Teglbjaerg CS, Zanchetta JR, et al. Denosumab significantly increases DXA BMD at both trabecular and cortical sites: results from the FREEDOM study. J Clin Densitom 2013;16(2):147–53.
10. McClung MR, Zanchetta JR, Hoiseth A, et al. Denosumab densitometric changes assessed by quantitative computed tomography at the spine and hip in postmenopausal women with osteoporosis. J Clin Densitom 2013;16(2):250–6.
11. Guerrini MM, Takayanagi H. The immune system, bone and RANKL. Arch Biochem Biophys 2014;561:118–23.
12. Leibbrandt A, Penninger JM. RANK/RANKL: regulators of immune responses and bone physiology. Ann N Y Acad Sci 2008;1143:123–50.
13. Papapoulos S, Lippuner K, Roux C, et al. The effect of 8 or 5 years of denosumab treatment in postmenopausal women with osteoporosis: results from the FREEDOM Extension study. Osteoporos Int 2015;26(12):2773–83.
14. Brown JP, Prince RL, Deal C, et al. Comparison of the effect of denosumab and alendronate on BMD and biochemical markers of bone turnover in postmenopausal women with low bone mass: a randomized, blinded, phase 3 trial. J Bone Miner Res 2009;24(1):153–61.
15. Tsai JN, Uihlein AV, Burnett-Bowie SA, et al. Comparative effects of teriparatide, denosumab, and combination therapy on peripheral compartmental bone density, microarchitecture, and estimated strength: the DATA-HRpQCT Study. J Bone Miner Res 2015;30(1):39–45.
16. Tsai JN, Uihlein AV, Lee H, et al. Teriparatide and denosumab, alone or combined, in women with postmenopausal osteoporosis: the DATA study randomised trial. Lancet (London, England) 2013;382(9886):50–6.

17. Leder BZ, Tsai JN, Uihlein AV, et al. Denosumab and teriparatide transitions in postmenopausal osteoporosis (the DATA-Switch study): extension of a randomised controlled trial. Lancet (London, England) 2015;386(9999):1147–55.
18. Bone H, Brandi ML, Brown JP, et al. Ten years of denosumab treatment in postmenopausal women with osteoporosis: results from the FREEDOM Extension Trial. ASBMR 2015 Annual Meeting. Seattle (WA), October 9-12, 2015.
19. Miller PD, Bolognese MA, Lewiecki EM, et al. Effect of denosumab on bone density and turnover in postmenopausal women with low bone mass after long-term continued, discontinued, and restarting of therapy: a randomized blinded phase 2 clinical trial. Bone 2008;43(2):222–9.
20. Brown JP, Ferrari S, Gilchrist N, et al. Discontinuation of denosumab and associated fracture incidence: analysis from FREEDOM and its Extension. ASBMR 2016 Annual Meeting. Atlanta (GA), September 16-19, 2016.
21. Brown JP, Roux C, Torring O, et al. Discontinuation of denosumab and associated fracture incidence: analysis from the Fracture Reduction Evaluation of Denosumab in Osteoporosis Every 6 Months (FREEDOM) trial. J Bone Miner Res 2013; 28(4):746–52.
22. McClung MR. Cancel the denosumab holiday. Osteoporos Int 2016;27(5): 1677–82.
23. Costa AG, Cusano NE, Silva BC, et al. Cathepsin K: its skeletal actions and role as a therapeutic target in osteoporosis. Nat Rev Rheumatol 2011;7(8):447–56.
24. Hou WS, Li Z, Gordon RE, et al. Cathepsin k is a critical protease in synovial fibroblast-mediated collagen degradation. Am J Pathol 2001;159(6):2167–77.
25. Gelb BD, Shi GP, Chapman HA, et al. Pycnodysostosis, a lysosomal disease caused by cathepsin K deficiency. Science 1996;273(5279):1236–8.
26. Bone HG, McClung MR, Roux C, et al. Odanacatib, a cathepsin-K inhibitor for osteoporosis: a two-year study in postmenopausal women with low bone density. J Bone Miner Res 2010;25(5):937–47.
27. Eisman JA, Bone HG, Hosking DJ, et al. Odanacatib in the treatment of postmenopausal women with low bone mineral density: three-year continued therapy and resolution of effect. J Bone Miner Res 2011;26(2):242–51.
28. Langdahl B, Binkley N, Bone H, et al. Odanacatib in the treatment of postmenopausal women with low bone mineral density: five years of continued therapy in a phase 2 study. J Bone Miner Res 2012;27(11):2251–8.
29. Brixen K, Chapurlat R, Cheung AM, et al. Bone density, turnover, and estimated strength in postmenopausal women treated with odanacatib: a randomized trial. J Clin Endocrinol Metab 2013;98(2):571–80.
30. Engelke K, Fuerst T, Dardzinski B, et al. Odanacatib treatment affects trabecular and cortical bone in the femur of postmenopausal women: results of a two-year placebo-controlled trial. J Bone Miner Res 2015;30(1):30–8.
31. Bone HG, Dempster DW, Eisman JA, et al. Odanacatib for the treatment of postmenopausal osteoporosis: development history and design and participant characteristics of LOFT, the long-term odanacatib fracture trial. Osteoporos Int 2015; 26(2):699–712.
32. McClung M, Langdahl B, Papapoulos S, et al. Odanacatib efficacy and safety in postmenopausal women with osteoporosis: 5-year data from the extension of the phase 3 long-term odanacatib fracture trial (LOFT). ASBMR 2016 Annual Meeting. Atlanta (GA), September 16-19, 2016.
33. Papapoulos S, McClung M, Langdahl B, et al. Safety of odanacatib in postmenopausal women with osteoporosis: 5-year data from the extension of the phase 3

long-term odanacatib fracture trial (LOFT). ASBMR 2016 Annual Meeting. Atlanta (GA), September 16-19, 2016.
34. O'Donoghue M, Cavallari I, Bonaca M, et al. The long-term odanacatib fracture trial (LOFT): cardiovascular safety results. ASBMR Annual Meeting 2016. Atlanta (GA), September 16-19, 2016.
35. Mullard A. Merck &Co. drops osteoporosis drug odanacatib. Nat Rev Drug Discov 2016;15(10):669.
36. Merck. Merck Provides Update on Odanacatib Development Program. 2016. Available at: http://www.mercknewsroom.com/news-release/research-and-development-news/merck-provides-update-odanacatib-development-program. Accessed November 1, 2016.
37. Tanaka M, Hashimoto Y, Hasegawa C. An oral cathepsin K inhibitor ONO-5334 inhibits N-terminal and C-terminal collagen crosslinks in serum and urine at similar plasma concentrations in postmenopausal women. Bone 2015;81:178–85.
38. Nagase S, Ohyama M, Hashimoto Y, et al. Bone turnover markers and pharmacokinetics of a new sustained-release formulation of the cathepsin K inhibitor, ONO-5334, in healthy post-menopausal women. J Bone Miner Metab 2015; 33(1):93–100.
39. Eastell R, Nagase S, Small M, et al. Effect of ONO-5334 on bone mineral density and biochemical markers of bone turnover in postmenopausal osteoporosis: 2-year results from the OCEAN study. J Bone Miner Res 2014;29(2):458–66.
40. Engelke K, Nagase S, Fuerst T, et al. The effect of the cathepsin K inhibitor ONO-5334 on trabecular and cortical bone in postmenopausal osteoporosis: the OCEAN study. J Bone Miner Res 2014;29(3):629–38.
41. Dobnig H, Turner RT. The effects of programmed administration of human parathyroid hormone fragment (1-34) on bone histomorphometry and serum chemistry in rats. Endocrinology 1997;138(11):4607–12.
42. Neer RM, Arnaud CD, Zanchetta JR, et al. Effect of parathyroid hormone (1-34) on fractures and bone mineral density in postmenopausal women with osteoporosis. N Engl J Med 2001;344(19):1434–41.
43. Andrews EB, Gilsenan AW, Midkiff K, et al. The US postmarketing surveillance study of adult osteosarcoma and teriparatide: study design and findings from the first 7 years. J Bone Miner Res 2012;27(12):2429–37.
44. Elraiyah T, Gionfriddo MR, Murad MH. Acting on black box warnings requires a GRADE evidence table and an implementation guide: the case of teriparatide. J Clin Epidemiol 2015;68(6):698–702.
45. Cipriani C, Irani D, Bilezikian JP. Safety of osteoanabolic therapy: a decade of experience. J Bone Miner Res 2012;27(12):2419–28.
46. Rubin MR, Bilezikian JP. Parathyroid hormone as an anabolic skeletal therapy. Drugs 2005;65(17):2481–98.
47. Bilezikian JP. Combination anabolic and antiresorptive therapy for osteoporosis: opening the anabolic window. Curr Osteoporos Rep 2008;6(1):24–30.
48. Horwitz MJ, Tedesco MB, Gundberg C, et al. Short-term, high-dose parathyroid hormone-related protein as a skeletal anabolic agent for the treatment of postmenopausal osteoporosis. J Clin Endocrinol Metab 2003;88(2):569–75.
49. Stewart AF, Cain RL, Burr DB, et al. Six-month daily administration of parathyroid hormone and parathyroid hormone-related protein peptides to adult ovariectomized rats markedly enhances bone mass and biomechanical properties: a comparison of human parathyroid hormone 1-34, parathyroid hormone-related protein 1-36, and SDZ-parathyroid hormone 893. J Bone Miner Res 2000;15(8): 1517–25.

50. Stewart AF. PTHrP(1-36) as a skeletal anabolic agent for the treatment of osteoporosis. Bone 1996;19(4):303–6.
51. Hattersley G, Dean T, Corbin BA, et al. Binding selectivity of abaloparatide for PTH-type-1-receptor conformations and effects on downstream signaling. Endocrinology 2016;157(1):141–9.
52. Miller PD, Hattersley G, Riis BJ, et al. Effect of abaloparatide vs placebo on new vertebral fractures in postmenopausal women with osteoporosis: a randomized clinical trial. JAMA 2016;316(7):722–33.
53. Costa AG, Bilezikian JP. Sclerostin: therapeutic horizons based upon its actions. Curr Osteoporos Rep 2012;10(1):64–72.
54. Baron R, Kneissel M. WNT signaling in bone homeostasis and disease: from human mutations to treatments. Nat Med 2013;19(2):179–92.
55. Wei W, Zeve D, Suh JM, et al. Biphasic and dosage-dependent regulation of osteoclastogenesis by beta-catenin. Mol Cell Biol 2011;31(23):4706–19.
56. Moester MJ, Papapoulos SE, Lowik CW, et al. Sclerostin: current knowledge and future perspectives. Calcif Tissue Int 2010;87(2):99–107.
57. Stein SA, Witkop C, Hill S, et al. Sclerosteosis: neurogenetic and pathophysiologic analysis of an American kinship. Neurology 1983;33(3):267–77.
58. Van Buchem FS, Hadders HN, Ubbens R. An uncommon familial systemic disease of the skeleton: hyperostosis corticalis generalisata familiaris. Acta Radiol 1955;44(2):109–20.
59. Gardner JC, van Bezooijen RL, Mervis B, et al. Bone mineral density in sclerosteosis; affected individuals and gene carriers. J Clin Endocrinol Metab 2005; 90(12):6392–5.
60. Wergedal JE, Veskovic K, Hellan M, et al. Patients with Van Buchem disease, an osteosclerotic genetic disease, have elevated bone formation markers, higher bone density, and greater derived polar moment of inertia than normal. J Clin Endocrinol Metab 2003;88(12):5778–83.
61. Tella SH, Gallagher JC. Biological agents in management of osteoporosis. Eur J Clin Pharmacol 2014;70(11):1291–301.
62. Ominsky MS, Vlasseros F, Jolette J, et al. Two doses of sclerostin antibody in cynomolgus monkeys increases bone formation, bone mineral density, and bone strength. J Bone Miner Res 2010;25(5):948–59.
63. McClung MR, Grauer A, Boonen S, et al. Romosozumab in postmenopausal women with low bone mineral density. N Engl J Med 2014;370(5):412–20.
64. Lindsay R, Krege JH, Marin F, et al. Teriparatide for osteoporosis: importance of the full course. Osteoporos Int 2016;27(8):2395–410.
65. Genant HK, Engelke K, Bolognese MA, et al. Effects of romosozumab compared with teriparatide on bone density and mass at the spine and hip in postmenopausal women with low bone mass. J Bone Miner Res 2016;1–7.
66. Cosman F, Crittenden DB, Adachi JD, et al. Romosozumab treatment in postmenopausal women with osteoporosis. N Engl J Med 2016;375(16):1532–43.
67. Padhi D, Allison M, Kivitz AJ, et al. Multiple doses of sclerostin antibody romosozumab in healthy men and postmenopausal women with low bone mass: a randomized, double-blind, placebo-controlled study. J Clin Pharmacol 2014;54(2): 168–78.
68. Padhi D, Jang G, Stouch B, et al. Single-dose, placebo-controlled, randomized study of AMG 785, a sclerostin monoclonal antibody. J Bone Miner Res 2011; 26(1):19–26.
69. Langdahl B, Libanati C, Crittenden DB, et al. Superior gains in bone mineral density and estimated strength at the hip for romosozumab compared with

teriparatide in women with postmenopausal osteoporosis transitioning from bisphosphonate therapy: results of the phase 3 open-label structure study. Boston (MA): ENDO; 2016.
70. Recker RR, Benson CT, Matsumoto T, et al. A randomized, double-blind phase 2 clinical trial of blosozumab, a sclerostin antibody, in postmenopausal women with low bone mineral density. J Bone Miner Res 2015;30(2):216–24.
71. Recknor CP, Recker RR, Benson CT, et al. The Effect of discontinuing treatment with blosozumab: follow-up results of a phase 2 randomized clinical trial in postmenopausal women with low bone mineral density. J Bone Miner Res 2015;30(9):1717–25.
72. McColm J, Hu L, Womack T, et al. Single- and multiple-dose randomized studies of blosozumab, a monoclonal antibody against sclerostin, in healthy postmenopausal women. J Bone Miner Res 2014;29(4):935–43.
73. Lilly Clinical Development Pipeline 2016. 2016. Available at: https://www.lilly.com/_Assets/SiteCollectionDocuments/Pipeline/Clinical-Development-Pipeline/index.html#PhaseI. Accessed November 3, 2016.
74. Lilly hopes new drug delivery R&D center will prove useful in osteoporosis, diabetes arenas. 2015. Available at: http://www.fiercepharma.com/drug-delivery/lilly-hopes-new-drug-delivery-r-d-center-will-prove-useful-osteoporosis-diabetes. Accessed November 3, 2016.

Index

Note: Page numbers of article titles are in **boldface** type.

A

AAs. See *African Americans (AAs).*
Abdominal soft tissue, effect on TBS, 155
aBPs (amino-bisphosphonates). See *Bisphosphonates (BPs).*
Adenoma(s), parathyroid, primary hyperparathyroidism related to, 88–89
 differential diagnosis of, 93–94
 treatment of, 94–95
ADHR. See *Autosomal dominant hypophosphatemic rickets (ADHR).*
Adipocytes, bone marrow, 42–43. See also *Marrow adipose tissue (MAT).*
Adipokines, Roux-en-Y gastric bypass effect on, 108–109
Adiponectin, Roux-en-Y gastric bypass effect on, 108
Adipose tissue, regulation of, osteocyte role in, 6
 visceral, fracture risk and, 68
 white, 42
 yellow/marrow, 42. See also *Marrow adipose tissue (MAT).*
Adiposity, bone marrow and, **41–50**. See also *Bone–fat interaction.*
Adjustable gastric banding (AGB), description of, 110–111
 effects on bone metabolism, 110–112
 US statistics on, 106
Advanced glycation end products (AGEs), with diabetes, bone disease and, 66–67
Adverse events (AEs). See *Drug-related adverse events.*
AEs (adverse events). See *Drug-related adverse events.*
AFF. See *Atypical femur fracture (AFF).*
African Americans (AAs), vitamin D status and bone health in, **135–152**
 introduction to, 135–136
 markers of classical bioactivity, 143–144
 physiology of, 136–139
 skeletal phenotype of, 144–146
 status assessment of, 139–143
 summary of, 147
 supplementation for, 146
 vs. white Americans, 135–136
  markers of, 139–144. See also *25-Hydroxyvitamin D.*
AGB. See *Adjustable gastric banding (AGB).*
AGEs (advanced glycation end products), with diabetes, bone disease and, 66–67
Aging, diabetes and, 67
 MAT alterations and, 43, 45
 osteocyte role in, 3, 6–7
Amino-bisphosphonates (aBPs). See *Bisphosphonates (BPs).*
Amino-terminal PTH-related protein (PTHrP)(1–36), in postmenopausal osteoporosis, 212
Amylin, Roux-en-Y gastric bypass effect on, 108
Anabolic agents. See *Osteoanabolic agents.*

Endocrinol Metab Clin N Am 46 (2017) 221–246
http://dx.doi.org/10.1016/S0889-8529(16)30141-4
0889-8529/17

Anorexia nervosa, in premenopausal women, 121–122
MAT alterations and, 43–44
Antidiabetic medications, fracture risk with, 65–66
Anti–fibroblast growth factor 23 antibody (anti-FGF23 antibody), for bone disease, 9–10
Antiosteoporotic therapy, effect on TBS, 166–170
Anti–receptor activator of nuclear factor κB ligand antibody (anti-RANKL antibody), for bone disease, as targeting osteocytes, 9–10
with postmenopausal osteoporosis, 194–196
with primary hyperparathyroidism, 96–97
Antiresorptive agents, for bone disease, with diabetes, 74–75
current controversies of, 75–76
with postmenopausal osteoporosis, cathepsin K inhibitors, 209–211
denosumab, 208–209
teriparatide plus, 199, 202–203
Antisclerostin antibodies, for bone disease, as targeting osteocytes, 9
with postmenopausal osteoporosis, 212–214
Apoptosis, of osteocytes, in bone disease, 5–7, 10
ARHR (autosomal recessive hypophosphatemic rickets), FGF23 excess associated with, 23, 31
Arthritis, effect on TBS, osteoarthritis, 155–156
rheumatoid, 173
Atrial fibrillation, as adverse event, with bisphosphonates, 182
Atypical femur fracture (AFF), as adverse event, incidence of, 183
pathophysiology of, 184
risk factors of, 183
with bisphosphonates, 183–184
with denosumab, 208–209, 211, 214
Autosomal dominant hypophosphatemic rickets (ADHR), FGF23 excess associated with, 23, 30–31
description of, 30
differential diagnosis of, 26, 31
treatment of, 31
Autosomal recessive hypophosphatemic rickets (ARHR), FGF23 excess associated with, 23, 26, 31

B

Bariatric surgery, effects on bone metabolism, **105–116**
clinical considerations of, 113
early procedures and, 106
fracture risk and, 112–113
hormone level changes and, fat-derived, 108–109
gastrointestinal, 107–109
introduction to, 105–107
key points of, 105
limitations of current studies of, 110, 112
mechanical loading and, 107
procedure-specific, 109–112
adjustable gastric banding as, 110–111
Roux-en-Y gastric bypass as, 109–110
sleeve gastrectomy as, 111–112

US statistics on, 105–106, 109
summary of, 113
vitamin D status and, 106–107
Basic multicellular units (BMUs), in bone remodeling, 203
Biliopancreatic diversion, effects on bone metabolism, 106
Biopsy. See *Bone biopsy.*
Bisphosphonates (BPs), for bone disease, administration of, 182
adverse events with, 182–186
acute phase response, 182
atrial fibrillation as, 182
conjunctivitis as, 183
esophageal cancer as, 182–183
femoral fractures as, atypical, 183–184
gastroesophageal, 182
osteonecrosis of jaw as, 184–186
scleritis as, 183
uveitis as, 183
as targeting osteocytes, 6, 10
dosing of, 182
efficacy of, 182
indications for, 182
with bariatric surgery, 113
with diabetes, 74–75
current controversies of, 75–76
with premenopausal osteoporosis, 125
teriparatide plus, for postmenopausal osteoporosis, 198–199, 201–202
discussions on, 203–204
introduction to, 193–194
mechanisms of action, 194–196
Blood pressure, primary hyperparathyroidism and, 92
BMD. See *Bone mineral density (BMD).*
BMUs (basic multicellular units), in bone remodeling, 203
Body composition, for BMD, 67–68
bariatric surgery and, 108–109, 112
T1DM and, 69
T2DM and, 71
Body mass index (BMI), in obesity, 105–106
Bone, as dynamic tissue, 41–42
density of. See *Bone mineral density (BMD).*
disease of. See *Bone disease.*
disuse and unloading of, MAT alterations and, 43, 45–46
fatigue of, osteocytes apoptosis associated with, 5
growth and development of. See also *Bone mass.*
antidiabetic medications impact on, 65–66
ET1 signaling in, 52–55, 57
Wnt signaling in, 55–57
loading of. See *Mechanical loading.*
microarchitecture of. See *Microarchitecture.*
microdamage of. See *Microdamage.*
physiology of. See *Bone metabolism.*
repair of, osteocyte role in, 2, 5–6

Bone (*continued*)
structure deficits in, primary hyperparathyroidism related to, 91
Bone biopsy, for premenopausal osteoporosis, 119, 124
for primary hyperparathyroidism, 91
Bone disease, bone–fat interaction and, **41–50**
altered, clinical scenarios of, 43–46
controversies and questions of, 42–43
future considerations of, 46
introduction to, 41–42
diabetes and, **63–85**
current controversies of, 75–76
epidemiology of, 64–65
future considerations of, 76
introduction to, 63–64
management of, 72, 74–75
pathophysiology of, 66–67
risk assessment of, 67–73
risk factors of, 65–66
fibroblast growth factor 23–mediated, **19–39**
deficiency of, disorders associated with, 19, 33–34
summary of, 23, 27
excess of, disorders associated with, 19, 23–33
autosomal dominant hypophosphatemic rickets as, 23, 30–31
autosomal recessive hypophosphatemic rickets as, 31
miscellaneous other as, 31–33
summary of, 23
tumor-induced osteomalacia as, 23–28
X-linked hypophosphatemic rickets as, 23, 28–30
introduction to, 19–20
pathophysiology of, 20–23
summary of, 34
genetics of, 3, 7–8, 10. See also *specific disorder.*
obesity and, 106
diabetes with, 67
MAT alterations and, 43–45
surgical management of, 105–106. See also *Bariatric surgery.*
osteoblast role in, 1, 10
osteocyte role in, **1–18**
aging and, 3, 6–7
bone mass abnormalities and, 3, 7–8
genetics and, 3, 7–8, 10
hypophosphatemic rickets and, 3, 7, 9–10
anti-FGF23 antibody for, 9–10
introduction to, 1–2
nonbone disease vs., 3, 8–9
normal functions vs., 2, 4–6
osteoporosis and, 3, 6
other factors of, 10
summary of, 10
therapeutics targeting, 9–10, 194
with primary hyperparathyroidism, 92

Bone geometry, as skeletal parameter, 154
for BMD, 67–68
T1DM and, 68
T2DM and, 70
Bone loss, during pregnancy and lactation, 120–121
incidence of, 41
induced, effect on TBS, osteoporosis treatment monitoring and, 170
with antiosteoporotic therapy, 166–169
with breast cancer treatment, 169–170
MAT alterations and, 43, 46
Bone marrow, inflammation of, with diabetes, 67
Bone marrow adipocytes, 42–43. See also *Marrow adipose tissue (MAT).*
Bone mass, bone–fat interaction and, **41–50**. See also *Bone–fat interaction.*
ET system signaling and, 55–56
loss of. See *Bone loss.*
osteocyte role in, genetics of, 2–4, 7–8, 10
Bone metabolism. See also *Calcium homeostasis; Vitamin D homeostasis.*
bariatric surgery effects on, **105–116**
clinical considerations of, 113
fracture risk and, 112–113
GI hormone level changes and, 107–109
fat-derived, 108–109
introduction to, 105–107
limitations of current studies of, 110, 112
mechanical loading and, 107
procedure-specific, 109–112
summary of, 113
bone–fat interaction in, **41–50**
altered, clinical scenarios of, 43–46
bone marrow adipocytes and, 42–43
controversies and questions of, 42–43
future considerations of, 46
introduction to, 41–42
endothelin signaling in, **51–62**
future considerations of, 57
in bone physiology, 54–57
in development, 52–55, 57
in osteoblastic metastasis, 54, 57
introduction to, 51–53
QTL of, 55–56
Bone mineral density (BMD), as skeletal parameter, 154
bariatric surgery effect on, 113
adjustable gastric banding, 110–111
Roux-en-Y gastric bypass as, 109–110
sleeve gastrectomy, 111–112
DXA measurement of, 67–68
in trabecular bone score, **153–180**. See also *Trabecular bone score (TBS).*
limitations for, 65–66, 110, 112
primary hyperparathyroidism and, 96
ET system signaling and, 55–56
in premenopausal osteoporosis, diagnostic interpretations of, 118–119

Bone (*continued*)
dynamics of peak BMD accrual, 120
special considerations required for, 120–121
with idiopathic low BMD, 119
with pregnancy and lactation physiology, 120–121
with pregnancy and lactation–associated osteoporosis, 121
low, treatment considerations of, 124–126
idiopathic, 126
secondary, 126–127
in primary hyperparathyroidism, 91
treatment considerations of, 95–97
in WAs vs. AAs, vitamin D status and, 145
low, bariatric surgery and, 107
in premenopausal osteoporosis, 124–127
incidence of, 41
MAT alterations and, 43, 46
with diabetes, epidemiology of, 64–65
future considerations of, 76
pathophysiology of, 66–67
risk assessment of, 67–70
risk factors of, 65–66
measurement of. See *Fracture prediction tools; specific test.*
postmenopausal osteoporosis therapy and, combined agents in, 196–203
discussions on, 203–204, 214
introduction to, 193–194, 207–208
mechanisms of action, 194–196
novel therapies in, 208–214
volumetric, postmenopausal osteoporosis therapy and, 202–204, 210, 213
Bone remodeling, postmenopausal osteoporosis therapy and, discussions on, 203–204, 214
with combined agents, 203–204
with novel therapies, 208–214
Bone resorption/turnover, as skeletal parameter, 154
bariatric surgery effect on, 106
adjustable gastric banding, 110–111
Roux-en-Y gastric bypass, 109–110
sleeve gastrectomy, 111–112
postmenopausal osteoporosis therapy and, combined agents in, 196–203
discussions on, 203–204, 214
introduction to, 193–194, 207–208
mechanisms of action, 194–196
novel agents in, 208–214
premenopausal osteoporosis related to, 124
Bone strength, factors of, 154
TBS association with, 156–157
Bone turnover markers (BTMs). See *Bone remodeling; Bone resorption/turnover.*
Bone–fat interaction, **41–50**
altered, clinical scenarios of, 43–46
aging and, 43, 45
anorexia nervosa as, 43–44
bone loss as, 43, 46

disuse and unloading of skeleton in, 43, 45–46
fracture risk as, 43, 46
gonadal deficiency as, 43, 45
obesity as, 43–45
radiation therapy impact as, 46
T1DM as, 43–44
T2DM as, 43–45
bone marrow adipocytes and, function of, 42–43
lineage of, 42
controversies and questions of, 42–43
future considerations of, 46
introduction to, 41–42
key points of, 41
summary of, 46
B-protein–coupled receptors, in endothelin system, 51–54
Breast cancer, metastasis of, ET1 signaling and, 51, 54, 57
treatment-induced bone loss with, effect on TBS, 169–170
BTMs (bone turnover markers). See *Bone remodeling; Bone resorption/turnover.*

C

Calcitonin, for bone disease, 10, 195
Calcium homeostasis, bone health and, FGF23 disorders and, 23–34. See also *specific disorder.*
FGF23 role in, 21–22
osteocyte role in, 2–5
vitamin D role in, binding protein and, 136–139
classical, 136–138
in WAs vs. AAs, 143–144
nonclassical, 137–138
with primary hyperparathyroidism, 90–93
treatment of, 94, 96
Calcium intake, bone disease and, with bariatric surgery, 113
with diabetes, 73–74
for premenopausal osteoporosis, 124
Cancers, esophageal, as adverse event, with bisphosphonates, 182–183
osteoblastic metastasis of, ET1 signaling and, 51, 54, 57
parathyroid, primary hyperparathyroidism related to, 88–89
differential diagnosis of, 93–94
treatment of, 94–95
Canonical physiology, vs. noncanonical physiology, of FGFs, 20
of vitamin D, 136–137
Cardiac function, osteocyte role in, 3, 8
as therapeutic target, 10
Cardiovascular anomalies, abnormalities of, ET1 signaling and, 52–53, 55
CASR gene, in primary hyperparathyroidism, 89–91
β-Catenin, bone disease and, osteocyte role in, 7–8
bone health and, ET system signaling and, 57
mechanosensation and, 2–4, 107
Cathepsin K inhibitors, for bone disease, 10
for postmenopausal osteoporosis, 209–211

CCND1 gene, in primary hyperparathyroidism, 89–90
Celiac disease, in premenopausal women, 121–122
Cell death, in bone disease, 5–7, 10
Chronic kidney disease (CKD), FGF23 excess associated with, 23, 26, 32–33
  osteocyte role in, 3, 6, 8
Clinical studies, of bariatric surgery effects on bone metabolism, 110, 112
  of postmenopausal osteoporosis therapy, with combined agents, 193–203
    with novel agents, 207–214
  of trabecular bone score in fracture risk, cross-sectional, 157–160
    in vitro, 156
    in vivo, 156–157
    longitudinal, 158, 161–165
Combined pharmacologic therapy, for postmenopausal osteoporosis, **193–206**
    discussions on, 203–204
    FDA approved, 194–195
    introduction to, 193–194
    key points of, 193
    mechanisms of action of, 194, 196–199
    teriparatide plus bisphosphonates, 198–199, 201–202
    teriparatide plus denosumab, 199, 202–203
    teriparatide plus estrogen, 196–197, 200–201
    teriparatide plus SERM, 196–197, 200–201
Computed tomography, micro, in TBS, 156–157
  quantitative. See *Quantitative computed tomography (QCT).*
Conjunctivitis, as adverse event, with bisphosphonates, 183
Converting enzymes, in endothelin system, 51–54
  in vitamin D physiology, 136–139
Craniofacial defects, ET1 signaling and, 52–53
Crohn disease, in premenopausal women, 121–122
CTX marker, in bariatric surgery, 108
  in postmenopausal osteoporosis therapy, mechanisms of action, 196
    with combined agents, 194–203
    with novel agents, 208
    with novel therapies, 208, 210, 213–214
Cytokines, bone disease and, 6
    diabetes and, 67
  vascular remodeling and, 55

D

DBP. See *Vitamin D binding protein (DBP).*
Denosumab
  dosing and administration of, 186
  efficacy of, 186
  for postmenopausal osteoporosis, 208–209
    as novel therapy, 208–209
    teriparatide plus, 199, 202–203
      discussions on, 203–204
      introduction to, 193–194
      mechanisms of action, 194–196
  premenopausal osteoporosis and, 125

side effects of, 186
Development. See *Growth and development.*
Diabetes mellitus (DM). See also *specific type.*
bone disease and, **63–85**
current controversies of, 75–76
effect on TBS, 170–171
epidemiology of, 64–65
future considerations of, 76
introduction to, 63–64
key points of, 63
management of, 72, 74–75
pathophysiology of, 66–67
risk assessment of, 67–73
risk factors of, 65–66
1,25 Dihydroxyvitamin D_3, bone health and, 1. See also *Vitamin D entries.*
Disuse, of skeleton, MAT alterations and, 43, 45–46
Dmp1 gene, bone health and, osteocyte role in, 2, 4, 7
Drug-related adverse events, with osteoporosis therapy, **181–192**
future considerations of, 188
introduction to, 181–182
key points of, 181
summary of, 187–188
with bisphosphonates, 182–186
with denosumab, 186
with novel therapies, 209, 211, 214
with selective estrogen receptor modulators, 187
with teriparatide, 187
Dual-energy x-ray absorptiometry (DXA), for BMD, 67–68
in premenopausal osteoporosis, 118–119
in trabecular bone score, **153–180**. See also *Trabecular bone score (TBS).*
limitations of, 65–66, 110, 112
primary hyperparathyroidism and, 96
Duodenal switch, effects on bone metabolism, 106
US statistics on, 106

E

Ece1 gene, ET signaling in bone and, 51–54, 57
Edn1 gene, ET signaling in bone and, 51–52, 55, 57
Ednra gene, ET signaling in bone and, 51–55, 57
EDNRs. See *Endothelin receptors (EDNRs).*
Endocrine functions, bone health regulation and, 1–2
FGFs role in, 20
osteocyte role in, 2–3, 6
canonical, vs. noncanonical, of FGFs, 20
of vitamin D, 136–137
Endothelin 1 (ET1) signaling, in bone, **51–62**
future considerations of, 57
in development, 52–55, 57
in osteoblastic metastasis, 51, 54, 57
in physiology, 54–57

Endothelin (*continued*)
introduction to, 52–53
key points of, 51
overview of, 52–54
QTL of, 55–56
Endothelin receptors (EDNRs), in bone physiology, 51–52
in ET1 signaling, 52–54
Endothelin (ET) system, gene and protein abbreviations for, 51–52
signaling pathway of, 52–54
Epidemiology, of bone disease, with bone loss, 41
with diabetes, 64–65
with obesity, bariatric surgery and, 105–106, 109
with primary hyperparathyroidism, 87–88
X-linked hypophosphatemic rickets, 28
of drug-related adverse events, atypical femur fracture as, 183
osteonecrosis of jaw as, 184–185
of vitamin D status and bone health, in WAs vs. AAs, 136
Esophageal cancer, as adverse event, with bisphosphonates, 182–183
Estrogen deficiency, bone disease and, 6
in premenopausal women, 121–122
Estrogen receptor modulators. See *Selective estrogen receptor modulators (SERMs).*
Estrogen therapy
teriparatide plus, for postmenopausal osteoporosis, 196–197, 200–201
discussions on, 203–204
introduction to, 193–194
mechanisms of action, 194–196
ET. See *Endothelin (ET) system.*
ET1. See *Endothelin 1 (ET1) signaling.*
Exercise therapy, for premenopausal osteoporosis, 124
Exploratory surgery, for primary hyperparathyroidism, limited vs. bilateral (4-gland), 95–96

F

Fall risk, with obesity, 113
Familial hypocalciuric hypercalcemia (FHH), primary hyperparathyroidism related to, 90–91, 93
Familial isolated hyperparathyroidism, 88
Familial tumoral calcinosis (FTC), FGF23 deficiency associated with, 33–34
diagnostic tests for, 33
differential diagnosis of, 27, 34
pathophysiology of, 19, 23, 33
symptoms of, 33
treatment of, 34
Fat tissue. See *Adipose tissue.*
Fat-derived hormones, Roux-en-Y gastric bypass effect on, 108–109
Fatigue, of bone, osteocytes apoptosis associated with, 5
FD/MCAS (fibrous dysplasia/McCune-Albright syndrome), FGF23 excess associated with, 23, 26, 31–32
Femur fracture. See *Atypical femur fracture (AFF).*
FGF23. See *Fibroblast growth factor 23 (FGF23).*
FGF23 gene, mutations of. See *Fibroblast growth factor 23 (FGF23); specific disorder.*

FGFRs (fibroblast growth factor receptors), 20
FGFs (fibroblast growth factors), tissue functions of, 20
FHH (familial hypocalciuric hypercalcemia), primary hyperparathyroidism related to, 90–91, 93
Fibroblast growth factor 23 (FGF23), bone disease mediated by, **19–39**
deficiency of, disorders associated with, 19, 23, 33–34
familial tumoral calcinosis as, 27, 33–34
excess of, disorders associated with, 19, 23–33
autosomal dominant hypophosphatemic rickets as, 23, 30–31
autosomal recessive hypophosphatemic rickets as, 31
chronic kidney disease as, 23, 26, 32–33
fibrous dysplasia/McCune-Albright syndrome as, 23, 26, 31–32
hypophosphatemic rickets with hyperparathyroidism as, 23, 26, 32
linear nevus sebaceous syndrome as, 23, 26, 32
miscellaneous other as, 31–33
osteoglophonic dysplasia as, 23, 26, 32
summary of, 23
tumor-induced osteomalacia as, 23–28
X-linked hypophosphatemic rickets as, 23, 28–30
functions of, 21–22
introduction to, 20
key points of, 19
Klotho expression and, 20–21
functional interactions of, 21–22
pathophysiology of, 20–23
summary of, 34
bone health and, as therapeutic target, 9–10
osteocyte role in, 2, 4, 6–7
nonbone disease and, osteocyte role in, 8
production of, regulators of, 22–23
Fibroblast growth factor receptors (FGFRs), 20
Fibroblast growth factors (FGFs), tissue functions of, 20
Fibrous dysplasia/McCune-Albright syndrome (FD/MCAS), FGF23 excess associated with, 23, 26, 31–32
Fluid flow shear stress, bone health and, osteocyte role in, 3–4
4-Gland exploration, for primary hyperparathyroidism, limited exploration vs., 95–96
Fracture(s), atypical femoral. See *Atypical femur fracture (AFF).*
fragility, with primary hyperparathyroidism, 92
Fracture history, in premenopausal osteoporosis, diagnostic interpretations of, 118
low trauma, as secondary cause, 121–123
treatment considerations of, 124–126
secondary, treatment considerations of, 126–127
with low trauma, 121–123
treatment considerations of, 126
with low trauma, 124–126
with secondary cause, 126–127
Fracture prediction tools, 67
bariatric surgery and, 113
T1DM and, 69
T2DM and, 71–73
trabecular assessment with, **153–180**. See also *Trabecular bone score (TBS).*

Fracture risk, bariatric surgery and, 112–113
adjustable gastric banding, 110–111
Roux-en-Y gastric bypass as, 109–110
sleeve gastrectomy, 111–112
in African Americans, vitamin D status and, 144–145
bone microarchitecture component of, 145–146
MAT alterations and, 43, 46
postmenopausal osteoporosis therapy and, with combined agents, 193–203
with novel agents, 207–214
skeletal parameters of, 154
with diabetes, epidemiology of, 64–65
future considerations of, 76
management of, 72, 74–76
pathophysiology of, 66–67
risk assessment of, 67–75
risk factors of, 65–66
with primary hyperparathyroidism, 91–92, 96
Fracture risk assessment tool (FRAX), 67, 214
bariatric surgery and, 113
T1DM and, 69
T2DM and, 71–73
TBS association with, 165–167
Fragility fracture, with primary hyperparathyroidism, 92
Free hormone hypothesis, of vitamin D metabolism, 138–139
FTC. See *Familial tumoral calcinosis (FTC).*

G

GALNT3 gene, FGF23 and, 20
deficiency of, FTC associated with, 19, 23, 27, 33
Garvan fracture risk calculator, diabetes and, 67, 72–73
Gastroesophageal adverse events, with bisphosphonates, 182
Gastrointestinal hormones, Roux-en-Y gastric bypass effect on, 107–108
Genetics. See also *specific gene.*
of bone disease, 3, 7–8, 10. See also *specific disorder.*
of bone health, osteocyte role in, 2, 4
of bone mass, osteocyte role in, 3, 7–8, 10
of endothelin system, 51–52
of primary hyperparathyroidism, 88–91
Geometry. See *Bone geometry.*
GH (growth hormone), Roux-en-Y gastric bypass effect on, 107
Ghrelin, Roux-en-Y gastric bypass effect on, 107
GIP (glucose-dependent insulinotropic polypeptide), Roux-en-Y gastric bypass effect on, 107
GLP-1 (glucagonlike peptide-1), Roux-en-Y gastric bypass effect on, 107–108
Glucagonlike peptide-1 (GLP-1), Roux-en-Y gastric bypass effect on, 107–108
Glucocorticoids, bone disease and, 6, 154
long-term exposure to, effect on TBS, 171–172
premenopausal osteoporosis and, 121–122, 127
Glucose-dependent insulinotropic polypeptide (GIP), Roux-en-Y gastric bypass effect on, 107

Gonadal deficiency, MAT alterations and, 43, 45
Growth and development, of bone. See also *Bone mass.*
antidiabetic medications impact on, 65–66
ET1 signaling in, 52–55, 57
Wnt signaling in, 55–57
Growth hormone (GH), replacement of, effect on TBS, 173
Roux-en-Y gastric bypass effect on, 107

H

Hematopoietic cells, osteocyte cross-talk with, 6
Heterotopic ossifications, effect on TBS, 155–156
High-resolution peripheral quantitative computed tomography (HRpQCT), of bone
microarchitecture, 154, 156–157
of postmenopausal osteoporosis, 203
Histomorphometry, of TIO, 25
History taking, for premenopausal osteoporosis, 121–122. See also *Fracture history.*
Hormone replacement therapy (HRT)
for bone disease, 6
as targeting osteocytes, 10
effect on TBS, 173
osteoporosis and, 182
teriparatide plus, for postmenopausal osteoporosis, 196–197, 200–201
discussions on, 203–204
introduction to, 193–194
mechanisms of action, 194–196
Hormones. See also *specific hormone.*
free hormone hypothesis of, in vitamin D metabolism, 138–139
peptide, in endothelin system, 51–54
parathyroid, for bone disease, 6, 10
Roux-en-Y gastric bypass effect on, fat-derived, 108–109
gastrointestinal, 107–108
HPT. See *Hyperparathyroidism (HPT).*
HR. See *Hypophosphatemic rickets (HR).*
HRpQCT. See *High-resolution peripheral quantitative computed tomography (HRpQCT).*
HRPT2 gene, in primary hyperparathyroidism, 89–90
HRT. See *Hormone replacement therapy (HRT).*
24,25-Hydroxyvitamin D, and vitamin D metabolite ratio, in WAs vs. AAs, 142–143
25-Hydroxyvitamin D. See also *Vitamin D entries.*
as vitamin D status marker, 139–144
in WAs vs. AAs., 139–140
calcium economy and, 143
secondary hyperparathyroidism and, 144
summary of, 147
supplementation and, 146
total vs. free/bioavailable, 140–141
clinical utility of determining, 141–142
vitamin D metabolite ratio with, 142–143
Hypercalcemia, with primary hyperparathyroidism, 92
familial hypocalciuric, 90–91, 93
treatment of, 94

Hypercalciuria, in premenopausal women, 121–122
Hypercortisolism, in premenopausal women, 121–122
Hyperglycemia, with diabetes, bone disease and, 66–67
Hyperlipidemia, with diabetes, bone disease and, 66
Hyperparathyroidism (HPT), familial isolated, 88
  hypophosphatemic rickets and, FGF23 excess associated with, 23, 26, 32
  in premenopausal women, 121–122
  neonatal severe, 89
  primary, bone health and, **87–104**. See also *Primary hyperparathyroidism (PHPT).*
  secondary, as classical vitamin D bioactivity marker, in WAs vs. AAs, 143–144
Hyperplasia, parathyroid, primary hyperparathyroidism related to, 88–89
Hypertension, with primary hyperparathyroidism, 92
Hypocalciuric hypercalcemia, familial, primary hyperparathyroidism related to, 90–91, 93
Hypophosphatemic rickets (HR), anti-FGF23 antibody for, 9–10
  autosomal dominant, 23, 30–31
  autosomal recessive, 23, 26, 31
  osteocyte role in, 3, 7
  with hyperparathyroidism, FGF23 excess associated with, 23, 26, 32
  X-linked, 23, 28–30. See also *X-linked hypophosphatemic rickets (XLH).*

I

Idiopathic osteoporosis premenopausal (IOP), 119, 124, 126
Imaging studies, of parathyroid, for primary hyperparathyroidism, 94
  of TIO, 25
  quantitative. See *Quantitative computed tomography (QCT).*
Inflammation. See also *Cytokines.*
  of bone marrow, with diabetes, 67
Insulin secretion, Roux-en-Y gastric bypass effect on, 108
Insulin therapy, fracture risk with, 66
IOP (idiopathic osteoporosis premenopausal), 119, 124, 126

J

Jejunoileal bypass, effects on bone metabolism, 106
Jones band, in bariatric surgery, 110–111

K

Kidney disease. See *Chronic kidney disease (CKD).*
Kidney stones, with primary hyperparathyroidism, 91–92, 96
Kidney transplant, effect on TBS, 173
Klotho gene, FGF23 and, 20–21
    deficiency of, FTC associated with, 19, 23, 27, 33
    functional interactions of, 21–22

L

Laboratory evaluation, of premenopausal osteoporosis, 123
  of TIO, 24

Lactation physiology, premenopausal osteoporosis and, BMD diagnostic interpretations with, 120–121
Leptin, Roux-en-Y gastric bypass effect on, 108–109
Lifestyle modifications, for premenopausal osteoporosis, 124
Linear nevus sebaceous syndrome (LNSS), FGF23 excess associated with, 23, 26, 32
Lithium, primary hyperparathyroidism related to, 88
Loading, of skeleton. See *Mechanical loading.*
Lrp5 receptor, bone health and, osteocyte role in, 4, 8
Wnt signaling and, 56, 212–213

M

Marrow adipose tissue (MAT), altered, clinical scenarios of, 43–46
aging and, 43, 45
anorexia nervosa as, 43–44
bone loss as, 43, 46
disuse and unloading of skeleton in, 43, 45–46
fracture risk as, 43, 46
gonadal deficiency as, 43, 45
obesity as, 43–45
radiation therapy impact as, 46
T1DM as, 43–44
T2DM as, 43–45
cellular function of, 42–43
cellular lineage of, 42
types of, 42
McCune-Albright syndrome (MCAS), fibrous dysplasia, FGF23 excess associated with, 23, 26, 31–32
μCT (micro-computed tomography), in TBS, 156–157
Mechanical loading, bone health and, bariatric surgery and, 107
MAT alterations with, 43, 45–46
osteocyte role in, 2–4
Mechanosensation, bone health and, 5, 9–10, 107
osteocyte role in, 2–4, 41
Mechanotransduction, ET system signaling and, 51, 55–57
Medical history, in premenopausal osteoporosis, 121–122. See also *Fracture history.*
MEN1 gene, in primary hyperparathyroidism, 89–90
MEPE gene, bone health and, osteocyte role in, 2, 4, 7
Metastasis, osteoblastic, ET1 signaling and, 51, 54, 57
Microarchitecture, of bone, as skeletal parameter, 154
in premenopausal women, 119
in WAs vs. AAs, vitamin D status and, 145–146
TBS association with, 156–157
Micro-computed tomography (μCT), in TBS, 156–157
Microdamage, of bone, as skeletal parameter, 154
osteocytes apoptosis associated with, 5
Micropetrosis, 7
Micro-RNA, ET system signaling and, 51, 55–56
MLO-Y4 osteocyte-like cells, as therapeutic target, 9
bone mechanosensation and, 3, 5
anti-RANKL antibody for, 9–10

MLO-Y4 (*continued*)
nonbone disease and, 8–9
Muscle, ET system signaling and, 55
osteocyte cross-talk with, 6, 9
reduced, fracture risk and, 68
Myokines, 9

N

Neonatal severe hyperparathyroidism (NSHPT), 89
Neurocognitive manifestations, of primary hyperparathyroidism, 92–93
Nitric oxide (NO), ET system signaling and, 53
vascular remodeling and, 55
Nonbone disease, osteocyte role in, **1–18**
bone disease vs., 3, 6–10
cardiac function and, 3, 8
chronic kidney disease and, 3, 6, 8
introduction to, 1–2
normal functions vs., 2, 4–6
sarcopenia and, 3, 8–9
summary of, 10
Nonpharmacologic management, of bone disease, with diabetes, 73–74
of premenopausal osteoporosis, 124
Novel therapies, for postmenopausal osteoporosis, **207–219**
antiresorptive agents as, 208–211
cathepsin K inhibitors, 209–211
denosumab, 208–209
introduction to, 207–208
key points of, 207
osteoanabolic agents as, 211–214
antisclerostin antibodies, 9, 212–214
PTH and analogs, 211–212
summary of, 214
NSHPT (neonatal severe hyperparathyroidism), 89
NTx marker, in postmenopausal osteoporosis therapy, mechanisms of action, 196
with combined agents, 196–203
with novel therapies, 210
Nutrition/nutritional supplements. See *Calcium intake; Vitamin D intake.*

O

Obesity, bariatric surgery for, as mechanical unloading, 107, 112
epidemiology of, 105–106
BMI in, 105–106
diabetes with, bone disease and, 67
MAT alterations and, 43–45
OC. See *Osteocalcin (OC).*
OGD (osteoglophonic dysplasia), FGF23 excess associated with, 23, 26, 32
1,25$(OH)_2D_3$, bone health and. See also *Vitamin D entries.*
as vitamin D status marker, in WAs vs. AAs, 139–144. See also *25-Hydroxyvitamin D.*
FGF23 disorders and, 23–34

of deficiency, 19, 23, 33–34
of excess, 19, 23–33
FGF23 role in, 21–22
Oncogenes, in primary hyperparathyroidism, 89–90
176RXXR179 motif, of FGF23 and Klotho expression, 20–21
ONJ. See *Osteonecrosis of jaw (ONJ).*
Oral contraceptives, combination, premenopausal osteoporosis and, 124–125, 127
Ossifications, heterotopic, effect on TBS, 155–156
Osteitis fibrosa, with primary hyperparathyroidism, 92
Osteoanabolic agents, for postmenopausal osteoporosis, 211–214
antisclerostin antibodies, 212–214
in combined therapy. See *Teriparatide.*
PTH and analogs, 211–212
insulin as, 108
Osteoarthritis, effect on TBS, 155–156
Osteoblastic metastasis, ET1 signaling and, 51, 54, 57
Osteoblasts, bone health and, 1–2
diabetes and, 66–67
ET system signaling and, 55–57
osteocyte factors vs., 6, 10
in bone remodeling, 203
Osteocalcin (OC), as postmenopausal osteoporosis therapy marker, with combined agents, 197–203
bone disease and, diabetes and, 67
osteocyte role in, 10
with postmenopausal osteoporosis, 196
nonbone disease and, osteocyte role in, 8–9
Osteoclasts, bone health and, 1, 6
osteocyte factors vs., 2, 10
in bone remodeling, 203
Osteocytes, **1–18**
cross-talk with hematopoietic cells, 6
cross-talk with muscle, 6, 9
defective functions of, 2–3
in bone disease, 6–8
in nonbone disease, 8–9
in bone disease, 6–8
aging and, 3, 6–7
bone mass abnormalities and, 3, 7–8
genetics and, 3, 7–8, 10
hypophosphatemic rickets and, 3, 7, 9–10
osteoporosis and, 3, 6
other factors of, 10
therapeutics targeting, 9–10, 194
in nonbone disease, 8–9
cardiac function and, 3, 8
chronic kidney disease and, 3, 6, 8
sarcopenia and, 3, 8–9
introduction to, 1–2
key points of, 1
normal functions of, 2

Osteocytes (*continued*)
bone repair as, 2, 5–6
calcium homeostasis as, 2, 4–5
endocrine, 2, 6
mechanosensation as, 2–4, 41
summary of, 10
Osteocytic osteolysis, 4
Osteogenesis, ET1 signaling in, 52–55
Osteoglophonic dysplasia (OGD), FGF23 excess associated with, 23, 26, 32
Osteonecrosis of jaw (ONJ), as adverse event, with bisphosphonates, 184–186
definition of, 184
incidence of, 184–185
pathophysiology of, 185
prevention of, 185–186
with novel therapies, for postmenopausal osteoporosis, 208–209, 211
Osteopenia, with diabetes, 64
Osteoporosis, BMD and. See *Bone mineral density (BMD).*
bone–fat interaction and, **41–50**. See also *Bone–fat interaction.*
drug-related adverse events with therapy for, **181–192**
introduction to, 181–182
summary of, 187–188
with bisphosphonates, 182–186
with denosumab, 186
with selective estrogen receptor modulators, 187
with teriparatide, 187
incidence of, 41
osteocyte role in, 3, 6
postmenopausal. See also *Postmenopausal osteoporosis.*
combined pharmacologic therapy for, **193–206**
novel therapies for, **207–219**
premenopausal, **117–133**. See also *Premenopausal osteoporosis.*
diagnosis of, 118–121
introduction to, 117
key points of, 117
secondary causes of, 121–124
summary of, 127
treatment considerations of, with fractures, 124–127
with glucocorticoid exposure, 127
with low BMD, 124–127
treatment of, drug-related adverse events with, **181–192**
effect on TBS, 166–170
with postmenopausal disease, combined pharmacologic therapy for, **193–206**
novel therapies for, **207–219**
with premenopausal disease, 124–127
with diabetes, epidemiology of, 64–65
future considerations of, 76
management of, 72, 74–76
pathophysiology of, 66–67
risk assessment of, 67–75
risk factors of, 65–66
Oxidative stress, bone disease and, 6

P

Parathyroid hormone (PTH), bone health and, 1
elevated. See *Hyperparathyroidism (HPT).*
FGF23 disorders and, 23–34. See also *specific disorder.*
FGF23 role in, 21–22
osteocyte role in, 4–6
primary hyperparathyroidism related to, autonomous production of, 88–89
differential diagnosis of, 93–94
for postmenopausal osteoporosis, 211–212
Parathyroid hormone (PTH)(1–34), premenopausal osteoporosis and, 125–126
Parathyroid hormone peptides, for bone disease, 6, 10
Parathyroid lesions, primary hyperparathyroidism related to, 88–89
localization studies of, 94
surgical management of, 94–96
Parathyroidectomy, for primary hyperparathyroidism, as definitive, 94–95
exploration controversies of, 95–96
for asymptomatic patients, 96
Peak BMD, in premenopausal women, 120
Peptide hormones, in endothelin system, 51–54
parathyroid, for bone disease, 6, 10
Peptide YY (PYY), Roux-en-Y gastric bypass effect on, 108
Pharmacologic management, of bone disease, as targeting osteocyte factors, 9–10, 194
with bariatric surgery, 113
with diabetes, 74–76
of diabetes, bone disease and, 74–76
fracture risk with, 65–66
of osteoporosis, adverse events with, **181–192**
introduction to, 181–182
summary of, 187–188
with bisphosphonates, 182–186
with denosumab, 186
with selective estrogen receptor modulators, 187
with teriparatide, 187
postmenopausal, combined pharmacologic therapy for, **193–206**
novel therapies for, **207–219**
premenopausal, 124–127
of postmenopausal osteoporosis, combined pharmacologic therapy for, **193–206**
discussions on, 203–204
FDA approved, 194–195
introduction to, 193–194
key points of, 193
mechanisms of action of, 194, 196–199
teriparatide plus bisphosphonates, 198–199, 201–202
teriparatide plus denosumab, 199, 202–203
teriparatide plus estrogen, 196–197, 200–201
teriparatide plus SERM, 196–197, 200–201
novel therapies for, **207–219**
antiresorptive agents as, 208–211
cathepsin K inhibitors, 209–211
denosumab, 208–209

Pharmacologic (*continued*)
introduction to, 207–208
key points of, 207
osteoanabolic agents as, 211–214
antisclerostin antibodies, 9, 212–214
PTH and analogs, 211–212
summary of, 214
of premenopausal osteoporosis, 124–127
bisphosphonates, 125
combination oral contraceptives, 124–125, 127
denosumab, 125
glucocorticoids and, 121–122, 127
PTH(1–34), 125–126
selective estrogen receptor modulators, 125
teriparatide, 125–126
primary hyperparathyroidism related to, 88, 96
Phex gene, bone health and, osteocyte role in, 2, 4, 7
Phosphate homeostasis, bone health and, FGF23 disorders and, 23–34. See also *specific disorder.*
FGFs role in, 20–23
Phosphaturic mesenchymal tumor mixed connective tissue variant (PMTMCT), 24
PHPT. See *Primary hyperparathyroidism (PHPT).*
Physical examination, for premenopausal osteoporosis, 122–123
PINP/P1NP marker, in postmenopausal osteoporosis therapy, mechanisms of action, 196
with combined agents, 197–203
with novel therapies, 208, 213
PMTMCT (phosphaturic mesenchymal tumor mixed connective tissue variant), 24
Postmenopausal osteoporosis, combined pharmacologic therapy for, **193–206**
discussions on, 203–204
FDA approved, 194–195
introduction to, 193–194
key points of, 193
mechanisms of action of, 194, 196–199
teriparatide plus bisphosphonates, 198–199, 201–202
teriparatide plus denosumab, 199, 202–203
teriparatide plus estrogen, 196–197, 200–201
teriparatide plus SERM, 196–197, 200–201
novel therapies for, **207–219**
antiresorptive agents as, 208–211
cathepsin K inhibitors, 209–211
denosumab, 208–209
introduction to, 207–208
key points of, 207
osteoanabolic agents as, 211–214
antisclerostin antibodies, 212–214
PTH and analogs, 211–212
summary of, 214
PRAD1 gene, in primary hyperparathyroidism, 89–90
Pregnancy physiology, premenopausal osteoporosis and, BMD diagnostic interpretations of, 120–121
Premenopausal osteoporosis, **117–133**

diagnosis of, 118–121
BMD interpretations in, 118–119
dynamics of peak BMD accrual, 120
with pregnancy and lactation physiology, 120–121
with pregnancy and lactation–associated osteoporosis, 121
bone biopsy for, 119, 124
laboratory evaluation for, 123
with fracture history, 118
with idiopathic low BMD, 119
introduction to, 117
key points of, 117
medication considerations of, 124–127
bisphosphonates, 125
combination oral contraceptives, 124–125, 127
denosumab, 125
glucocorticoids and, 121–122, 127
PTH(1–34), 125–126
selective estrogen receptor modulators, 125
teriparatide, 125–126
secondary causes of, 121–124
bone turnover markers and, 124
idiopathic, 124
low trauma fracture as, 121–123
summary of, 121–122
summary of, 127
treatment considerations of, 124–127
medications in, 124–126
with fractures, history of, 126
low trauma, 124–126
secondary, 126–127
with glucocorticoid exposure, 127
with low BMD, 124–126
idiopathic, 126
secondary, 126–127
Primary hyperparathyroidism (PHPT), bone health and, **87–104**
biochemical diagnosis of, 93
confirmation of, 94
clinical features of, 91–93
common presentations of, 91–92
hypercalcemic manifestations as, 92, 94
nonclassical manifestations as, 92–93
renal manifestations as, 92, 96
skeletal manifestations as, 92
differential diagnosis of, 93–94
effect on TBS, 172–173
epidemiology of, 87–88
future considerations of, 96–97
introduction to, 87
key points of, 87
pathophysiology of, 88–91
autonomous parathyroid production in, 88–89

Primary (*continued*)
molecular, 89–91
skeletal, 91
prognosis of, 95
risk factors of, 88
summary of, 97
surgical treatment of, definitive procedure for, 94–95
exploration controversies of, 95–96
for asymptomatic patients, 96
treatment of, diagnosis confirmation in, 94
for hypercalcemia, 94
localization studies in, 94
surgical, 94–96
Prostaglandins, osteocyte role in, bone health and, 2–4
nonbone disease and, 8
Prostate cancer, metastasis of, ET1 signaling and, 51, 54, 57
Proteins, AGEs impact on, 66
amino-terminal PTH-related, in postmenopausal osteoporosis, 212
binding, in vitamin D physiology, 136–139, 143–144
in endothelin system, 51–52, 54
PTH. See *Parathyroid hormone (PTH).*
PTH analogs, for postmenopausal osteoporosis, 211–212
PYY (peptide YY), Roux-en-Y gastric bypass effect on, 108

Q

QFracture score, diabetes and, 67, 72–73
Quantitative computed tomography (QCT), for BMD, in postmenopausal osteoporosis, with combined pharmacologic therapy, 196, 202–203
with novel therapies, 209–211
with bariatric surgery, 110, 112
high-resolution peripheral, of bone microarchitecture, 154, 156–157
of postmenopausal osteoporosis, 203
Quantitative trait locus (QTL), for bone size, shape, and strength, 55–56

R

Radiation therapy, MAT alterations and, 46
primary hyperparathyroidism related to, 88
Receptor activator of nuclear factor κB ligand (RANKL), bone health and, as therapeutic target, 9, 96, 194–196, 208
osteocyte role in, 2, 4–5
Renal manifestations. See also *Kidney entries.*
of primary hyperparathyroidism, 91–92, 96
RET gene, in primary hyperparathyroidism, 89–90
Rheumatoid arthritis, effect on TBS, 173
Rickets. See *Hypophosphatemic rickets (HR).*
Roux-en-Y gastric bypass (RYGB), description of, 109
effects on bone metabolism, 107, 109–110, 113
GI hormone level changes with, 107–108
US statistics on, 105, 109

S

Sarcopenia, osteocyte role in, 3, 8–9
Scleritis, as adverse event, with bisphosphonates, 183
Sclerostin, bone health and, as therapeutic target, 9, 212–214
bariatric surgery impact on, 107
ET system signaling and, 55–57
genetic mutations in, 8
osteocyte role in, 2–4
Screening BMD, in premenopausal women, 118
Secondary hyperparathyroidism, as classical vitamin D bioactivity marker, in WAs vs. AAs, 143–144
Secondary premenopausal osteoporosis, causes of, 121–124
treatment considerations of, 126–127
Selective estrogen receptor modulators (SERMs)
for bone disease, as targeting osteocytes, 10, 194
dosing and administration of, 187
efficacy of, 187
side effects of, 187
with premenopausal osteoporosis, 125
teriparatide plus, for postmenopausal osteoporosis, 196–197, 200–201
discussions on, 203–204
introduction to, 193–194
mechanisms of action, 194–196
SG. See *Sleeve gastrectomy (SG).*
Shear stress, fluid flow, bone health and, osteocyte role in, 3–4
vascular remodeling and, 55
Skeleton. See *Bone.*
Sleeve gastrectomy (SG), description of, 111–112
effects on bone metabolism, 107, 111–112
US statistics on, 105
SOST gene, bone mass and, ET system signaling and, 55–57
osteocyte role in, 7–8
Wnt signaling and, 213
Stem cells, osteocyte cross-talk with, 6
Sunlight exposure, vitamin D homeostasis and, 136
with obesity, 106
Surgical treatment, of primary hyperparathyroidism, definitive procedure for, 94–95
exploration controversies of, 95–96
for asymptomatic patients, 96

T

T1DM. See *Type 1 diabetes mellitus (T1DM).*
T2DM. See *Type 2 diabetes mellitus (T2DM).*
TBS. See *Trabecular bone score (TBS).*
Teriparatide, dosing and administration of, 187
efficacy of, 187
for postmenopausal osteoporosis
discussions on, 203–204
introduction to, 193–194

Teriparatide (*continued*)
mechanisms of action, 194–196
plus bisphosphonates, 198–199, 201–202
plus denosumab, 199, 202–203
plus estrogen, 196–197, 200–201
plus SERM, 196–197, 200–201
premenopausal osteoporosis and, 125–126
side effects of, 187
Thalassemia, effect on TBS, 173
TIO. See *Tumor-induced osteomalacia (TIO).*
Trabecular bone score (TBS), as DXA-derived measurement of fracture risk, **153–180**
abdominal soft tissue impact on, 155
association with 3-D measurements, 156–157
in vitro studies of, 156
in vivo studies of, 156–157
association with FRAX, 165–167
clinical data on, 157–166
from cross-sectional studies, 157–160
from longitudinal studies, 158, 161–165
heterotopic ossifications impact on, 155–156
in bone microarchitecture assessment, 156–157
in bone strength assessment, 156–157
induced bone loss effect on, osteoporosis treatment monitoring and, 170
with antiosteoporotic therapy, 166–169
with breast cancer treatment, 169–170
introduction to, 153–154
key points of, 153
osteoarthritis impact on, 155–156
summary of, 174
technical aspects of, 154–156
with special conditions, 170–173
diabetes mellitus as, 170–171
GH replacement as, 173
kidney transplant as, 173
long-term glucocorticoid exposure as, 171–172
primary hyperparathyroidism as, 172–173
rheumatoid arthritis as, 173
thalassemia as, 173
for BMD, 67–68
primary hyperparathyroidism and, 91
T1DM and, 68
T2DM and, 70–71
Tumor suppressor genes, in primary hyperparathyroidism, 89–90
Tumor-induced osteomalacia (TIO), FGF23 excess associated with, 23–28
description of, 23–24
diagnostic tests for, 24–25
histomorphometry as, 25
imaging as, 25
laboratory evaluation as, 24
differential diagnosis of, 25–26
pathophysiology of, 24

symptoms of, 24
treatment of, 27–28
Type 1 diabetes mellitus (T1DM), bone disease and, **63–85**
management of, 72, 74–76
physiological perspectives of, 63–67
risk assessment of, 68–69
MAT alterations and, 43–44
Type 2 diabetes mellitus (T2DM), bone disease and, **63–85**
management of, 72, 74–76
physiological perspectives of, 63–67
risk assessment of, 69–73
MAT alterations and, 43–45

U

Ultraviolet B (UVB) radiation. See *Sunlight exposure.*
Unloading, of skeleton, MAT alterations and, 43, 45–46
Uveitis, as adverse event, with bisphosphonates, 183

V

Vascular remodeling, ET1 signaling and, 55
Vertebral fracture assessment (VFA), for BMD, 67–68
primary hyperparathyroidism and, 91, 96
T1DM and, 68–69
T2DM and, 71
Visceral adipose tissue (VAT), fracture risk and, 68
Vitamin D binding protein (DBP), in vitamin D physiology, 136–139
classical, 136–138
in WAs vs. AAs, 143–144
nonclassical, 137–139
Vitamin D homeostasis, bone health and, 1
FGF23 disorders and, 23–34. See also *specific disorder.*
FGFs role in, 20–22
in African Americans, **135–152**
introduction to, 135–136
markers of classical bioactivity, 143–144
physiology of, 136–139
skeletal phenotype of, 144–146
status assessment of, 139–143
summary of, 147
supplementation for, 146
in white Americans, vs. African Americans, 135–136
markers of, 139–144. See also *25-Hydroxyvitamin D.*
obesity and, 106
with primary hyperparathyroidism, 93
physiology of, 136–139
binding protein in, 136–139, 143–144
classical endocrine, 136–138
in WAs vs. AAs, 143–144
nonclassical, 137–138

Vitamin (*continued*)
sources of, 136
Vitamin D intake, bone disease and, in African Americans, 146
with bariatric surgery, 113
with diabetes, 74
for premenopausal osteoporosis, 124
sources of, dietary vs. nondietary, 136
Vitamin D metabolite ratio, 24,25-hydroxyvitamin D and, in WAs vs AAs., 142–143

W

WAs. See *White Americans (WAs).*
White adipose tissue, vs. marrow adipose tissue, 42
White Americans (WAs), vitamin D status and bone health in, vs. African Americans, 135–136
markers of, 139–144. See also *25-Hydroxyvitamin D.*
skeletal phenotype and, 144–146
Wnt signaling, in bone disease, antisclerostin antibodies and, 212–213
diabetes and, 67
in bone health, mechanosensation and, 2–4, 107
osteocyte role in, 7–8
prostaglandin release and, 3
in ET system, 51–52
bone physiology and, 56
future considerations of, 57
osteoblastic metastasis and, 54, 57

X

X-linked hypophosphatemic rickets (XLH), FGF23 excess associated with, 23, 28–30
diagnostic tests for, 29
differential diagnosis of, 26, 29
incidence of, 28
pathophysiology of, 28
symptoms of, 28–29
treatment of, 29–30

Y

Yellow adipose tissue, 42. See also *Marrow adipose tissue (MAT).*

Moving?

Make sure your subscription moves with you!

To notify us of your new address, find your **Clinics Account Number** (located on your mailing label above your name), and contact customer service at:

Email: journalscustomerservice-usa@elsevier.com

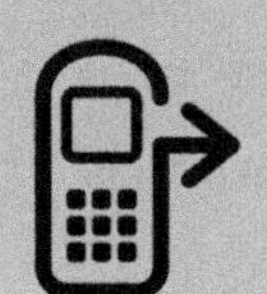

800-654-2452 **(subscribers in the U.S. & Canada)**
314-447-8871 **(subscribers outside of the U.S. & Canada)**

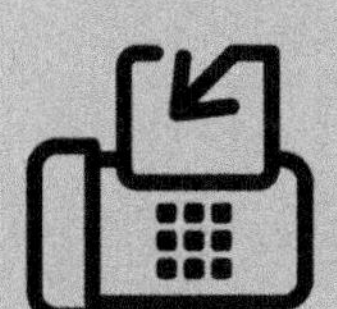

Fax number: 314-447-8029

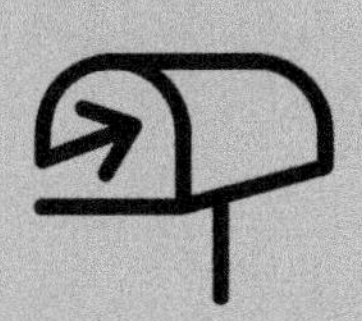

Elsevier Health Sciences Division
Subscription Customer Service
3251 Riverport Lane
Maryland Heights, MO 63043

*To ensure uninterrupted delivery of your subscription, please notify us at least 4 weeks in advance of move.

Printed and bound by CPI Group (UK) Ltd, Croydon, CR0 4YY
08/05/2025
01864698-0001